Dental Anatomy
COLORING BOOK

Dental Anatomy
COLORING BOOK

4th Edition

Edited by

MARGARET J. FEHRENBACH, RDH, MS

Oral Biologist and Dental Hygienist;
Adjunct Instructor, Bachelor of Applied Science Degree
Dental Hygiene Program
Seattle Central College;
Educational Consultant and Dental Science Technical Writer
Seattle, Washington

ELSEVIER

Elsevier
3251 Riverport Lane
St. Louis, Missouri 63043

DENTAL ANATOMY COLORING BOOK, FOURTH EDITION   ISBN: 978-0-323-81239-9
Copyright © 2023 Elsevier Inc. All Rights Reserved.

Notices

Practitioners and researchers must always rely on their own experience and knowledge in evaluating and using any information, methods, compounds, or experiments described herein. Because of rapid advances in the medical sciences, in particular, independent verification of diagnoses and drug dosages should be made. To the fullest extent of the law, no responsibility is assumed by Elsevier, authors, editors, or contributors for any injury and/or damage to persons or property as a matter of products liability, negligence or otherwise, or from any use or operation of any methods, products, instructions, or ideas contained in the material herein.

Previous editions copyrighted 2008, 2014, 2019

Senior Content Development Manager: Laura Schmidt
Senior Content Strategist: Kelly Skelton
Content Development Specialist: Kristen Helm/Casey Potter
Publishing Services Manager: Deepthi Unni
Project Manager: Nayagi Anandan
Design Direction: Bridget Hoette

Printed in the United States of America

Last digit is the print number: 9 8 7 6 5 4 3 2 1

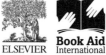

Working together
to grow libraries in
developing countries

www.elsevier.com • www.bookaid.org

A thorough understanding of anatomy related to dentistry is vital for today's dental professionals, and this fourth edition of the *Dental Anatomy Coloring Book* is an ideal companion for anyone studying dentally related anatomy. This latest edition has even more structures to color as well as more details added to previous structures. It will not only help you identify different structures, but also test your knowledge of all dentally related anatomy, with all its intricacies of embryologic background and histologic breakdown, using proven testing methods. Knowledge of related facial landmarks, veins, arteries, nerves, bones, and muscles of the head and neck region as well as dental anatomy is information that every dental professional needs to have to maintain clinical competence, and this resource enhances learning and memory retention in an easy-to-use, always FUN, format!

This fourth edition of the *Dental Anatomy Coloring Book* fully delivers complete anatomic coverage of the head and neck. Beginning with an overview of body systems and then moving on to specific regions of the head and neck as well as the oral cavity, the text follows the anatomic systems, including orofacial anatomy, dental anatomy, as well as the skeletal system, muscular system, vascular system, nervous system, and much more! This book will help you to visually understand the various parts of the head and neck as well as the oral cavity and how they relate to each other. In addition, the final chapter on fasciae and spaces will give the reader a better overall regional feel for the anatomy of the head and neck.

It has been noted that one of the most effective ways to learn about the intricacies of the body is by coloring detailed illustrations of various body parts. This coloring book is additionally helpful since it zeroes in on the specifics of the head and neck to allow focused learning for the dental professional. In addition, you do not have to be an expert artist to color!

Studies also show that adult coloring is therapeutic, reducing stress similarly to meditation. The gentle and repetitive motion of your hand bringing color to paper helps quiet your mind, bringing your usual rapid-fire thoughts down to a much slower pace while leaving the fast-paced digital world behind. We know we get a better night's sleep when avoiding engaging with electronics at night because exposure to the emitted light reduces your levels of the sleep hormone melatonin. Coloring is a relaxing and electronic-free bedtime ritual that will not disturb your level of melatonin and thus intrude on your sleep patterns.

Coloring also fosters creativity. This is because coloring requires the two hemispheres of the brain to communicate. While logic helps us stay inside the lines, choosing colors generates a creative thought process. So we invite you to take a break from your sometimes rote learning of your dental studies and find your creative center! Coloring also requires you to focus, but not so much that it is stressful. It opens up your frontal lobe, which controls organizing and problem solving, and allows you to put everything else aside and live in the moment, generating focus. Thus, regardless of your needs, there is so much to be gained by spending some time coloring.

HOW TO USE THE BOOK

Each page of the new edition contains a brief statement describing the body part featured and its orientation view, followed by a crisp easy-to-color illustration(s). Numbered leader lines clearly identify the structures to be colored and correspond to a numbered list appearing below the illustration. You can create your own "color code" by coloring in the boxed number appearing on the illustration and using the same color to fill in the corresponding numbered box on the list below. An example of a completed illustration can be found on the inside back cover. You can be distinctly creative with your color selections or go the classical route such as using red for arteries and blue for veins.

For review purposes for classroom or national board examination or certification, a numbered list appears at the page bottom or far right, which can be easily covered with a sheet of paper allowing self-examination. Additionally, included are 10 fully updated fill-in-the-blank review questions that appear on the back side of the page with the structures so that additional reviews can occur; the answers appear inverted below on the same page. In addition, textbook references for each figure are noted at the bottom of the page so the reader can easily obtain more information on each structure presented. Finally, there is a fully comprehensive test with 75 multiple-choice questions using the latest national board format with answers and rationale at the end that will help to summarize your study of dentally related anatomy and allow you to know which areas need more review!

It is suggested that you use colored pencils to avoid bleed through and after you are done coloring a page, carefully remove it from the textbook using its serrated edge and place it in a clear plastic three-hole cover sleeve. Add them to your class notes or purchase a three-ring binder to store them separately for easy reference. Then, take them with you and study while you're waiting for your clinical appointments or class to start, or eating on-the-run meals, etc. Enjoy; and learn!

CHAPTER 9   Lymphatic System   395

CHAPTER 10   Fasciae and Spaces   409

FIGURE 1.1 Anatomic position with body sections and planes

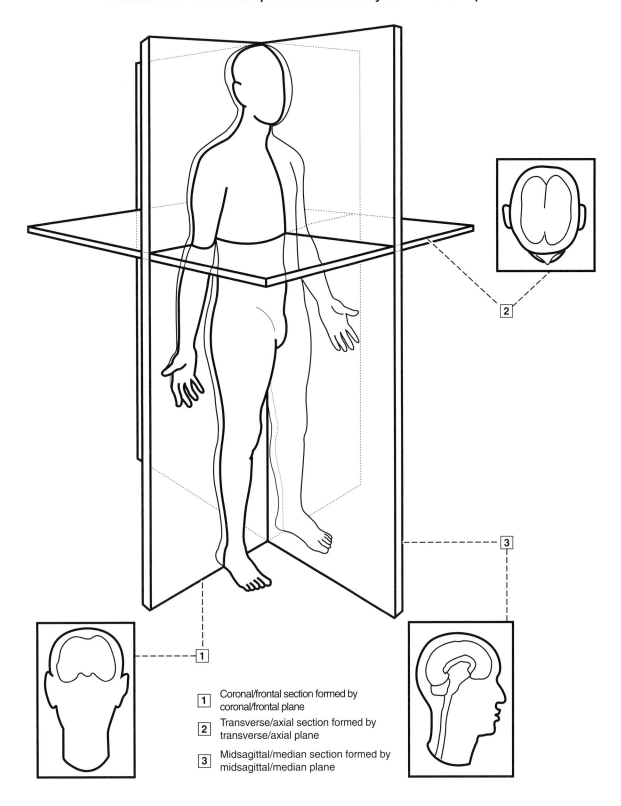

1 Coronal/frontal section formed by coronal/frontal plane

2 Transverse/axial section formed by transverse/axial plane

3 Midsagittal/median section formed by midsagittal/median plane

REVIEW QUESTIONS: Anatomic position with body sections and planes

Fill in the blanks by choosing the appropriate terms from the list below.

1. The anatomic nomenclature is a system of names for _____.

2. In _____ the body can be standing erect with the arms at the sides and the palms and toes directed forward as well as the eyes looking forward.

3. The _____ or *midsagittal section* is a division by the median or midsagittal plane.

4. The _____ or *frontal section* is a division by any coronal or frontal plane.

5. The _____ or *transverse section* is a division by any axial or transverse plane.

6. The _____ or *midsagittal plane* divides the body into equal right and left halves.

7. Dividing the body into anterior and posterior parts at any level is related to a(n) _____ or *coronal plane.*

8. A(n) _____ or *transverse plane* divides the body at any level horizontally into either superior and inferior parts and is always perpendicular to the midsagittal plane.

9. A sagittal plane divides the body parallel to the _____.

10. When the body in the anatomic position is lying down on its front, it is considered the _____, and when the body is lying down on its back, it is considered the supine position.

midsagittal plane	median section	frontal plane
coronal section	axial plane	axial section
anatomic position	median plane	prone position
anatomic structures		

Reference Chapter 1, Introduction to head and neck anatomy. In Fehrenbach MJ, Herring SW: *Illustrated anatomy of the head and neck,* ed 6, St. Louis, 2021, Saunders.

NOTES

FIGURE 1.2 Prenatal development overview

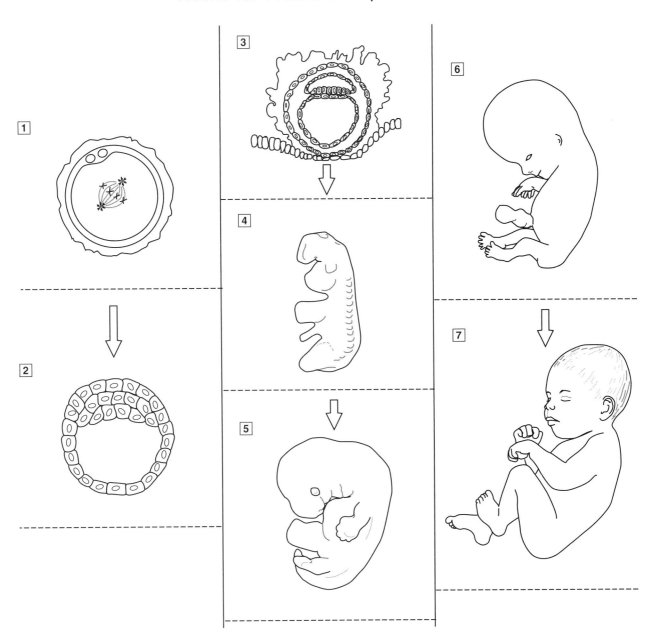

PREIMPLANTATION PERIOD: 1ST WEEK

1. Zygote
2. Blastocyst

EMBRYONIC PERIOD: 2ND-8TH WEEK

3. Disc
4. Embryo
5. Folded embryo

FETAL PERIOD: 3RD-9TH MONTH

6. Embryo
7. Fetus

REVIEW QUESTIONS: Prenatal development overview

Fill in the blanks by choosing the appropriate terms from the list below.

1. The process of _____ begins with the start of pregnancy and continues until the birth of the child.

2. The 9 months of gestation during prenatal development is usually divided into 3-month time spans or _____.

3. The study of prenatal development is also known as _____.

4. Each of the structures of the face, neck, and oral cavity has a(n) _____, the earliest indication of an organ or tissue during prenatal development.

5. At the beginning of the first week, conception takes place where a female's ovum is penetrated by and united with a male's sperm during fertilization; the union of the ovum and sperm subsequently forms a *fertilized egg* or _____.

6. The first period, the _____ of prenatal development, takes place during the first week after conception.

7. Because of the ongoing process of mitosis and secretion of fluid by the cells within the morula, the zygote becomes a(n) _____ (or blastula) that undergoes implantation.

8. During the second week of prenatal development within the embryonic period, a(n) _____ eventually develops from the blastocyst and appears as a three-dimensional but flattened circular plate of bilayered cells.

9. The second period of prenatal development, the embryonic period, extends from the beginning of the second week to the end of the eighth week, with the structure developing further and becoming a(n) _____.

10. The fetal period of prenatal development follows the embryonic period and encompasses the beginning of the ninth week or third month continuing to the ninth month, with the maturation of existing structures occurring as the embryo enlarges to become a(n) _____.

embryology	fetus	embryo
prenatal development	bilaminar embryonic disc	primordium
zygote	blastocyst	preimplantation period
trimesters		

Reference Chapter 3, Prenatal development. In Fehrenbach MJ, Popowics T: *Illustrated dental embryology, histology, and anatomy*, ed 5, St. Louis, 2020, Saunders.

ANSWER KEY   1. prenatal development, 2. trimesters, 3. embryology, 4. primordium, 5. zygote, 6. preimplantation period, 7. blastocyst, 8. bilaminar embryonic disc, 9. embryo, 10. fetus

FIGURE 1.3 Fertilization during prenatal development

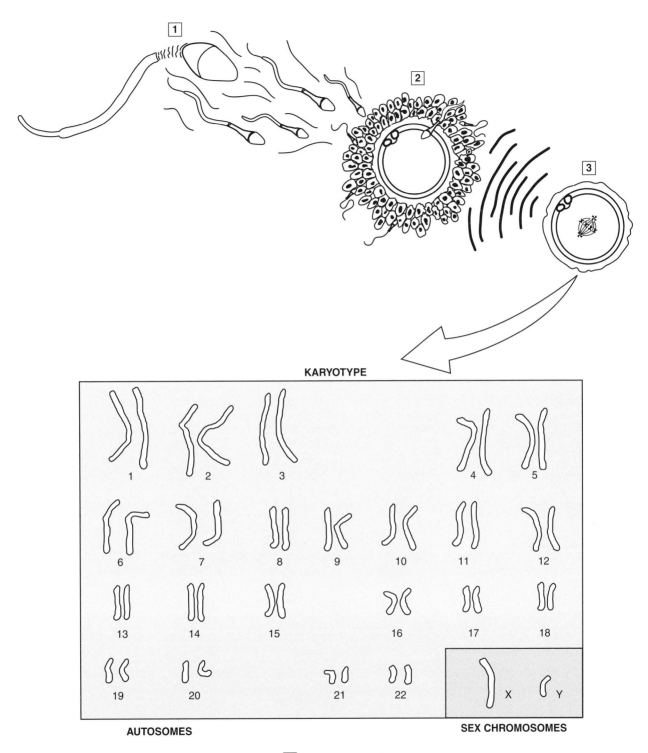

KARYOTYPE

1   2   3   4   5

6   7   8   9   10   11   12

13   14   15   16   17   18

19   20   21   22   X   Y

AUTOSOMES   SEX CHROMOSOMES

1 Sperm (enlarged)

2 Ovum

3 Zygote

REVIEW QUESTIONS: Fertilization during prenatal development

Fill in the blanks by choosing the appropriate terms from the list below.

1. At the beginning of the first week of prenatal development _____ takes place where a female's ovum is penetrated by and united with a male's sperm during fertilization.

2. The union of the ovum and sperm subsequently forms a(n) _____ or *zygote*.

3. During fertilization, the final stages of the process of _____ occur in the ovum, resulting in the joining of the ovum's chromosomes with those of the sperm; this joining of chromosomes from both biologic parents forms a new individual with "shuffled" chromosomes.

4. The zygote receives half its _____ from the female and half from the male, with the resultant genetic material a reflection of both biologic parents through the process of meiosis.

5. The photographic analysis or profile of a person's chromosomes is done in an orderly arrangement of the pairs in a(n) _____; with the sex known by the presence of either having *XX* chromosomes for female or *XY* chromosomes for male.

6. Each cell contains 46 chromosomes in the karyotype, with the number 46 being the _____ number for the cell.

7. Two of these are sex chromosomes in the karyotype; the remaining are _____.

8. Each chromosome is paired in the karyotype so that every cell has 22 _____ sets of paired autosomes, with one sex chromosome derived from the female and one from the male.

9. The _____ chromosomes, designated *X* and *Y* in the karyotype, are paired as *XX* in the female and *XY* in the male.

10. The ovum or sperm is required to have half as many chromosomes, which is the haploid number, so that on _____ the original complement of 46 chromosomes will be reestablished in the new cell.

fertilized egg	chromosomes	homologous
karyotype	diploid	sex
meiosis	autosomes	fertilization
conception		

References   Chapter 3, Prenatal development. In Fehrenbach MJ, Popowics T: *Illustrated dental embryology, histology, and anatomy,* ed 5, St. Louis, 2020, Saunders; Chapter 2, General embryology. In Nanci A, *Ten Cate's oral histology,* ed 9, St. Louis, 2018, Mosby.

NOTES

FIGURE 1.4 Preimplantation period to implantation during prenatal development (cross section)

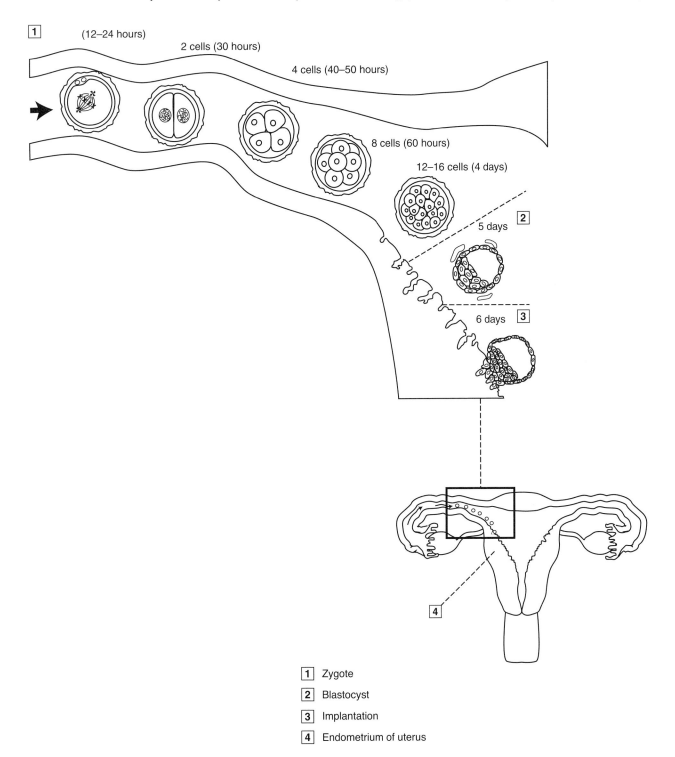

1 (12–24 hours)

2 cells (30 hours)

4 cells (40–50 hours)

8 cells (60 hours)

12–16 cells (4 days)

2 5 days

3 6 days

1 Zygote

2 Blastocyst

3 Implantation

4 Endometrium of uterus

REVIEW QUESTIONS: Preimplantation period to implantation during prenatal development

Fill in the blanks by choosing the appropriate terms from the list below.

1. The first period of prenatal development, the _____, takes place during the first week after conception, with the union of the ovum and sperm subsequently forming a fertilized egg or *zygote.*

2. After fertilization, the zygote undergoes _____ or individual cell division that splits it into many more cells due to cleavage.

3. After initial cleavage, the solid ball of cells becomes a(n) _____.

4. Because of the ongoing process of mitosis and secretion of fluid by the cells within the morula, the zygote becomes a(n) _____ (or blastula).

5. By the end of the first week, the blastocyst stops traveling and undergoes _____ and thus becomes embedded in the prepared endometrium, the innermost lining of the uterus on its back wall.

6. The process of _____ is key in prenatal development from the initial axial (head-to-tail) specification of the embryo through its segmentation and ultimately to the development of the dentition.

7. Patterning is a spatial and temporal event as exemplified by regional prenatal development of incisors, canines, premolars, and molars, which occurs at different times and involves the processes of _____, competence, and differentiation.

8. All the cells of an individual during prenatal development come from the _____; these cells have differentiated into populations that have assumed particular functions, shapes, and rates of turnover.

9. The process that initiates _____ is induction during prenatal development; an inducer is an agent that provides cells with the signal to enter this process; each compartment of cells must be competent to respond to the induction process.

10. After fertilization, prenatal development involves a phase of rapid _____ and migration of cells, with little or no differentiation; this phase lasts until three embryonic cell layers (or germ layers) have formed.

patterning	induction	morula
preimplantation period	differentiation	proliferation
mitosis	implantation	zygote
blastocyst		

References Chapter 3, Prenatal development. In Fehrenbach MJ, Popowics T: *Illustrated dental embryology, histology, and anatomy,* ed 5, St. Louis, 2020, Saunders; Chapter 2, General embryology. In Nanci A, *Ten Cate's oral histology,* ed 9, St. Louis, 2018, Mosby.

FIGURE 1.5 Implantation during prenatal development (internal view and cross section)

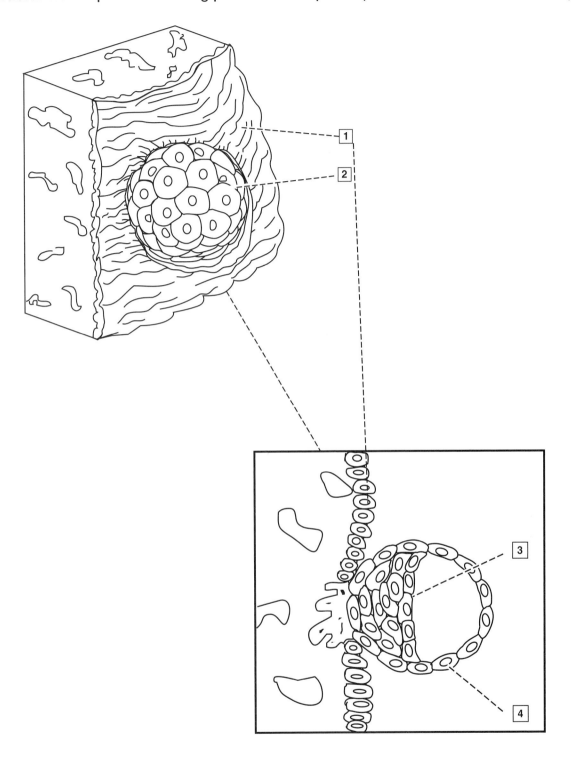

1	Endometrium of uterus	**3**	Embryoblast layer
2	Implanted blastocyst	**4**	Trophoblast layer

REVIEW QUESTIONS: Implantation during prenatal development

Fill in the blanks by choosing the appropriate terms from the list below.

1. Because of the ongoing process of _____ and secretion of fluid by the cells within the morula, the zygote becomes a blastocyst (or blastula).

2. The latter part of the first week of prenatal development is characterized by further mitotic _____, in which the blastocyst splits into smaller and more numerous cells as it undergoes successive cell divisions by mitosis.

3. By the end of the first week, the blastocyst stops traveling and undergoes implantation and thus becomes embedded in the prepared _____, the innermost lining of the uterus on its back wall.

4. After a week of cleavage, the blastocyst consists of a layer of peripheral cells, the trophoblast layer, and a small inner mass of embryonic cells or _____.

5. The trophoblast layer later gives rise to important prenatal support tissue and the embryoblast layer gives rise to the _____ during the embryonic period.

6. After fertilization, prenatal development involves a phase of rapid proliferation and _____ of cells, with little or no differentiation.

7. This proliferative phase of prenatal development lasts until three _____ (or germ layers) have formed.

8. Embryoblast cells form the embryo, whereas the _____ cells are associated with implantation of the embryo and formation of the placenta.

9. Over time, populations of embryonic cells vary their _____ from no response to maximum response and then back to no response during prenatal development; this is defined as the ability of an embryonic cell to react to the stimulation of an inductor, allowing continued growth or differentiation of the embryo.

10. Windows of embryonic competence of varying duration exist for different populations of cells; the concepts of induction, competence, and also _____ apply in the development of the tooth and its supporting tissue as well as development of the head and neck.

migration	embryonic cell layers	trophoblast
embryoblast layer	embryo	differentiation
endometrium	mitosis	embryonic competence
cleavage		

References Chapter 3, Prenatal development. In Fehrenbach MJ, Popowics T: *Illustrated dental embryology, histology, and anatomy,* ed 5, St. Louis, 2020, Saunders; Chapter 2, General embryology. In Nanci A, *Ten Cate's oral histology,* ed 9, St. Louis, 2018, Mosby.

ANSWER KEY 1. mitosis, 2. cleavage, 3. endometrium, 4. embryoblast layer, 5. embryo, 6. migration, 7. embryonic cell layers, 8. trophoblast, 9. embryonic competence, 10. differentiation

FIGURE 1.6 Second week of prenatal development during embryonic period (cross section)

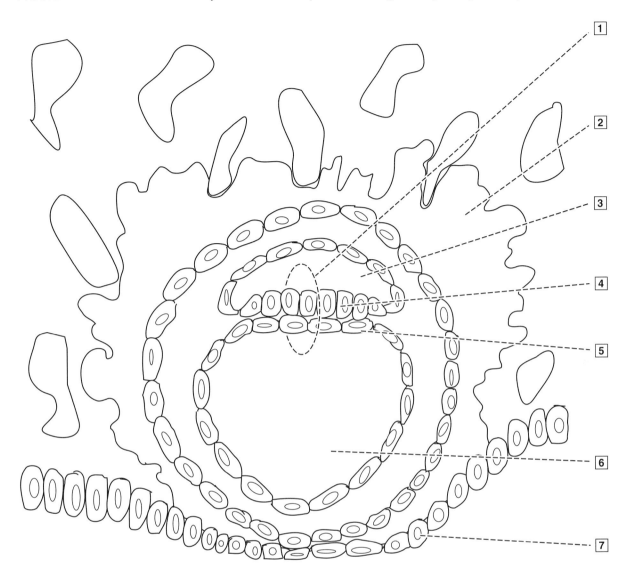

1	Bilaminar embryonic disc	5	Hypoblast layer
2	Placenta	6	Yolk sac
3	Amniotic cavity	7	Endometrium of uterus
4	Epiblast layer		

REVIEW QUESTIONS: Second week of prenatal development during embryonic period

Fill in the blanks by choosing the appropriate terms from the list below.

1. The second period of prenatal development, the _____, extends from the beginning of the second week to the end of the eighth week; it includes most of the latter part of the first trimester.

2. Certain physiologic processes or spatial and temporal events called *patterning* occur during the embryonic period, which are considered key to further development during prenatal development; these physiologic processes include _____, proliferation, differentiation, morphogenesis, and maturation.

3. During the second week of prenatal development, within the embryonic period, the implanted blastocyst grows by increased proliferation of the embryonic cells, with differentiation also occurring resulting in changes in cellular morphogenesis; the increased number of embryonic cells creates the _____ (or germ layers) within the blastocyst.

4. A(n) _____ is eventually developed from the blastocyst and appears as a three-dimensional but flattened circular plate of bilayered cells.

5. The bilaminar embryonic disc has both a superior layer and inferior layer, with the superior _____ composed of high columnar cells and the inferior hypoblast layer composed of small cuboidal cells.

6. After its creation, the bilaminar embryonic disc is suspended in the uterus's endometrium between two fluid-filled cavities, the _____, which faces the epiblast layer, and the yolk sac, which faces the hypoblast layer and serves as initial nourishment for the disc.

7. The bilaminar embryonic disc later develops into the _____ as prenatal development continues.

8. The _____, a prenatal organ that joins together the pregnant female and developing embryo, develops from the interactions of the trophoblast layer and endometrial tissue.

9. The formation of the placenta and the developing _____ permit selective exchange of soluble bloodborne substances between them, which includes oxygen and carbon dioxide as well as nutritional and hormonal substances.

10. During the embryonic period of prenatal development, differentiation occurs at various rates in the embryo affecting cells, tissue types, organs, and systems; this overall process includes different types of differentiation such as cytodifferentiation and _____.

embryo	bilaminar embryonic disc	embryonic period
umbilical circulation	epiblast layer	amniotic cavity
histodifferentiation	placenta	embryonic cell layers
induction		

Reference   Chapter 3, Prenatal development. In Fehrenbach MJ, Popowics T: *Illustrated dental embryology, histology, and anatomy,* ed 5, St. Louis, 2020, Saunders.

FIGURE 1.7 Third week of prenatal development during embryonic period (superior view and cross section)

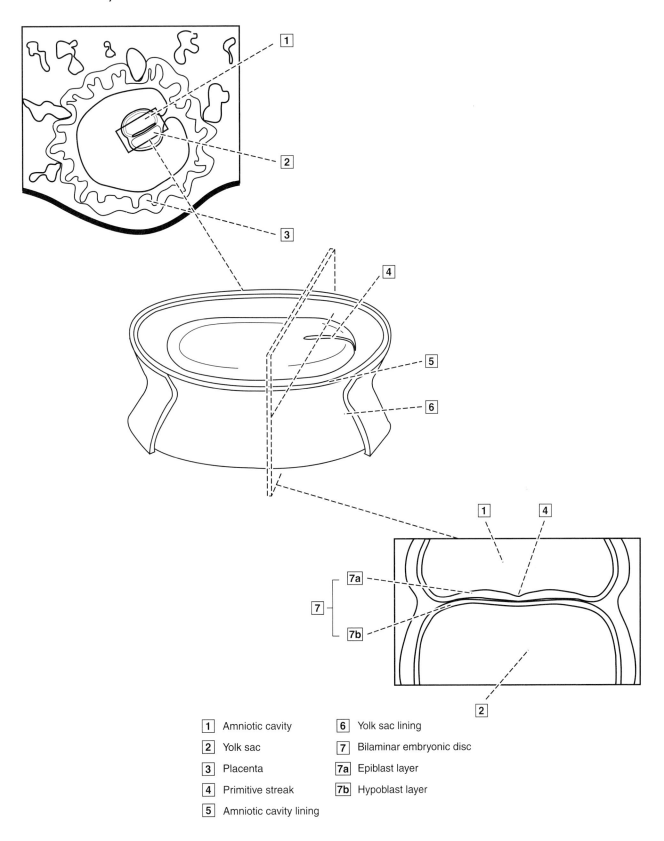

1 Amniotic cavity	6 Yolk sac lining
2 Yolk sac	7 Bilaminar embryonic disc
3 Placenta	7a Epiblast layer
4 Primitive streak	7b Hypoblast layer
5 Amniotic cavity lining	

REVIEW QUESTIONS: Third week of prenatal development during embryonic period

Fill in the blanks by choosing the appropriate terms from the list below.

1. During the beginning of the third week of prenatal development within the embryonic period, the _____ forms within the bilaminar embryonic disc; it is a furrowed rod-shaped thickening in the middle of the disc that results from increased proliferation of cells in the midline area.

2. The primitive streak causes the bilaminar embryonic disc to have _____, with a right half and left half; most of the further development of each half of the embryo mirrors the other half.

3. During the beginning of the third week, some cells from the _____ move or migrate toward the hypoblast layer only in the area of the primitive streak of the bilaminar embryonic disc.

4. The migratory cells from the epiblast layer into the hypoblast layer of the bilaminar embryonic disc are located in the middle between the two layers and become _____, an embryonic connective tissue as well as embryonic endoderm.

5. Mesodermal cells have the potential to proliferate and differentiate into diverse types of _____, forming cells such as fibroblasts, chondroblasts, and osteoblasts.

6. When three layers are present, the bilaminar embryonic disc becomes thickened into a(n) _____ during the third week of prenatal development.

7. With the creation of a new embryonic cell layer of mesoderm within the trilaminar embryonic disc, the epiblast layer is now considered _____, and the hypoblast layer has been displaced by the cells migrating into the primitive streak and now becomes extraembryonic endoderm.

8. Because the trilaminar embryonic disc undergoes so much growth during the first 3 weeks, certain anatomic structures of the disc become apparent, and the trilaminar embryonic disc now has a(n) _____ or *head end*.

9. At the cephalic end of the trilaminar embryonic disc, the _____ forms; it consists of only ectoderm externally and endoderm internally without any intermediate mesoderm, which is the location of the future primitive mouth or stomodeum of the embryo and thus the beginning of the digestive tract.

10. The trilaminar embryonic disc has a(n) _____ or *tail end*, which is where the cloacal membrane forms that is the location of the future anus or terminal end of the digestive tract.

connective tissue	trilaminar embryonic disc	primitive streak
bilateral symmetry	ectoderm	epiblast layer
cephalic end	oropharyngeal membrane	caudal end
mesoderm		

Reference Chapter 3, Prenatal development. In Fehrenbach MJ, Popowics T: *Illustrated dental embryology, histology, and anatomy,* ed 5, St. Louis, 2020, Saunders.

FIGURE 1.8 Central nervous system and muscular system development during embryonic period (transverse section and posterior and lateral views)

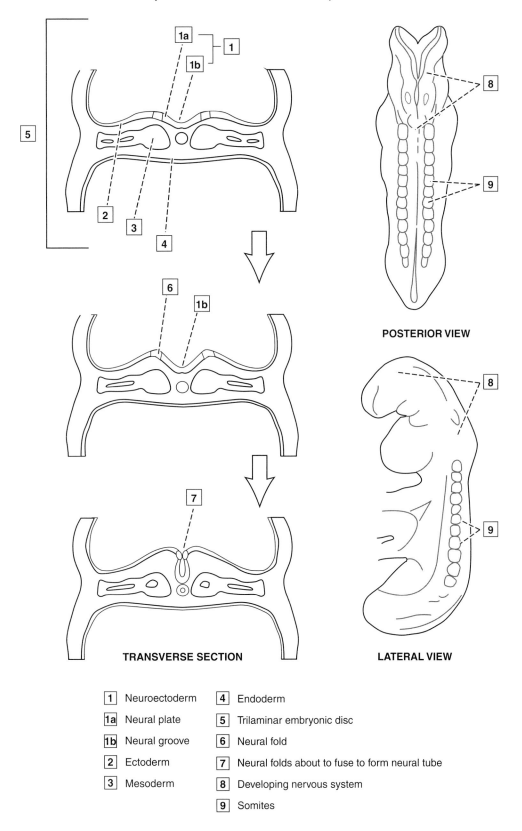

POSTERIOR VIEW

TRANSVERSE SECTION

LATERAL VIEW

1 Neuroectoderm	4 Endoderm
1a Neural plate	5 Trilaminar embryonic disc
1b Neural groove	6 Neural fold
2 Ectoderm	7 Neural folds about to fuse to form neural tube
3 Mesoderm	8 Developing nervous system
	9 Somites

REVIEW QUESTIONS: Central nervous system and muscular system development during embryonic period

Fill in the blanks by choosing the appropriate terms from the list below.

1. During the latter part of the third week of prenatal development, the _____ begins to develop in the embryo; many steps occur during this week to form the beginnings of the spinal cord and brain.

2. A specialized group of cells differentiates from the ectoderm during the latter part of the third week of prenatal development and is now considered _____.

3. The neuroectoderm is localized to the _____ of the embryo, which is a central band of cells that extends the length of the embryo, from the cephalic end to the caudal end.

4. The neural plate of the embryo undergoes further growth and thickening within the third week of prenatal development, which causes it to deepen and invaginate inward, forming the _____.

5. Near the end of the third week of prenatal development, the neural groove deepens further and is surrounded by the _____.

6. As further growth of the neuroectoderm occurs, the _____ is formed during the fourth week by the neural folds undergoing fusion at the most superior part; in the future, this structure forms into the spinal cord as well as other neural tissue of the central nervous system.

7. In addition, during the third week of prenatal development, another specialized group of cells, the _____, develop from neuroectoderm; these cells migrate from the crests of the neural folds and then join the mesoderm to form mesenchyme.

8. The _____ is involved in the development of many face and neck structures, such as the pharyngeal or branchial arches, because they differentiate to form most of the connective tissue of the head.

9. By the end of the third week of prenatal development, the _____ additionally differentiates and begins to divide on each side of the tube within the embryo into 38-paired cuboidal segments of mesoderm forming the somites.

10. The _____ appear as distinct elevations on the surface of the sides of the embryo and continue to develop in the following weeks of prenatal development, giving rise to most of the skeletal structures of the head, neck, and trunk as well as the associated muscles and dermis of the skin.

neural tube	neural groove	central nervous system
mesenchyme	somites	neural folds
mesoderm	neural plate	neuroectoderm
neural crest cells		

Reference Chapter 3, Prenatal development. In Fehrenbach MJ, Popowics T: *Illustrated dental embryology, histology, and anatomy,* ed 5, St. Louis, 2020, Saunders.

ANSWER KEY 1. central nervous system, 2. neuroectoderm, 3. neural plate, 4. neural groove, 5. neural folds, 6. neural tube, 7. neural crest cells, 8. mesenchyme, 9. mesoderm, 10. somites

FIGURE 1.9 Fourth week of prenatal development with embryonic folding and organ development during embryonic period (lateral view with midsagittal sections)

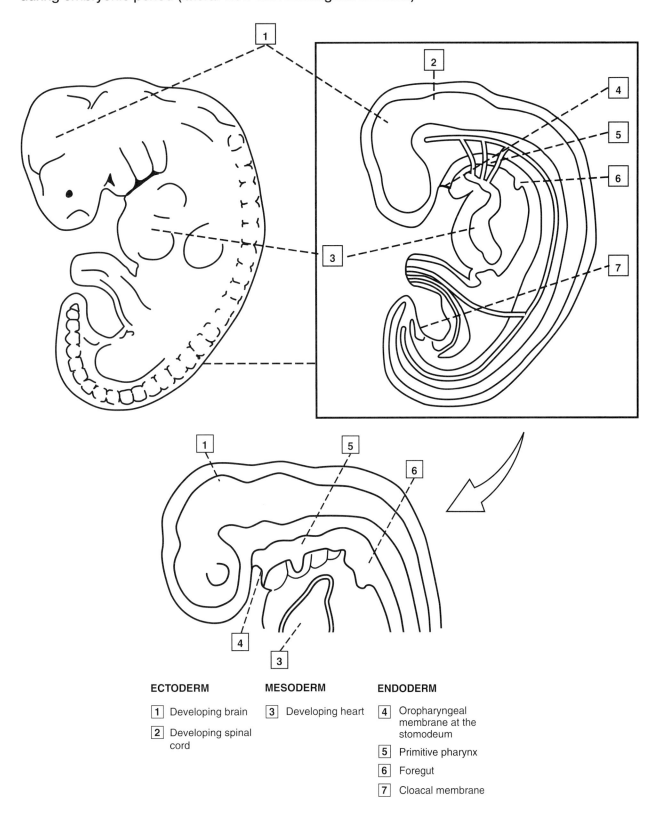

ECTODERM	**MESODERM**	**ENDODERM**
1 Developing brain	3 Developing heart	4 Oropharyngeal membrane at the stomodeum
2 Developing spinal cord		5 Primitive pharynx
		6 Foregut
		7 Cloacal membrane

REVIEW QUESTIONS: Fourth week of prenatal development with embryonic folding and organ development during embryonic period

Fill in the blanks by choosing the appropriate terms from the list below.

1. During the fourth week of prenatal development within the embryonic period, the trilaminar embryonic disc undergoes anterior (cephalic) and lateral _____, which places forming tissue types into their proper positions for further embryonic development as well as producing a tubular embryo.

2. After folding of the embryonic disc into the embryo, the endoderm now lies inside the _____, with mesoderm filling in the areas between these two layers forming one long hollow tube lined by endoderm from the cephalic end to the caudal end of the embryo; specifically, the tube runs from the oropharyngeal membrane to the cloacal membrane.

3. The tube formed during embryonic folding is the future _____ and is separated into three major regions, the foregut, midgut, and hindgut.

4. The anterior part of the tube in the embryo when it becomes folded is the foregut, which forms the _____ or *primitive throat* and includes a part of the primitive yolk sac as it becomes enclosed with folding; the two more posterior parts, the midgut and hindgut, respectively, go on to form the rest of the mature pharynx as well as the remainder of the digestive tract.

5. During development of the digestive tract, four pairs of _____ form from evaginations on the lateral walls lining the pharynx during the fourth week of prenatal development.

6. A crucial prenatal developmental event is the folding of the _____ in two planes, along the rostrocaudal axis and along the lateral axis.

7. The head fold is critical to the formation of a(n) _____ (or stomatodeum) or primitive mouth, which will form the future oral cavity; the ectoderm comes through this fold to line the stomodeum, with this structure separated from the gut by the oropharyngeal membrane.

8. The lateral folding of the embryo during prenatal development determines the disposition of the middle layer or _____.

9. As another result of embryonic folding, the ectoderm of the floor of the _____ now encapsulates the embryo and forms the surface epithelium.

10. In addition, after folding of the embryo, the paraxial mesoderm remains adjacent to the future _____ and notochord.

embryo	mesoderm
primitive pharynx	digestive tract
pharyngeal pouches	embryonic folding
ectoderm	amniotic cavity
stomodeum	neural tube

References   Chapter 3, Prenatal development. In Fehrenbach MJ, Popowics T: *Illustrated dental embryology, histology, and anatomy,* ed 5, St. Louis, 2020, Saunders; Chapter 2, General embryology. In Nanci A, *Ten Cate's oral histology,* ed 9, St. Louis, 2018, Mosby.

ANSWER KEY 1. embryonic folding, 2. ectoderm, 3. digestive tract, 4. primitive pharynx, 5. pharyngeal pouches, 6. embryo, 7. stomodeum, 8. mesoderm, 9. amniotic cavity, 10. neural tube

FIGURE 1.10   Fetal period of prenatal development

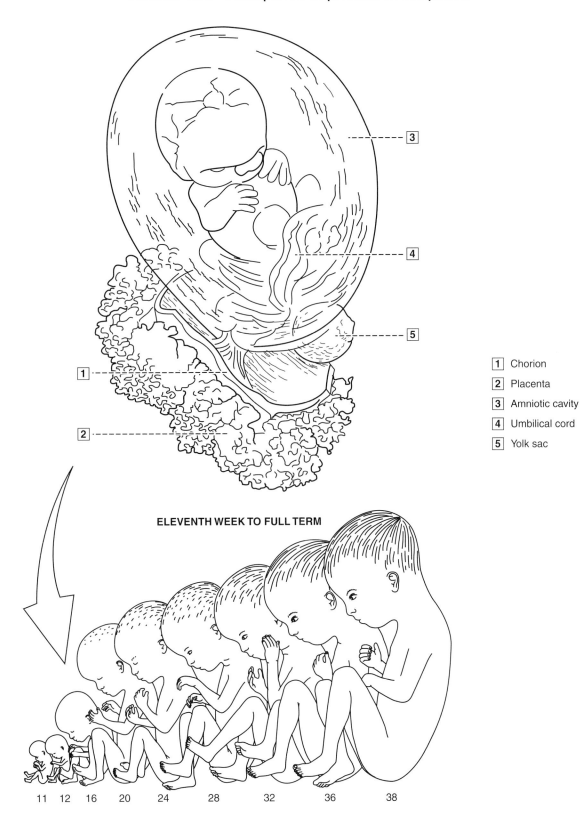

1 Chorion
2 Placenta
3 Amniotic cavity
4 Umbilical cord
5 Yolk sac

ELEVENTH WEEK TO FULL TERM

11 12 16 20 24 28 32 36 38

REVIEW QUESTIONS: Fetal period of prenatal development

Fill in the blanks by choosing the appropriate terms from the list below.

1. As the third and final period of prenatal development, the _____ follows the embryonic period.

2. The fetal period of prenatal development encompasses the beginning of the ninth week or third month continuing to the ninth month; thus, this period includes both the second and third _____.

3. During the fetal period of prenatal development there is maturation of existing structures occurring as the embryo enlarges to become a(n) _____.

4. During the fetal period of prenatal development, the changes involve not only the physiologic process of _____ the individual tissue types and organs but also further proliferation, differentiation, and morphogenesis, similar to the processes occurring before the development of the embryo.

5. Although developmental changes with the fetus during the fetal period of prenatal development are not as dramatic as those that occur earlier during the _____, they are important because they allow the newly formed tissue types and organs to begin to function.

6. The _____ of the fetus during prenatal development is linear up to 37 weeks of gestation, after which it begins to level until birth.

7. The growth rate of an embryo, fetus, or infant can be reflected as the _____ per gestational age and is often given as in relation to what would be expected by the gestational age.

8. An infant born within the usual range of weight at that time is considered appropriate for _____.

9. The growth rate during prenatal development can be roughly correlated with the fundal height, which can be estimated with the _____ of the pregnant female.

10. More exact measurements of either the embryo or fetus and its growth rate can be performed with obstetric _____ using sound waves.

gestational age	maturation	weight
embryonic period	fetus	abdominal palpation
trimesters	growth rate	ultrasonography
fetal period		

References   Chapter 3, Prenatal development. In Fehrenbach MJ, Popowics T: *Illustrated dental embryology, histology, and anatomy,* ed 5, St. Louis, 2020, Saunders; Chapter 2, General embryology. In Nanci A, *Ten Cate's oral histology,* ed 9, St. Louis, 2018, Mosby.

ANSWER KEY   1. fetal period, 2. trimesters, 3. fetus, 4. maturation, 5. embryonic period, 6. growth rate, 7. weight, 8. gestational age, 9. abdominal palpation, 10. ultrasonography

FIGURE 1.11 Cell with cell membrane and organelles

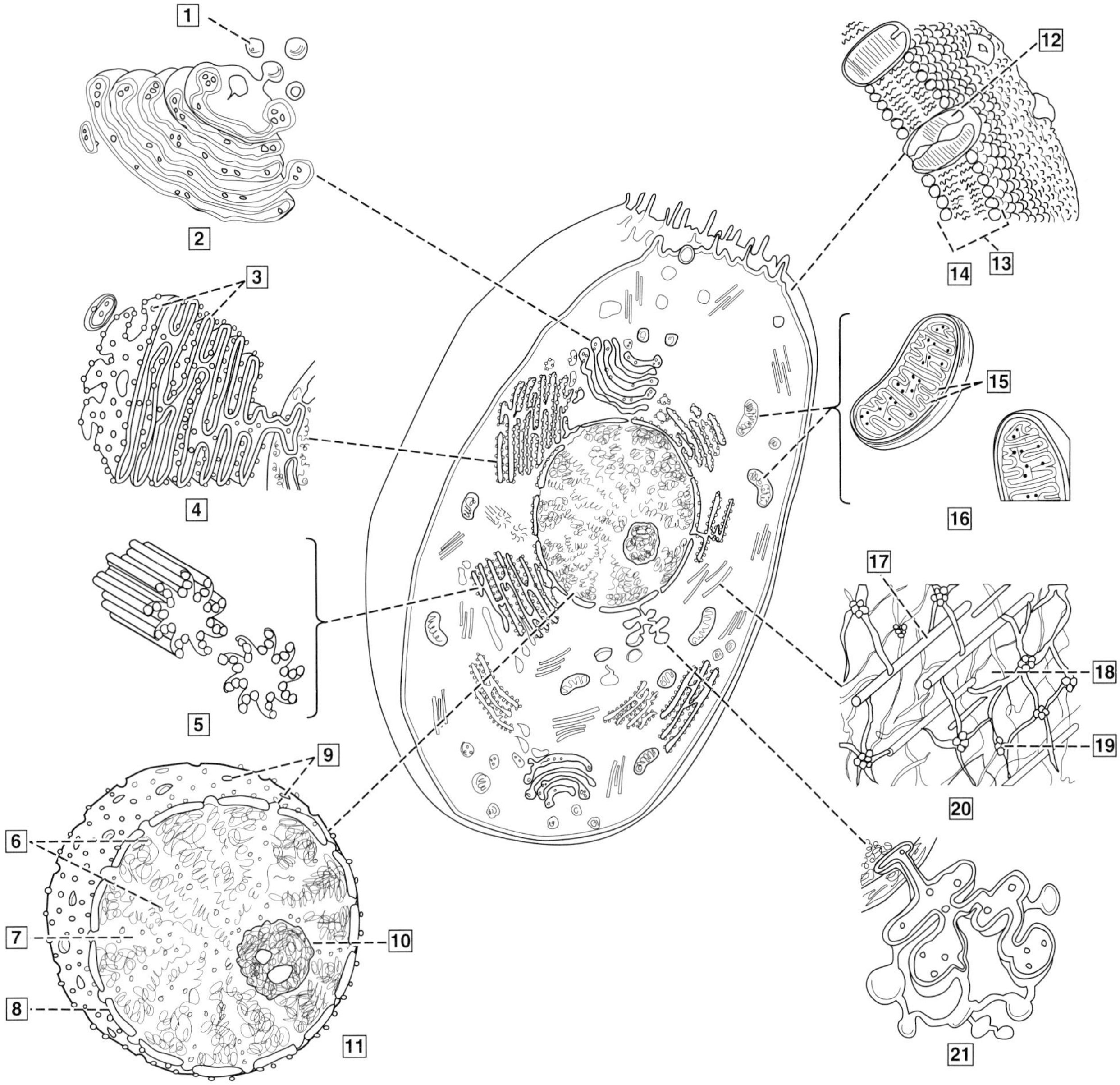

1 Lysosome	8 Nuclear envelope	15 Cristae
2 Golgi complex	9 Nuclear pore	16 Mitochondria
3 Ribosomes	10 Nucleolus	17 Microtubule
4 Rough endoplasmic reticulum	11 Nucleus	18 Cytoplasm
5 Centrioles of centrosome	12 Protein	19 Microfilament
6 Chromatin	13 Phospholipid bilayer	20 Cytoskeleton
7 Nucleoplasm	14 Cell membrane	21 Smooth endoplasmic reticulum

REVIEW QUESTIONS: Cell with cell membrane and organelles

Fill in the blanks by choosing the appropriate terms from the list below.

1. The smallest living unit of organization in the body is the _____ because each is capable of performing any necessary functions without the aid of others; each has a cell membrane, cytoplasm, organelles, and inclusions.

2. The _____ (or plasma membrane) surrounds the cell; usually, it is an intricate bilayer, consisting mostly of phospholipids and proteins.

3. The _____ of the cell includes the semifluid part contained within the cell membrane boundary as well as the skeletal system of support or cytoskeleton.

4. The _____ are metabolically active specialized structures within the cell that allow each cell to function according to its genetic code; these structures include the nucleus, mitochondria, ribosomes, endoplasmic reticulum, Golgi complex, lysosomes, and cytoskeleton.

5. The _____ is the largest, densest, and most conspicuous organelle in the cell; it is found in all cells of the body except mature red blood cells, and most cells have a single one.

6. The fluid part within the nucleus is the _____, which contains important molecules used in the construction of ribosomes, nucleic acids, and other nuclear materials; the nucleus is also surrounded by the nuclear envelope, a membrane similar to the cell membrane except that it is double layered.

7. Contained within the nucleus is the _____, a prominent and rounded nuclear organelle that is centrally placed in the nucleoplasm, which mostly produces types of ribonucleic acid.

8. The _____ are the most numerous organelles in the cell and are associated with energy conversion since they are a major source of adenosine triphosphate.

9. The _____ consists of parallel membrane-bound channels that interconnect, forming a system of channels and folds and are continuous with the nuclear envelope so they can modify, store, segregate, and transport proteins; these structures can be classified as either smooth or rough, which is determined by the absence or presence of ribosomes.

10. Once the endoplasmic reticulum has modified a new protein, it is then transferred to the _____ (or apparatus) for subsequent segregation, packaging, and transport of the protein compounds; it is the second largest organelle after the nucleus and is composed of stacks of three to twenty flattened smooth-membrane vesicular sacs arranged parallel to one another.

nucleus	nucleoplasm	mitochondria
cytoplasm	organelles	nucleolus
Golgi complex	endoplasmic reticulum	cell membrane
Cell		

Reference   Chapter 7, Cells. In Fehrenbach MJ, Popowics T: *Illustrated dental embryology, histology, and anatomy,* ed 5, St. Louis, 2020, Saunders.

ANSWER KEY   1. cell, 2. cell membrane, 3. cytoplasm, 4. organelles, 5. nucleus, 6. nucleoplasm, 7. nucleolus, 8. mitochondria, 9. endoplasmic reticulum, 10. Golgi complex

FIGURE 1.12 Cell cycle

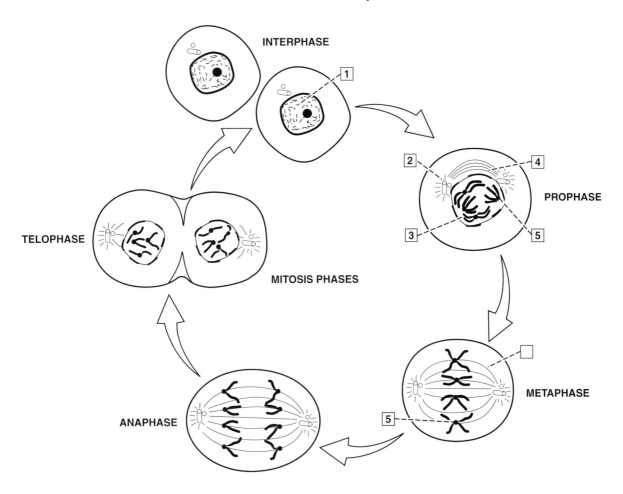

INTERPHASE

PROPHASE

TELOPHASE

MITOSIS PHASES

METAPHASE

ANAPHASE

1 Chromatin

2 Centrosome
with centrioles

3 Chromosomes

4 Spindle fibers

5 Centromere

REVIEW QUESTIONS: Cell cycle

Fill in the blanks by choosing the appropriate terms from the list below.

1. The main nucleic acid in the nucleoplasm is _____ in the form of chromatin, which looks like diffuse stippling; in an actively dividing cell, the chromatin condenses into visible and discrete rodlike chromosomes, with each chromosome having a centromere or a clear constricted area near the middle.

2. The _____ then become two filamentous or threadlike chromatids (or daughters) joined by a centromere during cell division; after cell division, major segments again become uncoiled and dispersed between the other components of the nucleoplasm as before.

3. The _____ is a dense somewhat oval-shaped organelle that contains a pair of cylindrical structures, the centrioles, which are always located near the nucleus; there are two centrioles within this organelle and each is composed of triplets of microtubules arranged in a cartwheel pattern.

4. Before cell division, deoxyribonucleic acid is replicated during _____ as part of the cell cycle.

5. Interphase has _____ phases, which include Gap 1 or *G1* (or initial resting phase with cell growth and functioning); Synthesis or *S* (or cell deoxyribonucleic acid synthesis by duplication); and Gap 2 or *G2* (or second resting phase that resumes cell growth and functioning).

6. The cell division that takes place during mitosis consists of _____ phases, which include prophase, metaphase, anaphase, and telophase; cell division is followed again by interphase continuing the overall cell cycle.

7. During _____ of cell division, the chromatin condenses into chromosomes in the cell, replicated centrioles migrate to opposite poles, and the nuclear membrane and nucleolus disintegrate.

8. During _____ of cell division, the chromosomes move so that their centromeres are aligned in the equatorial plane and the mitotic spindle forms.

9. During _____ of cell division, the centromeres split and each chromosome separates into two chromatids, while the chromatids migrate to opposite poles by the mitotic spindle.

10. During _____ of cell division, the division into two daughter cells that are identical to the parent cell as well as to each other occurs and the nuclear membrane reappears.

three	chromosomes	telophase
interphase	prophase	anaphase
deoxyribonucleic acid	four	centrosome
metaphase		

Reference   Chapter 7, Cells. In Fehrenbach MJ, Popowics T: *Illustrated dental embryology, histology, and anatomy*, ed 5, St. Louis, 2020, Saunders.

FIGURE 1.13 **Major body cavities (midsagittal section)**

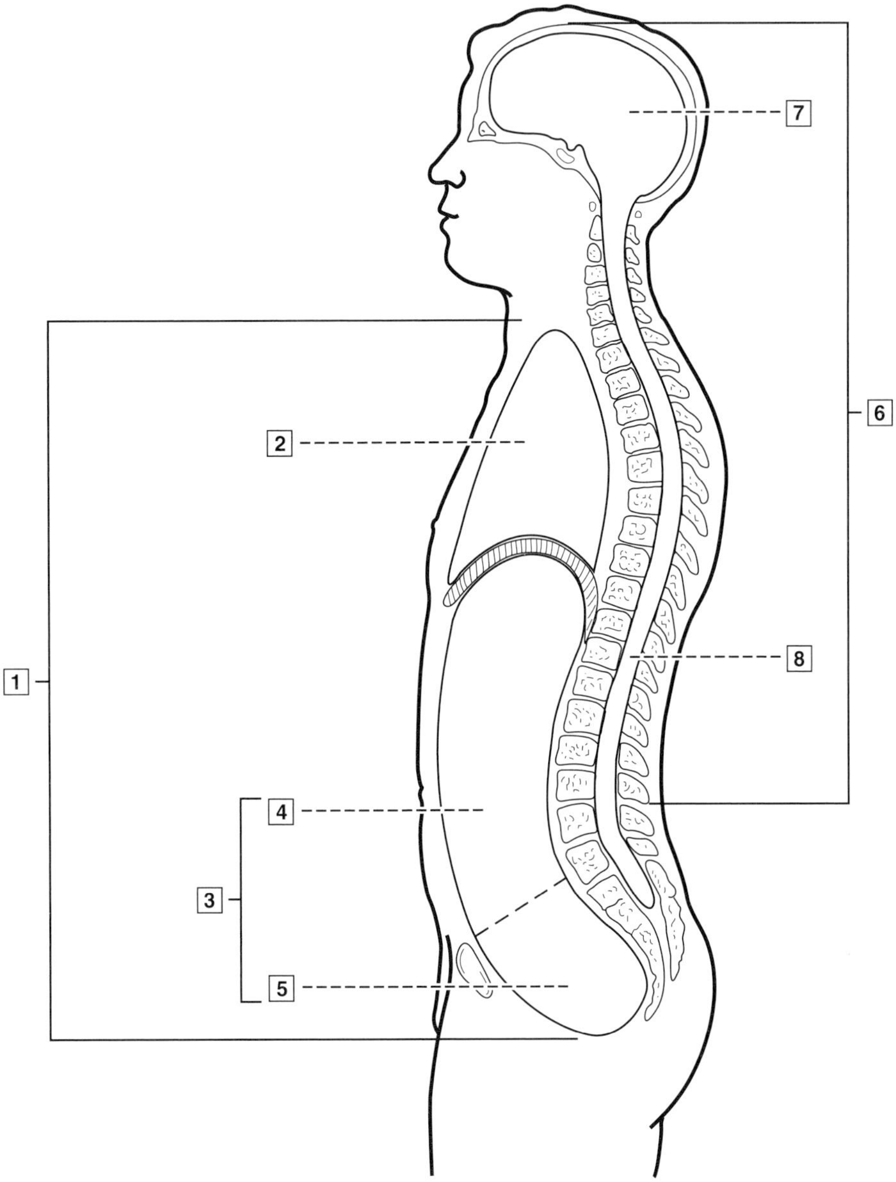

1	Ventral cavity	**5**	Pelvic cavity
2	Thoracic cavity	**6**	Dorsal cavity
3	Abdominopelvic cavity	**7**	Cranial cavity
4	Abdominal cavity	**8**	Spinal cavity

REVIEW QUESTIONS: Major body cavities

Fill in the blanks by choosing the appropriate terms from the list below.

1. A(n) _____ is a space in the body filled with fluid.

2. The _____ is a body cavity in the ventral or anterior aspect of the body; it has two subdivisions that include the thoracic cavity and the abdominopelvic cavity.

3. The _____ is a body cavity that is divided into the abdominal cavity and pelvic cavity, but there is no physical barrier between these two subdivisions, only an imaginary line from the inferior pubis to the superior sacrum dividing them.

4. The _____ is a body cavity that contains digestive organs, spleen, and kidneys, while the pelvic cavity is a body cavity that contains the urinary bladder, internal reproductive organs, and rectum; both of these body cavities are protected by a layer of the peritoneum.

5. The _____ is the body cavity formed by the ribcage; it is divided from the abdominopelvic cavity by the diaphragm muscle, which is then further divided into the pleural cavity that contains the lungs and the superior mediastinum that includes the pericardial cavity with the heart.

6. The _____ is a body cavity bounded by the pelvic bones that primarily contains reproductive organs, the urinary bladder, the pelvic colon, and the rectum.

7. The _____ is a body cavity in the dorsal or posterior aspect of the body that lies within the skull and vertebral column, having two subdivisions that include the cranial cavity and the spinal cavity.

8. The _____ or *intracranial space* is a body cavity within the cranium that contains the brain, proximal parts of the cranial nerves, blood vessels, and cranial venous sinuses as well as having the eyes and ears.

9. The _____ or *spinal canal* is a body cavity through which the spinal cord passes that is enclosed within the vertebral foramen of the vertebrae.

10. Both the cranial cavity and spinal cavity are lined by the _____.

abdominopelvic cavity	dorsal cavity	cranial cavity
body cavity	spinal cavity	ventral cavity
pelvic cavity	meninges	abdominal cavity
thoracic cavity		

Reference Various chapters. In Drake R, Vogl AW, Mitchell AWM: *Gray's anatomy for students,* ed 4, Philadelphia, 2020, Churchill Livingstone.

FIGURE 1.14 Major bones (anterior and posterior views)

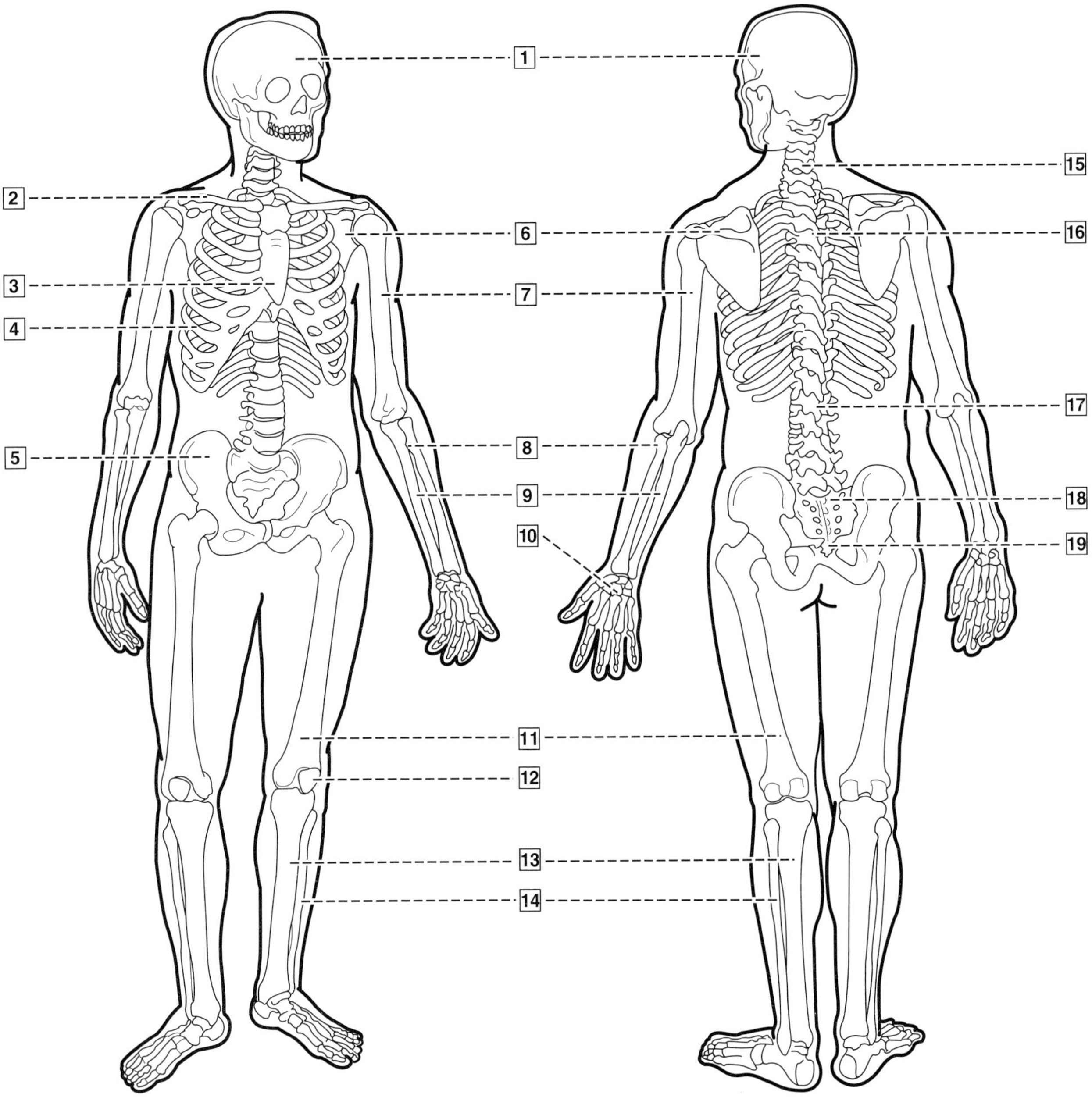

1 Skull	6 Scapula	11 Femur	16 Thoracic vertebrae
2 Clavicle	7 Humerus	12 Patella	17 Lumbar vertebrae
3 Sternum	8 Radius	13 Tibia	18 Sacrum
4 Ribs	9 Ulna	14 Fibula	19 Coccyx
5 Os coxae	10 Carpals	15 Vertebral column/ Cervical vertebrae	

REVIEW QUESTIONS: Major bones

Fill in the blanks by choosing the appropriate terms from the list below.

1. Adults have 206 bones, although at birth there are about 300 bones; however, many of the bones _____ together with growth.

2. The _____ is composed of the cranium and mandible.

3. The _____ or *backbone* is composed of 24 bones and includes the vertebrae, sacrum, and coccyx.

4. The top seven vertebrae, the _____, compose the neck, with the next twelve, thoracic vertebrae attaching to the ribs, with the last five vertebrae being the lumbar vertebrae; the sacrum is directly inferior to the lumbar vertebrae and is attached to the pelvic bone or *hipbone*, and the coccyx or *tailbone* is located further inferior to it, with the os coxa of an adult pelvic girdle formed by the fusion of the ilium, ischium, and pubis.

5. The _____ create a bony cage protecting internal organs such as the heart, lungs, and liver; although there are usually twelve pairs of ribs, occasionally there is one extra pair or one missing pair.

6. The superior seven ribs connect to the _____ or *breastbone*; they also attach to the clavicle or *collarbone*, and the more inferior thoracic vertebrae hold all twelve ribs in place.

7. The arms each contain one _____, which is the large bone at the superior part of the arm, and two long bones of the forearm, which are the ulna and radius; the carpals are the bones of the wrist.

8. The long bone of the thigh is the _____; the patella or *kneecap* articulates with this bone.

9. The two long bones running from the knee to the ankle, the _____ and the fibula, compose the bones of the legs.

10. The bones of the ankle are the _____; the metacarpals and metatarsals are bones of the hand and foot, respectively, with the phalanges being the bones of the fingers and toes.

fuse	tibia	skull
cervical vertebrae	femur	humerus
tarsals	sternum	vertebral column
ribs		

Reference   Various chapters. In Drake R, Vogl AW, Mitchell AWM: *Gray's anatomy for students,* ed 4, Philadelphia, 2020, Churchill Livingstone.

FIGURE 1.15 Bone and cartilage anatomy (external and microanatomic views)

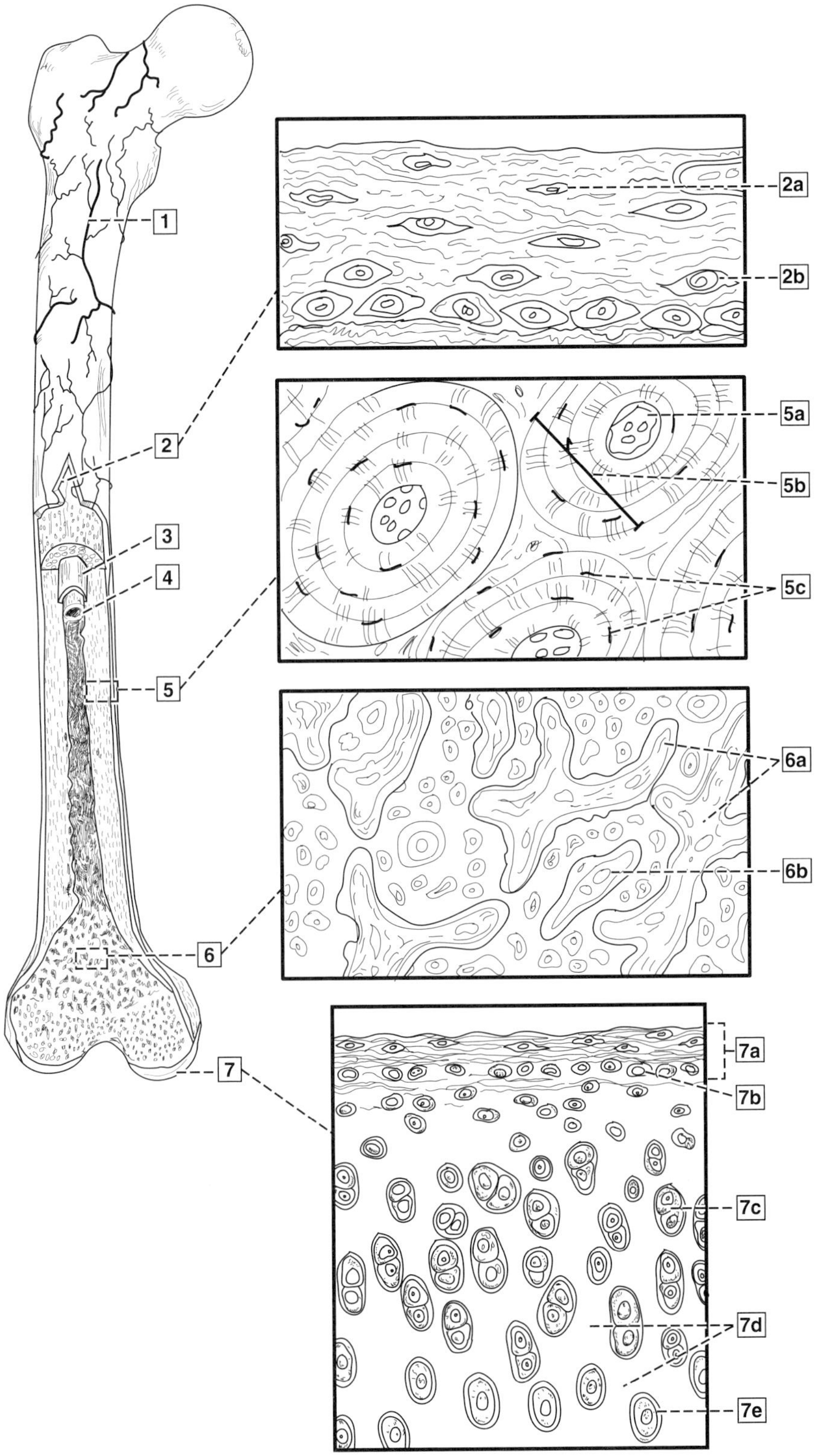

1 Blood vessel
2 Periosteum
2a Fibroblast
2b Osteoblast
3 Endosteum
4 Bone marrow
5 Compact bone
5a Haversian canal
5b Osteon
5c Lamellae

6 Cancellous bone
6a Trabeculae
6b Blood vessel
7 Articular cartilage
7a Perichondrium
7b Chondroblast
7c Daughter chondrocytes in lacuna
7d Cartilage matrix
7e Singular chondrocyte in lacuna

REVIEW QUESTIONS: Bone and cartilage anatomy

Fill in the blanks by choosing the appropriate terms from the list below.

1. The _____ is a hard rigid form of connective tissue that constitutes most of the mature skeleton; thus, it serves as protective and structural support for soft tissue and as an attachment mechanism.

2. The outer part of bone is covered by the _____, which is a double-layered dense connective tissue sheath.

3. The outer layer of the periosteum contains blood vessels and nerves; the inner layer contains a single layer of cells that gives rise to bone-forming cells, the _____.

4. Deep to the periosteum is a dense layer of _____, which is that part of a bone composed of densely packed bone tissue; and deep to compact bone is the spongy bone or cancellous bone that is that part of a bone composed of less dense bone tissue.

5. Lining the medullary cavity of bone on the inside of the layers of compact bone and cancellous bone is the _____, which has the same composition as the periosteum but is thinner; on the innermost part of bone in the medullary cavity is the bone marrow that is a gelatinous substance where the stem cells of the blood are located, the lymphocytes are created, and B cells mature.

6. Bone matrix is initially formed as _____, which later undergoes mineralization; this is produced by osteoblasts that are cuboidal cells arising from fibroblasts.

7. The process of _____ involves the formation of osteoid between two dense connective tissue sheets, which then eventually replaces the outer connective tissue; this type of process contrasts with the process of endochondral ossification that involves the formation of the osteoid within a hyaline cartilage model that subsequently becomes mineralized and dies.

8. The _____ is a firm but flexible nonmineralized connective tissue that serves as a temporary skeletal tissue in the embryo and then serves as structural support for certain soft tissue after birth; it can also serve as a model or template in which certain bones of the body subsequently develop as well as be present at articular surfaces of most freely movable joints, such as the temporomandibular joint.

9. The connective tissue surrounding most cartilage is the _____, a fibrous connective tissue sheath containing blood vessels.

10. Two types of cells found in cartilage are the immature chondroblasts, which lie internal to the perichondrium and produce cartilage matrix, and the _____, which are mature chondroblasts maintaining the cartilage matrix within their lacunae.

osteoblasts	cartilage	chondrocytes
compact bone	bone	periosteum
endosteum	osteoid	intramembranous ossification
perichondrium		

Reference   Chapter 8, Basic tissue. In Fehrenbach MJ, Popowics T: *Illustrated dental embryology, histology, and anatomy,* ed 5, St. Louis, 2020, Saunders.

FIGURE 1.16 Bone (transverse section with microanatomic views)

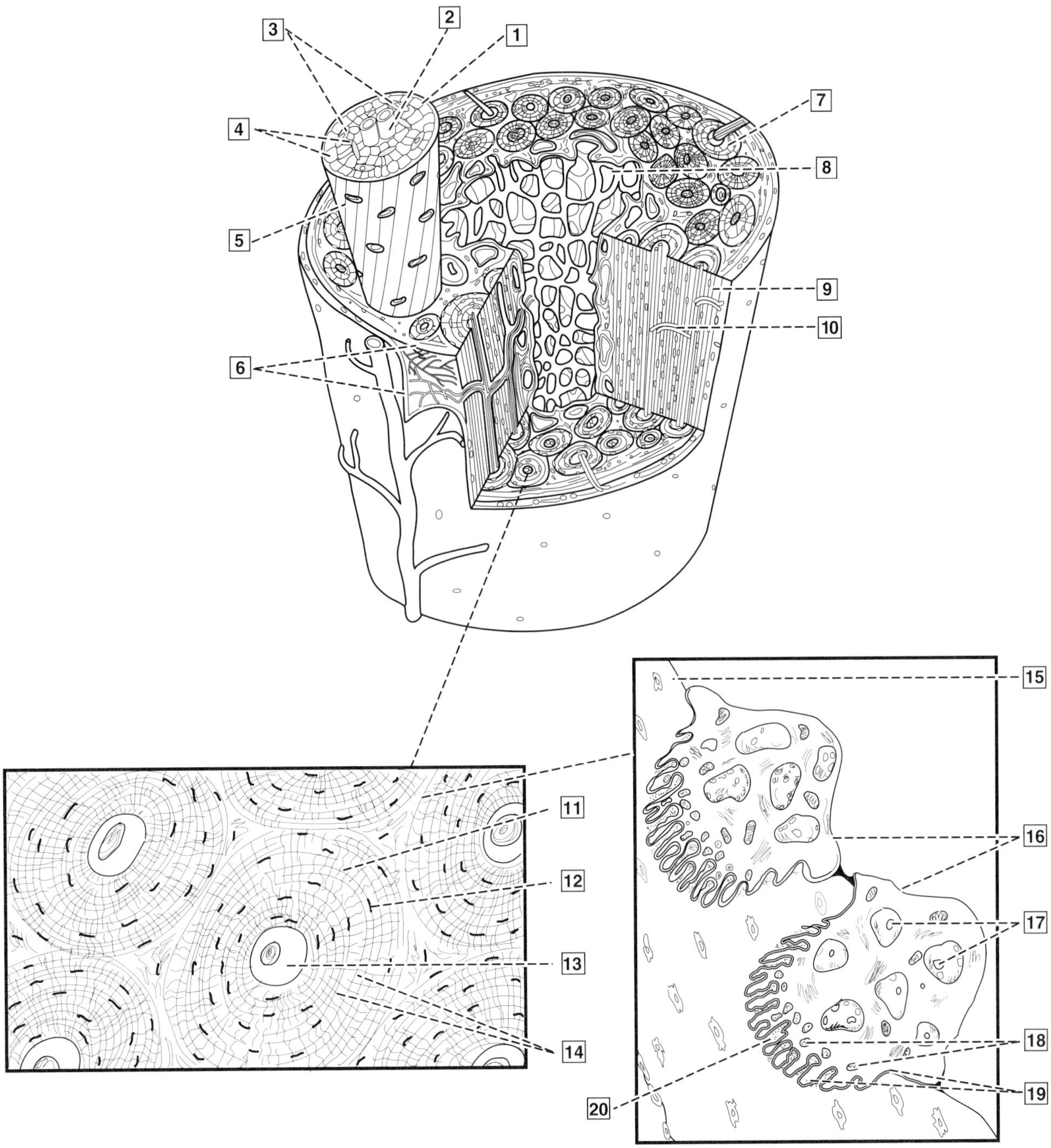

1 Lamellae	**6** Periosteum	**11** Canaliculi	**16** Osteoclasts
2 Haversian canal	**7** Osteon of compact bone	**12** Osteocyte in lacuna	**17** Nuclei
3 Lacunae containing osteocytes	**8** Trabeculae of cancellous bone	**13** Haversian canal	**18** Lysosomes
4 Canaliculi	**9** Haversian canal	**14** Concentric lamellae	**19** Howship lacuna
5 Osteon	**10** Volkmann canal	**15** Mineralized bone	**20** Area of bone resorption

REVIEW QUESTIONS: Bone

Fill in the blanks by choosing the appropriate terms from the list below.

1. Bone consists of cells and a partially mineralized matrix that is composed of inorganic or mineralized material, which is a crystalline formation of mainly _____ that gives bone its hardness.

2. Within fully mineralized bone are _____, which are entrapped mature osteoblasts; similar to the chondrocyte, the cell body is surrounded by bone, except for the space immediately around it, the lacuna.

3. Unlike chondrocytes, _____ never undergo mitosis during tissue formation and thus only one osteocyte is ever found in its lacuna.

4. The cytoplasmic processes of the osteocyte radiate outward in all directions in the bone and are located in tubular canals of matrix or _____; these canals provide for interaction between the osteocytes.

5. Bone matrix in compact bone is formed into closely apposed sheets or _____; within and between them are embedded osteocytes with their cytoplasmic processes in the canals.

6. The highly organized arrangement of concentric lamellae in compact bone is the _____; within it, the lamellae form concentric layers of matrix into cylinders or osteons.

7. The _____ (or central canal) is a central vascular canal within each osteon surrounded by the lamellae; it contains longitudinally running blood vessels, nerves, and a small amount of connective tissue that is overall lined by endosteum.

8. Located on the periphery of the Haversian system in compact bone are _____, which are similar nutrient canals to the Haversian canals, and are also lined by endosteum.

9. The cell in mature bone that causes resorption of bone is the _____.

10. The osteoclast is a large multinucleated giant cell located on the surface of secondary bone in a large shallow pit created by this resorption, a(n) _____.

osteocytes	osteoblasts	lamellae
calcium hydroxyapatite	Haversian system	Haversian canal
Howship lacuna	Volkmann canals	osteoclast
canaliculi		

Reference   Chapter 8, Basic tissue. In Fehrenbach MJ, Popowics T: *Illustrated dental embryology, histology, and anatomy,* ed 5, St. Louis, 2020, Saunders.

FIGURE 1.17   Joint types

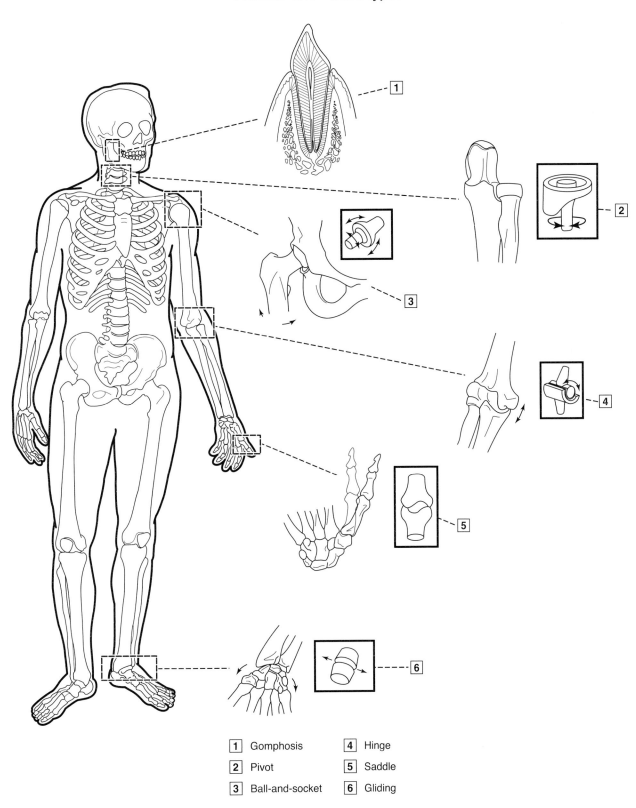

1 Gomphosis	**4** Hinge
2 Pivot	**5** Saddle
3 Ball-and-socket	**6** Gliding

REVIEW QUESTIONS: Joint types

Fill in the blanks by choosing the appropriate terms from the list below.

1. Joints are areas where usually two _____ structures that come together and can be categorized according to function or structure.

2. Joints that do not allow mobility in adults, such as the _____ of the skull are synarthrosis joints, with most being fibrous joints.

3. Other joints that allow slight mobility are amphiarthrosis joints, with most being cartilaginous joints, such as the _____ of the spinal column.

4. Joints that allow a variety of types of mobility are _____ joints, which are the most common type of joints.

5. All diarthrosis joints are _____ joints and include ball-and-socket, hinge, pivot, gliding, or ellipsoidal joints.

6. The _____ joint, such as the shoulder and hip joints, allows backward, forward, sideways, and rotating movements, including flexion, extension, and rotation.

7. The _____ joint, such as in the humeroulnar joint of the elbow, allows only bending and straightening movements, all within one direction.

8. The _____ joint, such as the neck joints, including the atlantoaxial joint, allows limited rotating movements as with the head; the gliding or *plane joint* allows sliding movement when one bone moves across the surface of another such as the radioulnar joint.

9. The _____ or *condylar joint*, such as the wrist joint, allows all types of movement except pivotal movements; the saddle joint is noted with the carpometacarpal joint of the thumb when touching the fingers, which allows flexion, extension, abduction, adduction, and circumduction.

10. The gomphosis (plural, *gomphoses*) is a(n) _____ joint involving the root of the tooth to the bony socket (or *dental alveolus*) in either the maxillae or mandible that usually allow only slight mobility; the fibrous connection between a tooth and its socket is the periodontal ligament, with the connection made to the bony jaw by way of the cementum of the tooth.

ball-and-socket	hinge	sutures
diarthrosis	pivot	synovial
ellipsoid	skeletal	vertebrae
fibrous		

Reference Various chapters. In Drake R, Vogl AW, Mitchell AWM: *Gray's anatomy for students,* ed 4, Philadelphia, 2020, Churchill Livingstone.

ANSWER KEY 1. skeletal, 2. sutures, 3. vertebrae, 4. diarthrosis, 5. synovial, 6. ball-and-socket, 7. hinge, 8. pivot, 9. ellipsoid, 10. fibrous

FIGURE 1.18 Skeletal muscle (transverse sections with microanatomic views)

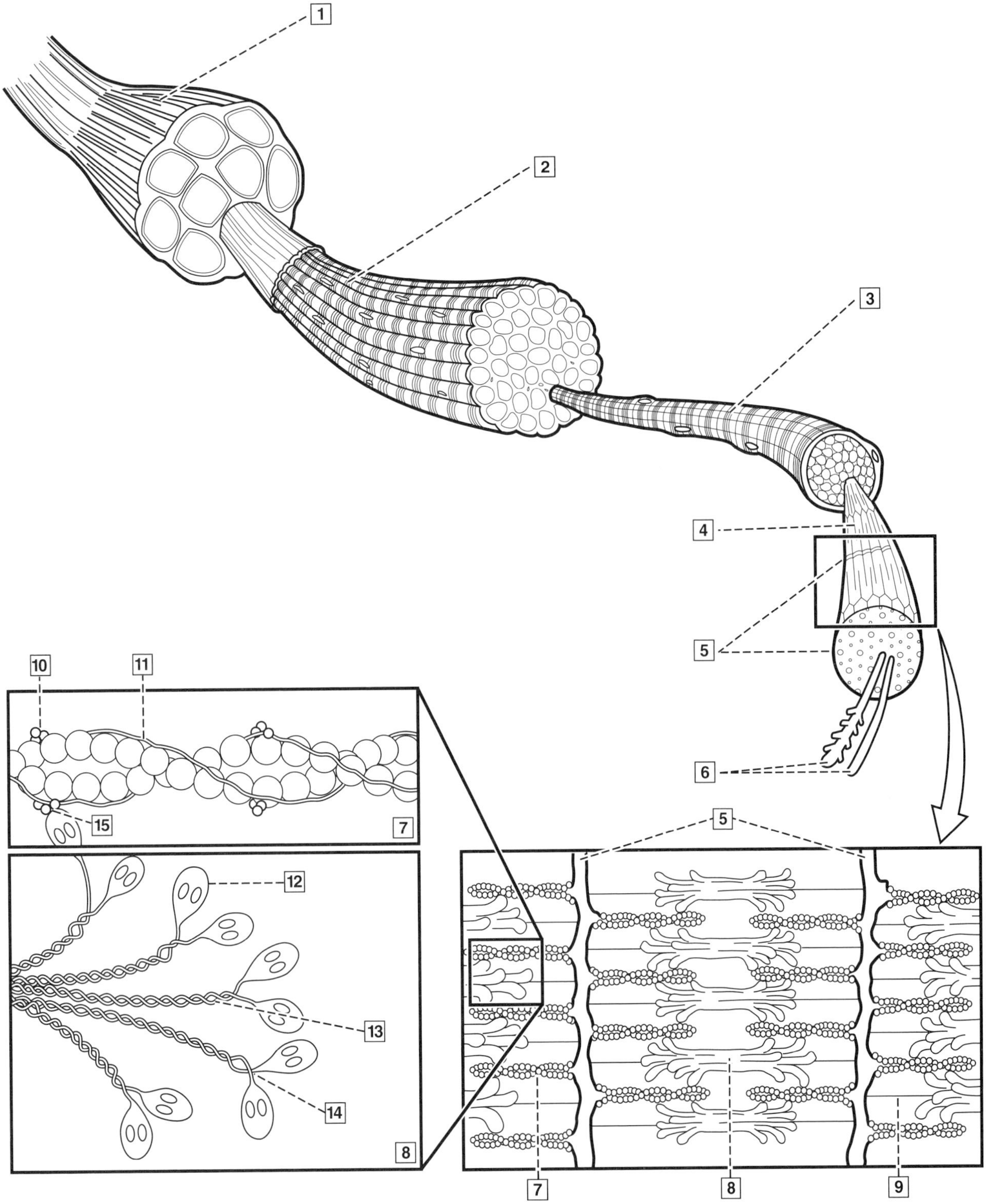

1 Muscle	**5** Sarcomere	**9** Elastic (titin) myofilament	**13** Stalk
2 Muscle fascicle	**6** Myofilaments	**10** Troponin	**14** Hinge
3 Myofiber	**7** Thin (actin) myofilament	**11** Tropomyosin	**15** Actin-myosin crossbridge
4 Myofibril	**8** Thick (myosin) myofilament	**12** Myosin head	

REVIEW QUESTIONS: Skeletal muscle

Fill in the blanks by choosing the appropriate terms from the list below.

1. The muscle tissue in the body is part of the _____ and is similar to connective tissue; most muscles are derived from somites.

2. Each muscle _____ under neural control, causing soft tissue and bony structures of the body to move.

3. The _____ types of muscle are classified according to structure, function, and innervation, and include skeletal, smooth, and cardiac muscles.

4. Skeletal muscles are considered _____ because they are under voluntary control, and involve the somatic nervous system.

5. The skeletal muscles in the head and neck include the muscles of _____, which give the face its expression as well as the muscles of the tongue, pharynx, upper esophagus, and mastication that assist the temporomandibular joint in the actions involved in mastication.

6. The skeletal muscles are usually attached to _____ of the skeleton.

7. The skeletal muscles are also considered _____ because the muscle cells appear striped microscopically.

8. Each muscle is composed of numerous muscle bundles or fascicles, which then are composed of numerous muscle cells or _____.

9. Each myofiber in muscle extends the entire length of the muscle and is composed of smaller subunits of _____ surrounded by the other organelles of the cell.

10. Each myofibril in muscle is composed of even smaller subunits of _____.

shortens	facial expression	voluntary muscles
muscular system	bones	striated muscles
myofilaments	myofibrils	myofibers
three		

Reference   Chapter 8, Basic tissue. In Fehrenbach MJ, Popowics T: *Illustrated dental embryology, histology, and anatomy,* ed 5, St. Louis, 2020, Saunders.

NOTES

ANSWER KEY 1. muscular system, 2. shortens, 3. three, 4. voluntary muscles, 5. facial expression, 6. bones, 7. striated muscles, 8. myofibers, 9. myofibrils, 10. myofilaments

FIGURE 1.19   Major body muscles (anterior view)

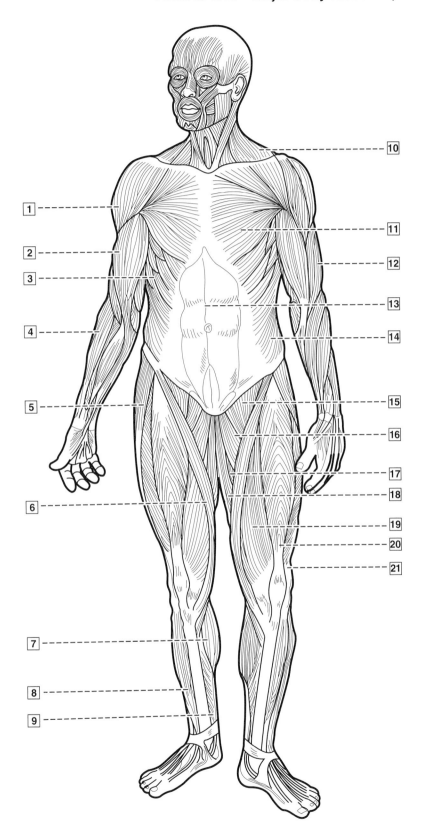

1 Deltoid

2 Biceps brachii

3 Serratus anterior

4 Brachioradialis

5 Tensor fasciae latae

6 Sartorius

7 Gastrocnemius

8 Tibialis anterior

9 Soleus

10 Trapezius

11 Pectoralis major

12 Brachialis

13 Linea alba

14 External abdominal oblique

15 Iliopsoas

16 Adductor longus

17 Adductor magnus

18 Gracilis

19 Vastus medialis

20 Rectus femoris

21 Vastus lateralis

REVIEW QUESTIONS: Major body muscles (anterior view)

Fill in the blanks by choosing the appropriate terms from the list below.

1. The _____ enables the arm to draw away from the median axis of the body to direct it toward the anterior and posterior until it is horizontal.

2. The _____ mainly enables the forearm to flex on the arm.

3. The _____ enables the thigh to flex and to rotate outside the median axis; it also allows the leg to flex.

4. The _____ forms the curve of the calf and enables the foot to extend; it also enables the knee to extend.

5. The _____ enables the foot to flex on the leg and to draw near the median axis of the body; the posterior tibial muscle enables the foot to extend.

6. The _____ enables various arm movements, such as drawing the arm near the median axis of the body and rotating it toward the median axis; it also aids in inhalation.

7. The _____ located on the inner thigh mainly enables the knee to extend as it stabilizes the knee; the vastus lateralis muscle in the outer thigh also mainly enables the knee to extend as it stabilizes the knee.

8. The _____ enables the forearm to flex and to rotate outwardly with the palm toward the anterior; the biceps contracts while the triceps brachii muscle relaxes.

9. The _____ enables the knee to extend and the thigh to flex on the pelvis.

10. The _____ enables the thigh to draw near the median axis of the body as well as rotating outside the median axis and to flex.

vastus medialis muscle	biceps brachii muscle	adductor longus muscle
sartorius muscle	pectoralis major muscle	anterior tibialis muscle
deltoid muscle	gastrocnemius muscle	brachioradialis muscle
rectus femoris muscle		

Reference Various chapters. In Drake R, Vogl AW, Mitchell AWM: *Gray's anatomy for students,* ed 4, Philadelphia, 2020, Churchill Livingstone.

NOTES

FIGURE 1.20 **Major body muscles (posterior view)**

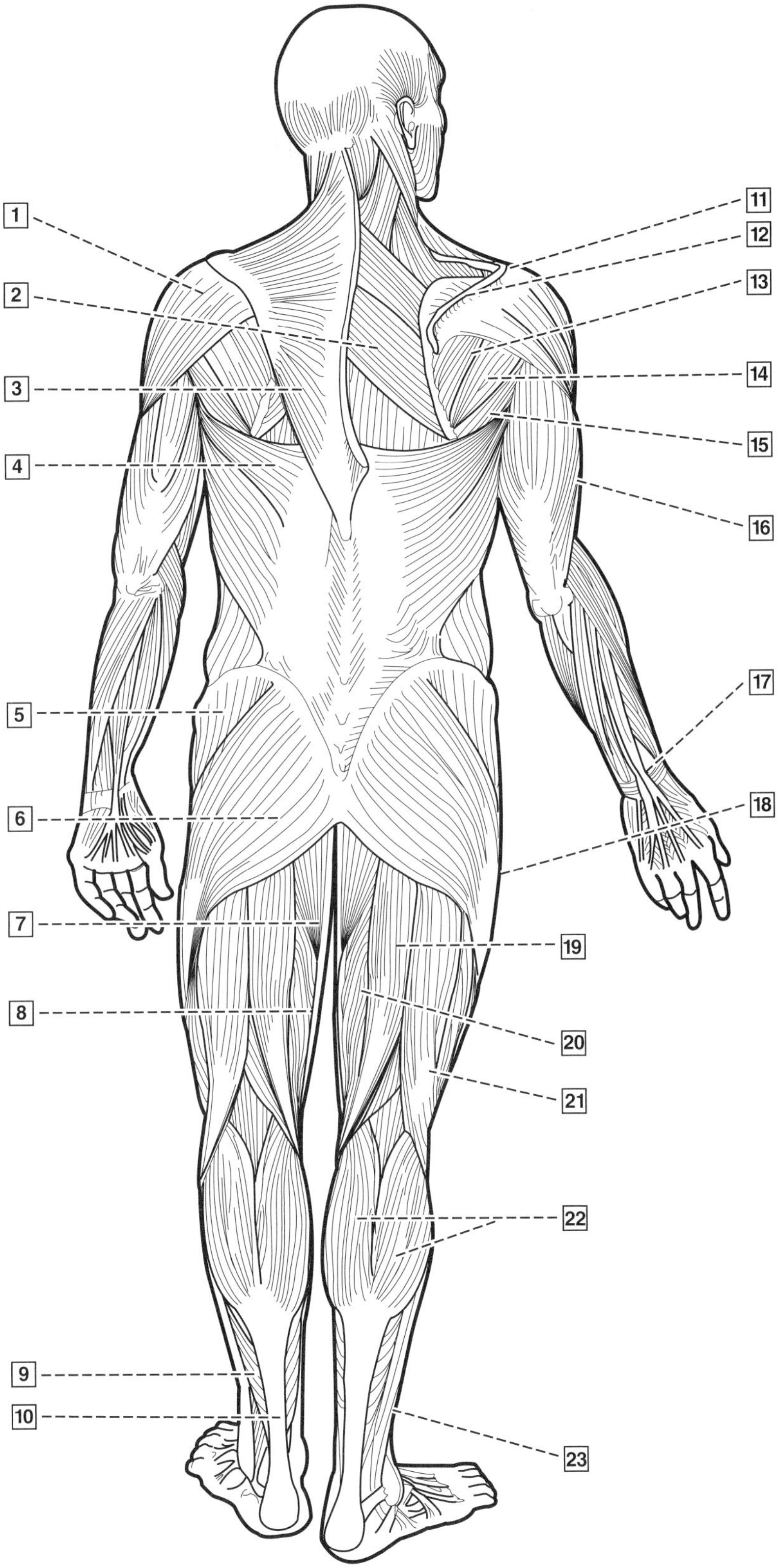

1	Deltoid
2	Rhomboideus major
3	Trapezius
4	Latissimus dorsi
5	Gluteus medius
6	Gluteus maximus
7	Adductor magnus
8	Gracilis
9	Soleus
10	Calcaneal tendon
11	Cut edge of trapezius
12	Supraspinatus
13	Infraspinatus
14	Teres minor
15	Teres major
16	Triceps brachii
17	Extensor digitorum
18	Tensor fasciae latae
19	Semitendinosus
20	Semimembranosus
21	Biceps femoris
22	Gastrocnemius
23	Peroneus longus

REVIEW QUESTIONS: Major body muscles (posterior view)

Fill in the blanks by choosing the appropriate terms from the list below.

1. The _____ especially enables the arm to draw near the median axis of the body, to extend, and to rotate inwardly.

2. The _____ enables the hip to extend and to rotate outside the median axis; it also allows the trunk to return to a vertical position.

3. The _____ enables the thigh to draw near the median axis of the body and the leg to flex on the thigh and rotate toward the median axis.

4. The _____ enables the thigh to draw near the median axis of the body, to rotate outside the median axis, to flex, and to extend.

5. The _____ enables the arm to rotate outside the median axis; it also stabilizes the shoulder joint.

6. The _____ enables the arm to rotate outside the median axis as it stabilizes the shoulder joint; the teres major muscle enables the arm to draw near the median axis of the body and also rotate toward the median axis.

7. The _____ enables the forearm to extend on the arm; it contracts, whereas the biceps brachii muscle relaxes.

8. The _____ especially enables the leg to stretch and the thigh to flex and draw away from the median axis of the body; it also stabilizes the hip and the knee.

9. The _____ enables the thigh to extend on the pelvis, the knee to flex, and the thigh and the leg to rotate toward the median axis.

10. The _____ enables the leg to flex on the thigh and to rotate outside the median axis as well as the thigh to extend on the pelvis.

latissimus dorsi muscle	infraspinatus muscle	gluteus maximus muscle
gracilis muscle	biceps femora muscle	tensor of fascia latae muscle
teres minor muscle	triceps brachii muscle	semimembranosus muscle
adductor magnus muscle		

Reference Various chapters. In Drake R, Vogl AW, Mitchell AWM: *Gray's anatomy for students,* ed 4, Philadelphia, 2020, Churchill Livingstone.

NOTES

ANSWER KEY 1. latissimus dorsi muscle, 2. gluteus maximus muscle, 3. gracilis muscle, 4. adductor magnus muscle, 5. infraspinatus muscle, 6. teres minor muscle, 7. triceps brachii muscle, 8. tensor of fascia latae muscle, 9. semimembranosus muscle, 10. biceps femora muscle

FIGURE 1.21   Blood components (with microanatomic views)

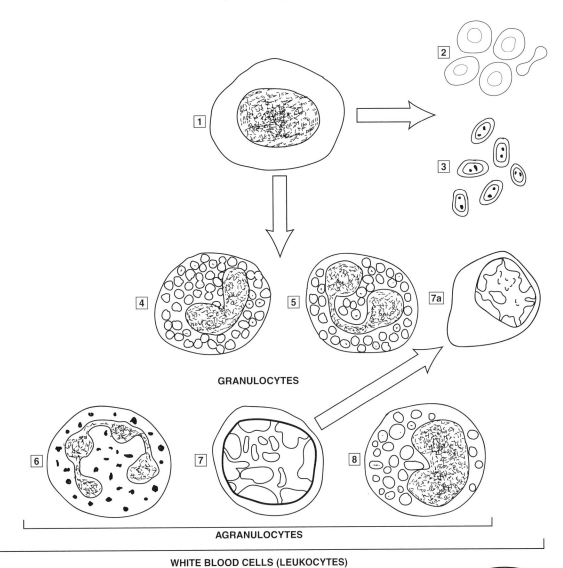

GRANULOCYTES

AGRANULOCYTES

WHITE BLOOD CELLS (LEUKOCYTES)

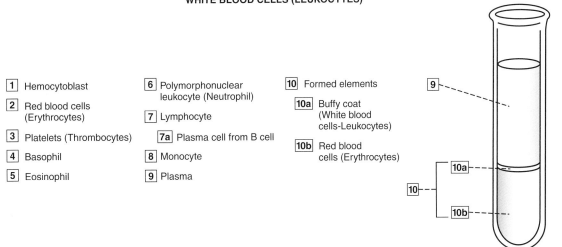

1 Hemocytoblast	**6** Polymorphonuclear leukocyte (Neutrophil)	**10** Formed elements
2 Red blood cells (Erythrocytes)	**7** Lymphocyte	**10a** Buffy coat (White blood cells-Leukocytes)
3 Platelets (Thrombocytes)	**7a** Plasma cell from B cell	**10b** Red blood cells (Erythrocytes)
4 Basophil	**8** Monocyte	
5 Eosinophil	**9** Plasma	

REVIEW QUESTIONS: Blood components

Fill in the blanks by choosing the appropriate terms from the list below.

1. The most common cell in the blood is the _____ or erythrocyte, which is a biconcave disc that contains hemoglobin that binds and then transports oxygen and carbon dioxide; it has no nucleus and does not undergo mitosis because it is formed from the bone marrow's stem cells.

2. The blood contains _____ or thrombocytes, which are smaller than red blood cells, disc-shaped, and also have no nucleus; however, these formed elements are not considered true blood cells but instead fragments of bone marrow cells (or megakaryocytes) and are found in fewer numbers than red blood cells and function in the clotting mechanism.

3. In lesser numbers in the blood is the _____ or leukocyte and like a red blood cell, it forms from bone-marrow stem cells and later matures in the bone marrow or in various lymphatic organs; it is involved in the defense mechanisms of the body, including the inflammatory and immune responses.

4. The most common white blood cell in the blood is the _____ or neutrophil, which is the first cell to appear at an injury site when the inflammatory response is triggered; it has a short life span, contains lysosomal enzymes, is active in phagocytosis, and responds to chemotactic factors.

5. The second most common white blood cell in the blood is the _____, which has three functional types that include the B cell, T cell, and natural killer (NK) cell; cytokines are produced by both B and T cells and are one of the major chemical mediators of the immune response.

6. The B-cell lymphocytes divide during the immune response to form _____, which when mature produce an immunoglobulin, which is also considered an antibody and one of the blood proteins; there are five distinct classes, which include IgA (serum or secretory types), IgD, IgE, IgG, and IgM.

7. The most common white blood cell in the connective tissue proper is the _____, which is considered a monocyte before it migrates from the blood into the tissue; like neutrophils, it contains lysosomal enzymes and is involved in phagocytosis, is actively mobile, and has the ability to respond to chemotactic factors and cytokines; however, unlike a neutrophil, it also assists in the immune response to facilitate immunoglobulin production, has a longer life span, and is only in a small percentage of the leukocyte count.

8. In certain disease states, numbers of macrophages may fuse together, forming _____ with multiple nuclei; in bone connective tissue, these are considered osteoclasts that will resorb bone.

9. The _____ is usually found only as a small percentage of the leukocyte count, but its percentage is increased during a hypersensitivity response (allergy) and in parasitic diseases because its primary function seems to be the phagocytosis of immune complexes.

10. The _____ is usually found as a very small percentage of the leukocyte count and is involved in the hypersensitivity response (allergy) releasing bioactive products.

Platelets
red blood cell
polymorphonuclear leukocyte
giant cells

lymphocyte
white blood cell
macrophage

eosinophil
basophil
plasma cells

Reference Chapter 8, Basic tissue. In Fehrenbach MJ, Popowics T: *Illustrated dental embryology, histology, and anatomy,* ed 5, St. Louis, 2020, Saunders.

FIGURE 1.22 Blood vessels (transverse sections with microanatomic views)

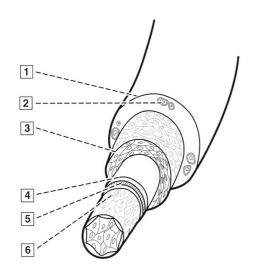
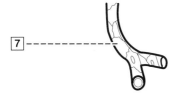
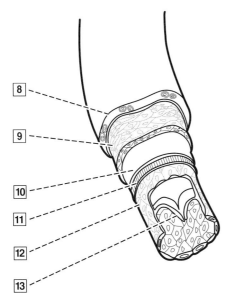

ARTERY

Tunica externa (adventitia)

| 1 | Connective tissue |
| 2 | Vasa vasorum |

Tunica media

| 3 | Smooth muscle |

Tunica intima

4	Elastic fibers
5	Basement membrane
6	Endothelium

CAPILLARY

| 7 | Endothelium |

VEIN

Tunica externa

| 8 | Connective tissue |

Tunica media

| 9 | Smooth muscle |

Tunica intima

10	Elastic fibers
11	Basement membrane
12	Endothelium
13	Venous valve

REVIEW QUESTIONS: Blood vessels

Fill in the blanks by choosing the appropriate terms from the list below.

1. The _____ is a type of blood vessel that begins at the heart and carries blood away from the heart; most of the blood in this type of vessel is usually oxygenated, except for the blood in the pulmonary and umbilical ones.

2. The outermost layer of the artery is the _____ or *tunica adventitia*, which is composed of connective tissue as well as the vasa vasorum, a network of small blood vessels that supply large blood vessels.

3. The _____, which is the middle layer of smooth muscle cells with varying amounts of elastic fibers.

4. The inner layer of the artery in direct contact with the flow of blood is the _____; it is composed of mainly endothelial cells and elastic fibers.

5. The _____ has the smallest diameter of the other blood vessels and is part of the microcirculation because it forms groups in a type of bed format for a larger area; at the same time, the arteries branch and narrow into the arterioles and then branch further still into large numbers of these blood vessels.

6. The _____ is a type of blood vessel that travels to the heart and carries blood toward it; most of these vessels carry deoxygenated blood from the tissue back to the heart; it is important to note that the exceptions are the pulmonary and umbilical ones, both of which carry oxygenated blood to the heart.

7. The thick outermost layer of a vein is composed of connective tissue and is the _____ or *tunica externa.*

8. The middle layer of smooth muscle in a vein is the tunica media, which in general is thin because veins do not function primarily as a(n) _____ structure.

9. The inner layer of the vein of the tunica intima is lined with elastic fibers and _____ as well as a venous valve.

10. The _____ has a very small diameter and drains the capillaries in the area of the microcirculation that allows deoxygenated blood to return from the capillary beds to the larger diameter veins.

tunica media	tunica externa	contractile
artery	capillary	tunica intima
tunica adventitia	venule	vein
endothelium		

References Chapter 6, Vascular system. In Fehrenbach MJ, Herring SW: *Illustrated anatomy of the head and neck,* ed 6, St. Louis, 2021, Saunders; Various chapters. In Drake R, Vogl AW, Mitchell AWM: *Gray's anatomy for students,* ed 4, Philadelphia, 2020, Churchill Livingstone.

ANSWER KEY 1. artery, 2. tunica externa, 3. tunica media, 4. tunica intima, 5. capillary, 6. vein, 7. tunica adventitia, 8. contractile, 9. endothelium, 10. venule

FIGURE 1.23 Major systemic arteries (frontal view)

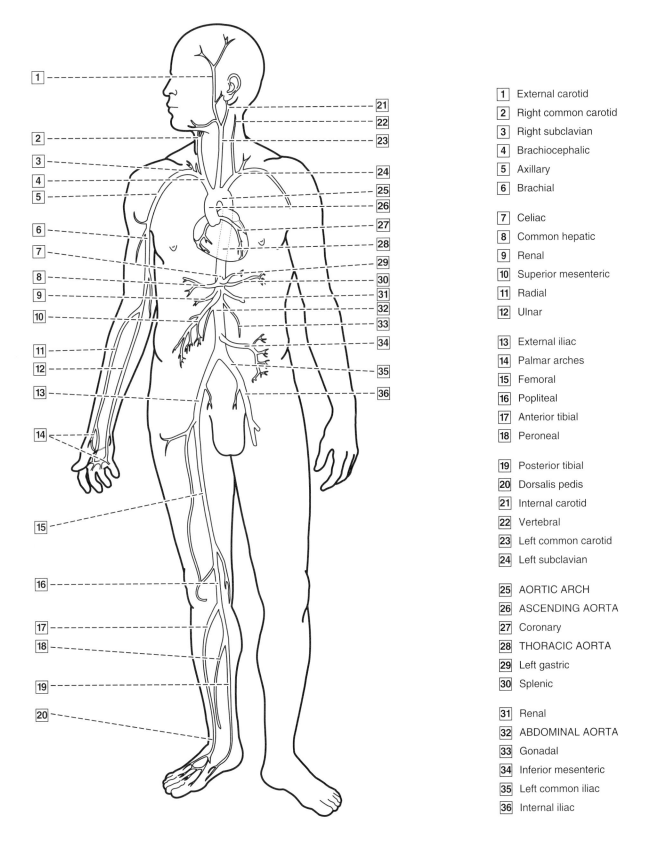

1	External carotid
2	Right common carotid
3	Right subclavian
4	Brachiocephalic
5	Axillary
6	Brachial
7	Celiac
8	Common hepatic
9	Renal
10	Superior mesenteric
11	Radial
12	Ulnar
13	External iliac
14	Palmar arches
15	Femoral
16	Popliteal
17	Anterior tibial
18	Peroneal
19	Posterior tibial
20	Dorsalis pedis
21	Internal carotid
22	Vertebral
23	Left common carotid
24	Left subclavian
25	AORTIC ARCH
26	ASCENDING AORTA
27	Coronary
28	THORACIC AORTA
29	Left gastric
30	Splenic
31	Renal
32	ABDOMINAL AORTA
33	Gonadal
34	Inferior mesenteric
35	Left common iliac
36	Internal iliac

REVIEW QUESTIONS: Major systemic arteries

Fill in the blanks by choosing the appropriate terms from the list below.

1. The _____ are arteries that travel along the neck entering the cranial cavity through the foramen magnum after beginning from the subclavian arteries; these arteries then converge within the cranial cavity forming the basilar artery, which is one of the arteries that supplies the brain.

2. The _____ ends by dividing in the neck into the internal and external carotid arteries; it is important to note that the left common carotid artery and subclavian artery begin directly from the aorta and travel along the left side of the neck, whereas the right common carotid artery and subclavian artery are both branches from the brachiocephalic artery; the brachiocephalic artery is a direct branch of the aorta.

3. The _____ is a major artery that supplies the brain and also supplies the orbital region; it branches into the ophthalmic artery, anterior cerebral artery, and middle cerebral artery.

4. The _____ is a major artery that supplies the more superficial structures of the head and neck, with the exception of the orbital region; it branches into several arteries, including the superior thyroid artery, lingual artery, facial artery, occipital artery, maxillary artery, and superficial temporal artery.

5. The _____ begins from the relatively short brachiocephalic artery (trunk) when it divides into the subclavian and the right common carotid artery; the left subclavian artery begins from the aortic arch.

6. The _____ originates along the first rib bone, beginning from the subclavian artery and branches into the brachial artery; the brachial artery supplies the muscles of the arm.

7. Originating in the elbow, the _____ begins from the brachial artery; later it follows along the ulnar bone of the forearm and it supplies the forearm, wrist, and hand; within the elbow, at the same point at which the brachial artery branches into this artery, the brachial artery also branches into the parallel radial artery, which travels along the radial bone supplying the forearm, wrist, and hand but is smaller than the ulnar artery.

8. The _____ courses along the femoral bone of the lower extremities; it supplies the lower extremities and is one of the largest arteries in the body.

9. The _____ extends from the femoral artery and ends near the knee; similar to the femoral artery, the artery supplies the leg.

10. The _____ are composed of two arteries, the anterior tibial artery and the posterior tibial artery; these arteries course along the tibial bone of the leg, eventually ending in the foot.

popliteal artery	vertebral arteries	axillary artery
common carotid artery	external carotid artery	internal carotid artery
right subclavian artery	ulnar artery	tibial arteries
femoral artery		

Reference Various chapters. In Drake R, Vogl AW, Mitchell AWM: *Gray's anatomy for students,* ed 4, Philadelphia, 2020, Churchill Livingstone.

ANSWER KEY 1. vertebral arteries, 2. common carotid artery, 3. internal carotid artery, 4. external carotid artery, 5. right subclavian artery, 6. axillary artery, 7. ulnar artery, 8. femoral artery, 9. popliteal artery, 10. tibial arteries

FIGURE 1.24   Major systemic veins (frontal view)

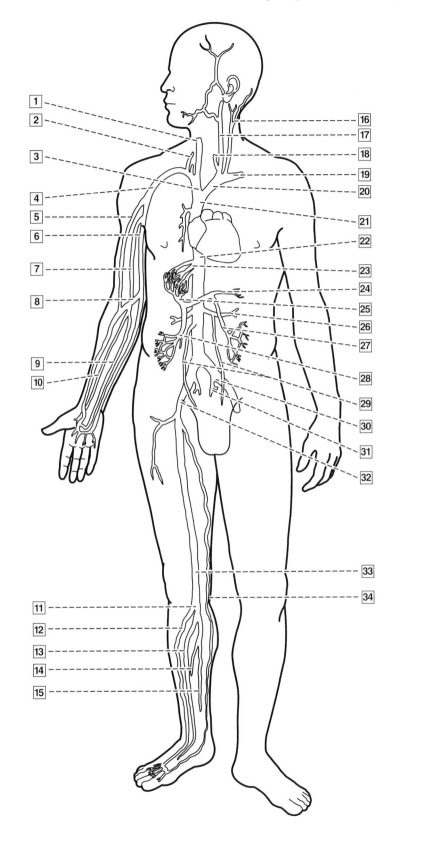

1 Right internal jugular
2 Right external jugular
3 Right brachiocephalic
4 Axillary
5 Cephalic
6 Basilic

7 Brachial
8 Median cubital
9 Ulnar
10 Radial
11 Popliteal
12 Small saphenous

13 Anterior tibial
14 Peroneal
15 Posterior tibial
16 Left external jugular
17 Left internal jugular
18 Vertebral

19 Subclavian
20 Left brachiocephalic
21 Superior vena cava
22 Inferior vena cava
23 Hepatic
24 Splenic

25 Hepatic portal
26 Renal
27 Inferior mesenteric
28 Superior mesenteric
29 Gonadal
30 Common iliac

31 Internal iliac
32 External iliac
33 Femoral
34 Great saphenous

REVIEW QUESTIONS: Major systemic veins

Fill in the blanks by choosing the appropriate terms from the list below.

1. The _____ is a major vein that travels along the neck and drains the more superficial structures of the head and neck; it is the more superficial of the two jugular veins and terminates in the subclavian vein.

2. The _____ is a major vein that travels along the neck and lies deep to the external jugular vein and drains the brain and neck; this vein terminates in the subclavian vein similar to the external jugular vein.

3. The _____ is a vein that lies parallel to the brachial artery along the arm and drains the arm.

4. The _____ is a major vein that lies deep to the clavicle bone and drains the upper extremities of the body; it has a right and left branch.

5. The _____ is a vein that runs along the axillary artery and begins from the basilic vein that eventually becomes the subclavian vein; it drains the axillary division of the body.

6. The _____ is a vein that lies along the ulnar bone parallel to the ulnar artery, and drains the forearm, wrist and hand; the radial vein lies along the radial bone of the forearm parallel to the radial artery and similar to the ulnar vein, it drains the forearm, wrist and hand.

7. The _____ is a vein formed by the convergence of the internal and external iliac veins along the superior part of the pelvis; the popliteal vein runs parallel to the popliteal artery of the upper leg and drains the knee and surrounding tissue.

8. The _____ is a vein that lies parallel to the femoral artery, traveling along the femoral bone of the thigh; it is one of the larger veins and drains the lower extremities of the body.

9. The _____ is a vein that lies posterior to the tibial bone and drains the lower leg, ankle, and foot.

10. The _____ is a vein of the leg running from the foot to the pelvis; it drains the lower extremities of the body and delivers it to the femoral vein.

external jugular vein	axillary vein	common iliac vein
brachial vein	femoral vein	posterior tibial vein
internal jugular vein	great saphenous vein	ulnar vein
subclavian vein		

Reference   Various chapters. In Drake R, Vogl AW, Mitchell AWM: *Gray's anatomy for students,* ed 4, Philadelphia, 2020, Churchill Livingstone.

FIGURE 1.25 Major blood vessels and heart (frontal view)

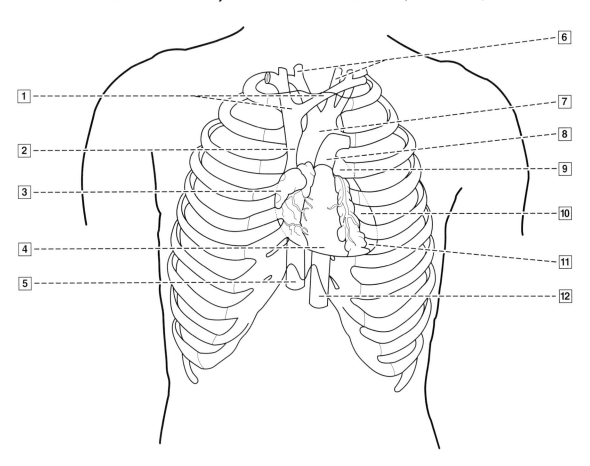

1	Brachiocephalic veins	7	Aorta (arch)
2	Superior vena cava	8	Pulmonary trunk
3	Right atrium	9	Left atrial appendage
4	Right ventricle	10	Left ventricle
5	Inferior vena cava	11	Apex
6	Common carotid arteries	12	Aorta (thoracic)

REVIEW QUESTIONS: Major blood vessels and heart

Fill in the blanks by choosing the appropriate terms from the list below.

1. The _____ is the largest artery in the body and the artery from which most major arteries branch off; it originates from the left ventricle of the heart and extends down to the abdomen, where it divides into the two smaller common iliac arteries.

2. The _____ or *brachiocephalic trunk* or *innominate artery* carries oxygenated blood from the aorta (arch) to the head, neck, and arm regions of the body.

3. The _____ supply oxygenated blood to the head and neck regions of the body.

4. The _____ carry oxygenated blood from the aorta (abdominal) to the legs and feet.

5. The _____ carry deoxygenated blood from the right ventricle to the lungs.

6. The _____ are two large veins that join to form the superior vena cava.

7. The _____ are veins that join to form the inferior vena cava.

8. The _____ transport oxygenated blood from the lungs to the heart.

9. The _____, both inferior and superior, transport deoxygenated blood from various regions of the body to the heart.

10. The _____ is a muscular pouch connected to the left atrium of the heart and has a distinct embryologic origin.

common iliac arteries	common iliac veins	pulmonary veins
aorta	brachiocephalic veins	venae cavae
brachiocephalic artery	pulmonary arteries	left atrial appendage
common carotid arteries		

Reference Various chapters. In Drake R, Vogl AW, Mitchell AWM: *Gray's anatomy for students,* ed 4, Philadelphia, 2020, Churchill Livingstone.

NOTES

FIGURE 1.26 **Heart (internal views)**

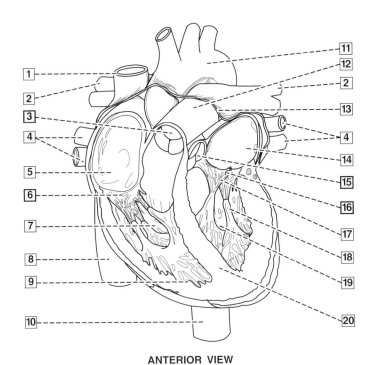

ANTERIOR VIEW

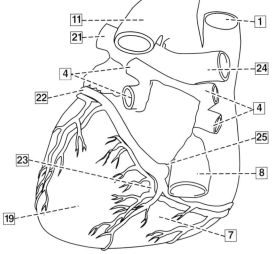

POSTERIOR VIEW

1 Superior vena cava	8 Inferior vena cava		
2 Pulmonary arteries	9 Trabeculae carneae		
3 Pulmonic valve	10 Aorta (thoracic)		
4 Pulmonary veins	11 Aorta (arch)		
5 Right atrium	12 Pulmonary trunk		
6 Tricuspid valve	13 Cut edge of pericardium		
7 Right ventricle	14 Left atrium		

15 Aortic valve	**22 Coronary vein**
16 Mitral valve	23 Coronary artery
17 Chordae tendineae	24 Right pulmonary artery
18 Papillary muscle	25 Carotid sinus
19 Left ventricle	
20 Interventricular septum	
21 Left pulmonary artery	

REVIEW QUESTIONS: Heart

Fill in the blanks by choosing the appropriate terms from the list below.

1. The heart has four main chambers, the two superior atria and the two _____ and is divided into separate right and left sections by the interventricular septum.

2. The _____ are the receiving chambers for the heart; the inferior ventricles are the discharging chambers for the heart.

3. The _____ is a double-walled sac that contains the heart and the roots of the great vessels.

4. Deoxygenated blood flows through the heart in one direction, entering through the _____ and left subclavian artery into the right atrium and is pumped through the tricuspid valve into the right ventricle before being pumped out through the pulmonary valve to the pulmonary arteries into the lungs.

5. The oxygenated blood returns from the lungs through the _____ to the left atrium where it is pumped through the mitral valve into the left ventricle before leaving through the aortic valve to the aorta.

6. The aortic and pulmonic valves are the _____, whereas the tricuspid and mitral valves are the *atrioventricular valves;* all the valves are trileaflet, with the exception of the mitral valve, which has two leaflets.

7. The tricuspid valve separates the right atrium from the right ventricle; the _____ or *pulmonary valve* separates the right ventricle from the pulmonary artery.

8. The _____ or *bicuspid valve* separates the left atrium from the left ventricle; the aortic valve separates the left ventricle from the ascending aorta.

9. The _____ are rounded or irregular muscular columns that project from the inner surface of the right and left ventricles of the heart; the chordae tendineae or *heartstrings* are cord-like tendons that connect the papillary muscles to the tricuspid valve and the mitral valve in the heart.

10. The aorta is usually divided into _____ segments or sections that include the ascending aorta, the arch of the aorta, the descending aorta, the thoracic aorta, and the abdominal aorta.

five	pulmonic valve	mitral valve
pericardium	trabeculae carneae	superior atria
pulmonary veins	semilunar valves	superior vena cava
inferior ventricles		

Reference Various chapters. In Drake R, Vogl AW, Mitchell AWM: *Gray's anatomy for students,* ed 4, Philadelphia, 2020, Churchill Livingstone.

ANSWER KEY 1. inferior ventricles, 2. superior atria, 3. pericardium, 4. superior vena cava, 5. pulmonary veins, 6. semilunar valves, 7. pulmonic valve, 8. mitral valve, 9. trabeculae carneae, 10. five

FIGURE 1.27 Respiratory system (midsagittal section with frontal and microanatomic views)

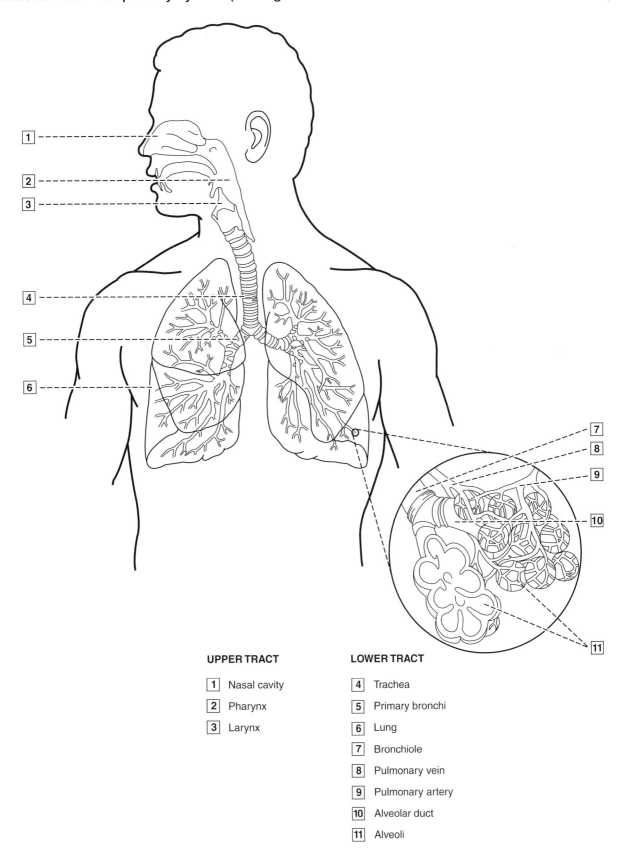

UPPER TRACT

1	Nasal cavity
2	Pharynx
3	Larynx

LOWER TRACT

4	Trachea
5	Primary bronchi
6	Lung
7	Bronchiole
8	Pulmonary vein
9	Pulmonary artery
10	Alveolar duct
11	Alveoli

REVIEW QUESTIONS: Respiratory system

Fill in the blanks by choosing the appropriate terms from the list below.

1. The primary function of the _____ is to supply the blood with oxygen by way of breathing for the blood to deliver oxygen to all parts of the body; with breathing, there is mainly the inhaling of oxygen and exhaling of carbon dioxide.

2. The needed oxygen initially enters the respiratory system through the oral cavity and the _____ and then into the pharynx or *throat.*

3. The oxygen then passes through the _____ or *voice box,* which is where speech sounds are produced via the vocal folds or *vocal cords,* and then into the trachea, which filters the air.

4. In the chest cavity, the _____ or *windpipe* splits into two smaller tubes, the *primary bronchi,* which enter the roots of the two lungs; the epiglottis covers it so that food does not go down it when eating.

5. The _____ then divide again and again into secondary and tertiary ones, finally forming the bronchioles in the lungs.

6. The _____ terminate in air-filled sacs of the alveoli in the lungs.

7. The inhaled oxygen passes into the very small _____ in the lungs and then diffuses through the surrounding capillaries into the arterial blood; the waste-rich blood from the veins releases its carbon dioxide into them; the carbon dioxide follows the same path out of the lungs when exhaling.

8. The two _____, the main organs of the respiratory system are located in two somewhat similar cavities on either side of the heart; both are separated into lobes by fissures, with three lobes on the right and two on the left, with the lobes further divided into segments and then into lobules; each lobe is surrounded by a pleural cavity.

9. The _____ are two large veins that carry oxygenated blood from the lungs to the left atrium of the heart, which is unusual since almost all other veins of the body carry deoxygenated blood.

10. The _____ are two large arteries that carry deoxygenated blood from the heart to the lungs; they are the only arteries of the body (other than umbilical arteries in the fetus) that carry deoxygenated blood.

lungs	primary bronchi	nasal cavity
pulmonary arteries	bronchioles	respiratory system
alveoli	larynx	pulmonary veins
trachea		

Reference Various chapters. In Drake R, Vogl AW, Mitchell AWM: *Gray's anatomy for students,* ed 4, Philadelphia, 2020, Churchill Livingstone.

ANSWER KEY 1. respiratory system, 2. nasal cavity, 3. larynx, 4. trachea, 5. primary bronchi, 6. bronchioles, 7. alveoli, 8. lungs, 9. pulmonary veins, 10. pulmonary arteries

FIGURE 1.28   Endocrine system (midsagittal sections with frontal and posterior views)

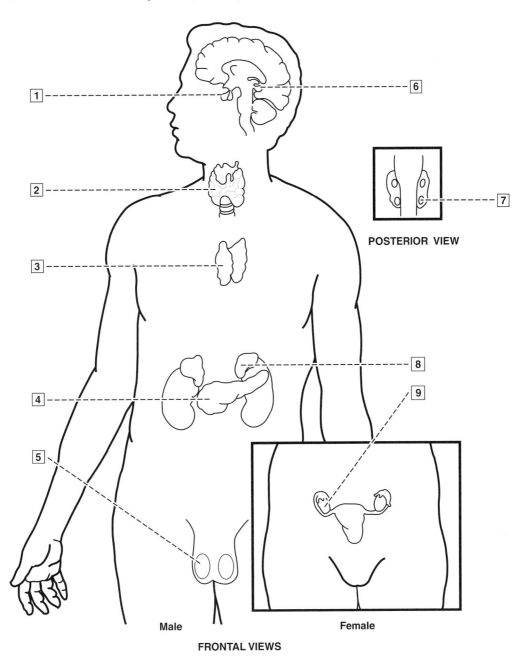

POSTERIOR VIEW

Male

Female

FRONTAL VIEWS

1	Pituitary gland	6	Pineal gland
2	Thyroid gland	7	Parathyroid gland (on posterior surface of thyroid gland)
3	Thymus		
4	Pancreas	8	Adrenal gland
5	Testis	9	Ovary

REVIEW QUESTIONS: Endocrine system

Fill in the blanks by choosing the appropriate terms from the list below.

1. The _____ is the system of glands, each of which secretes a type of hormone directly into the bloodstream to regulate the body; this system is in contrast to the exocrine system, which secretes hormones into the blood stream to also regulate the body by instead using ducts.

2. The _____ of the endocrine system are the hypothalamus, pituitary, thyroid, parathyroids, adrenals, pineal body, and the reproductive organs (ovaries and testes); the pancreas is also a part of this system because it has a role in hormone production as well as in the process of digestion.

3. In addition to the specialized endocrine organs that secrete _____, many other organs that are part of other body systems, such as the kidney, liver, and heart, have secondary endocrine functions; for example, the kidney secretes erythropoietin and renin.

4. The _____ belongs to the endocrine system, but it is under the control of the hypothalamus, the true *master gland;* it is important to note that together they secrete several hormones, such as those that control the female's menstrual cycle, pregnancy, and birth of a child; this includes follicle-stimulating hormone, which stimulates development and maturation of a follicle in one of the ovaries and luteinizing hormone, which causes the bursting of that follicle during ovulation with the formation of a corpus luteum from the remains of the follicle.

5. One non-sex hormone secreted by the pituitary gland located at the base of the skull between the optic nerves is the _____, which helps prevent excess water excretion by the kidneys; the same gland releases thyroid-stimulating hormone under influence of hypothalamic thyrotropin-releasing hormone.

6. The _____ can serve both as a ducted exocrine gland, secreting digestive enzymes into the small intestine as well as a ductless endocrine gland, in that the islets of Langerhans secrete insulin and glucagon to regulate the blood sugar level; they can secrete glucagon, which informs the liver to take carbohydrate out of storage to raise a low blood sugar level, and they can secrete insulin to inform the liver to take excess glucose out of circulation to lower a blood sugar level that is too high.

7. The _____ of the endocrine system that are located superior to the kidneys secrete epinephrine or *adrenalin* and other similar hormones in response to stressors such as fright, anger, caffeine, or low blood sugar as well as cortisone that can be involved in the inflammatory response.

8. The _____ or *sex organs* of the endocrine system, the female's ovaries and the male's testes also secrete sex hormones through pituitary gland hormones in addition to producing gametes for conception; both sexes make some of the hormones with the male's testes secreting primarily androgens including testosterone and the female's ovaries secreting estrogen and progesterone in varying amounts depending on the time of the female's cycle.

9. The _____ of the endocrine system is located near the center of the brain and is stimulated by nerves from the eyes, which enables it to secrete melatonin to promote sleep; it also affects reproductive functions by depressing the activity of the gonads as well as affecting the thyroid and adrenal cortex functions.

10. The endocrine system uses cycles as well as _____ mechanisms to regulate physiologic functions; cycles of secretion maintain homeostatic control and can range from hours to months in duration within the blood system.

gonads	pineal gland	pituitary gland
adrenal glands	antidiuretic hormone	endocrine system
negative feedback	pancreas	major glands
hormones		

Reference Various chapters. In Drake R, Vogl AW, Mitchell AWM: *Gray's anatomy for students,* ed 4, Philadelphia, 2020, Churchill Livingstone.

FIGURE 1.29 Digestive system (midsagittal section and frontal view)

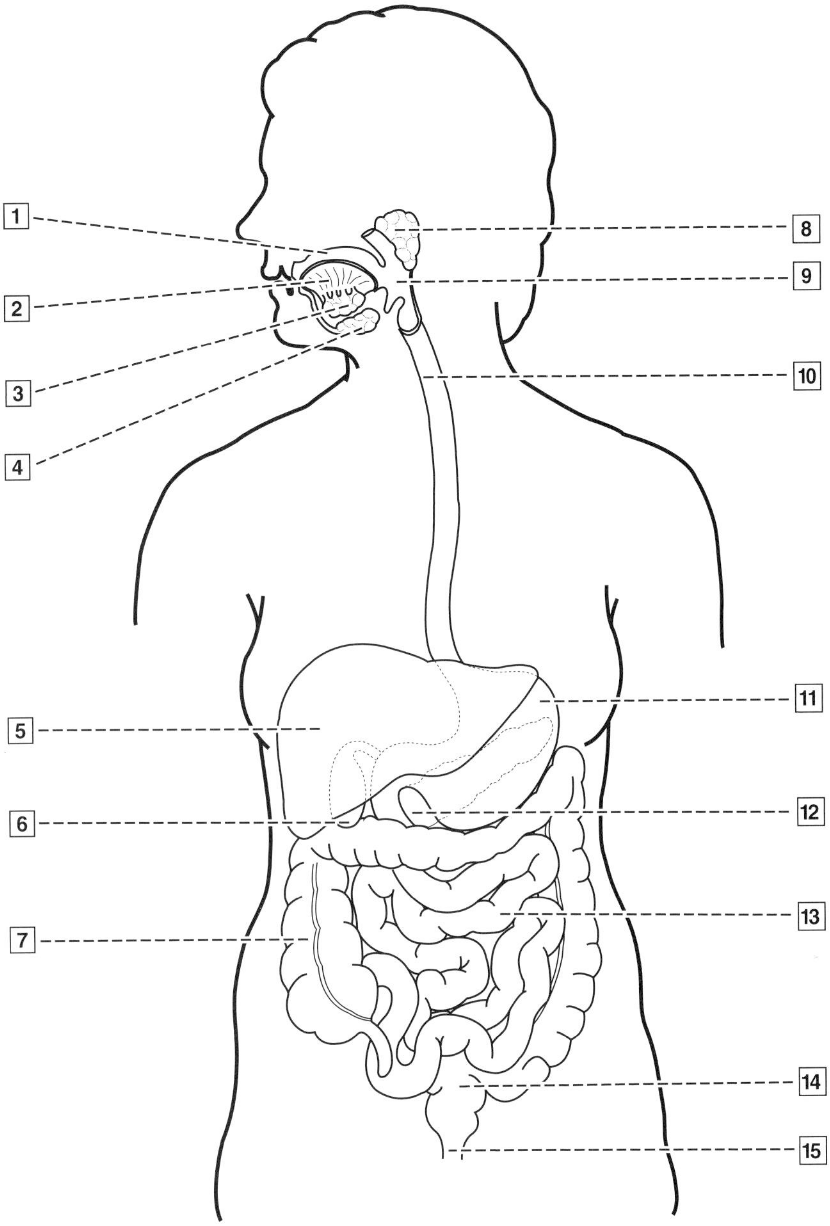

1	Mouth (oral cavity)	6	Gallbladder	11	Stomach
2	Tongue	7	Large intestine	12	Pancreas
3	Sublingual salivary gland	8	Parotid salivary gland	13	Small intestine
4	Submandibular salivary gland	9	Pharynx	14	Rectum
5	Liver	10	Esophagus	15	Anus

REVIEW QUESTIONS: Digestive system

Fill in the blanks by choosing the appropriate terms from the list below.

1. The _____ is composed of the digestive tract, a series of hollow organs joined in a long twisting tube from the oral cavity to the anus as well as other organs that help the body break down and absorb food; the organs that are included along the digestive tract include the oral cavity, esophagus, stomach, small intestine, large intestine, and anus with parts of the nervous and vascular systems also playing roles.

2. Inside these hollow digestive system organs is a lining of _____; the digestive tract also contains a layer of smooth muscle in the mucosa that helps break down food and move it along the tract.

3. In the oral cavity, stomach, and small intestine, the mucosa contains glands that produce _____ to help digest food; saliva produced by the salivary glands contains amylase that begins to digest the starch from food into smaller molecules, and the stomach has pepsin that begins to digest the protein.

4. In the oral cavity, the teeth, jaws, and the tongue begin the mechanical breakdown of food into smaller particles; the mixture of food and saliva or *bolus* is pushed into the pharynx or *throat*, and then through the _____, which is a muscular tube whose muscular contractions of peristalsis propel the bolus to the stomach along with the moisture and lubrication provided by the mucus.

5. The _____ produces not only the enzyme pepsin but also hydrochloric acid for the gastric juice found in it that does not directly function in digestion but activates the enzyme; the organ also mechanically churns the food into chyme along with the mucus.

6. Two of the digestive organs, the _____ and the pancreas, produce bile and pancreatic juice that neutralizes the chyme, respectively; it is important to note that substances reach the intestine through small tubes called *ducts;* the gallbladder stores the bile until it is needed in the intestine.

7. Digestion of carbohydrates, proteins, and fats continues in the _____; starch and glycogen are broken down into maltose by enzymes and proteases, which are enzymes secreted by the pancreas that continue the breakdown of protein into small peptide fragments and amino acids.

8. Most digested molecules of food, as well as water and minerals, are absorbed through the small intestine, because the mucosa contains many folds that are covered with tiny fingerlike projections, the _____, which have their own microscopic projections, the *microvilli.*

9. The _____ produced by the liver dissolve fat into tiny droplets and allow pancreatic and intestinal enzymes to break the large fat molecules into smaller ones such as fatty acids and cholesterol; these then combine with these smaller molecules to help move them into the cells of the mucosa.

10. The _____ is composed of the colon, cecum, appendix, and rectum and is involved in the recovery of water and electrolytes from digested food as well as the formation and storage of feces.

small intestine	large intestine	mucosa
liver	enzymes	esophagus
villi	bile acids	stomach
digestive system		

Reference   Various chapters. In Drake R, Vogl AW, Mitchell AWM: *Gray's anatomy for students,* ed 4, Philadelphia, 2020, Churchill Livingstone.

ANSWER KEY 1. digestive system, 2. mucosa, 3. enzymes, 4. esophagus, 5. stomach, 6. liver, 7. small intestine, 8. villi, 9. bile acids, 10. large intestine

FIGURE 1.30 Urinary system (frontal view) and kidney (sagittal section)

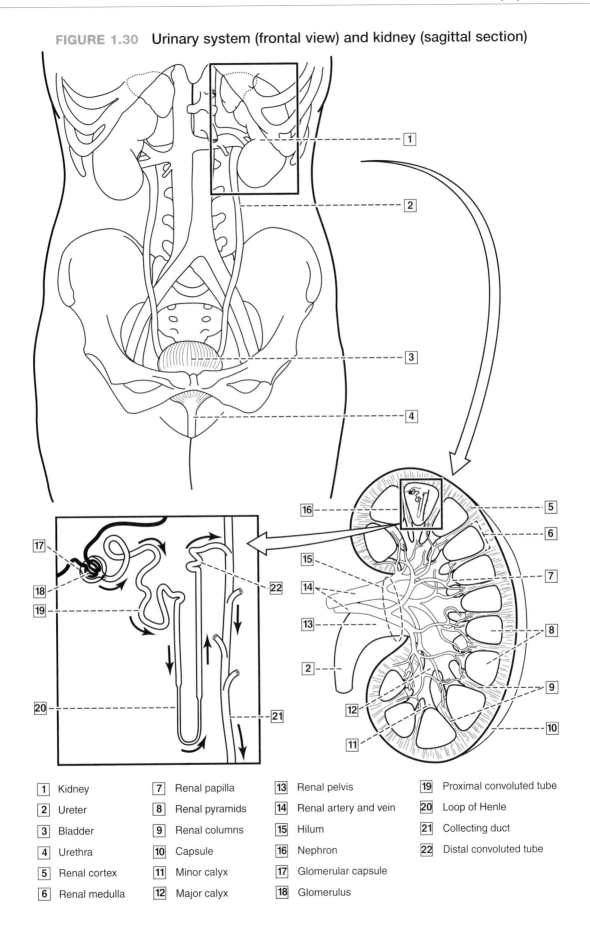

1	Kidney	7	Renal papilla	13	Renal pelvis	19	Proximal convoluted tube
2	Ureter	8	Renal pyramids	14	Renal artery and vein	20	Loop of Henle
3	Bladder	9	Renal columns	15	Hilum	21	Collecting duct
4	Urethra	10	Capsule	16	Nephron	22	Distal convoluted tube
5	Renal cortex	11	Minor calyx	17	Glomerular capsule		
6	Renal medulla	12	Major calyx	18	Glomerulus		

REVIEW QUESTIONS: Urinary system and kidney

Fill in the blanks by choosing the appropriate terms from the list below.

1. The _____ or *urinary tract* includes two kidneys, two ureters, the bladder, and the urethra that together produce, store, and eliminate urine; this system also eliminates waste products from the body in the urine as well as maintains fluid and salt balance (including potassium and sodium).

2. The _____ of the urinary system are bean-shaped organs that lie within the abdomen, retroperitoneal to the organs of digestion, around or just inferior to the ribcage and close to the lumbar spine; each organ consists of an outer cortex and medullary pyramid or *papillae,* and within these two regions are found the components of the structural and functional unit of the organ, the nephron.

3. The _____ has a glomerulus, a tuft of capillaries that produce the glomerular filtrate, housed in the renal corpuscle; this structure is followed by a series of tubules specialized for both excretion and reabsorption.

4. The kidney also includes, besides the glomerulus, the _____, the descending and ascending loop of Henle, and the distal convoluted tubule.

5. Each nephron drains into a collecting tubule, which serves as a duct system to conduct the urine out of the kidney; the urine in the collecting tubules is collected in the renal pelvis and exits the kidney in the _____.

6. The ureter of the urinary system travels to the _____ where the urine can be stored.

7. The bladder of the urinary system is drained by the _____, which leads to the external orifice.

8. The tubule of the nephron functions to reabsorb most of the glomerular filtrate; the cells of the tubule reabsorb vital nutrients and water back into the blood, while retaining the _____ that the body needs to eliminate.

9. The plexus formed by the efferent arteriole from the glomerulus passes closely to the proximal convoluted tubule, allowing direct transfer into the blood; in the _____, the filtrate is further concentrated.

10. The amount of water reabsorbed within the kidney is controlled by the _____ secreted by the pituitary gland, and the amount of salts reabsorbed is controlled by aldosterone secreted by the adrenal gland; these hormones are increased or decreased according to the needs of the body.

bladder	urethra	loop of Henle
proximal convoluted tubule	ureter	kidneys
nephron	antidiuretic hormone	waste products
urinary system		

Reference Various chapters. In Drake R, Vogl AW, Mitchell AWM: *Gray's anatomy for students,* ed 4, Philadelphia, 2020, Churchill Livingstone.

ANSWER KEY 1. urinary system, 2. kidneys, 3. nephron, 4. proximal convoluted tubule, 5. ureter, 6. bladder, 7. urethra, 8. waste products, 9. loop of Henle, 10. antidiuretic hormone

FIGURE 1.31   **Major lymphatics (sagittal section with explanatory view)**

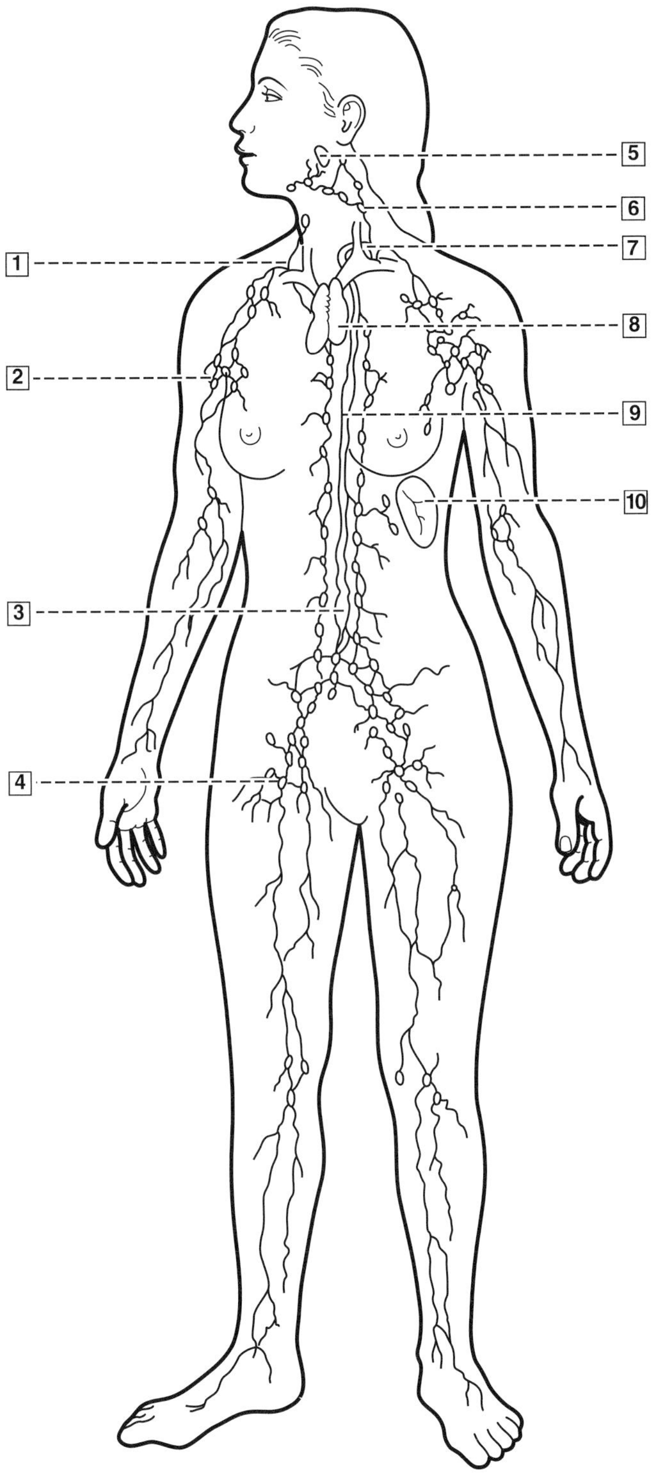

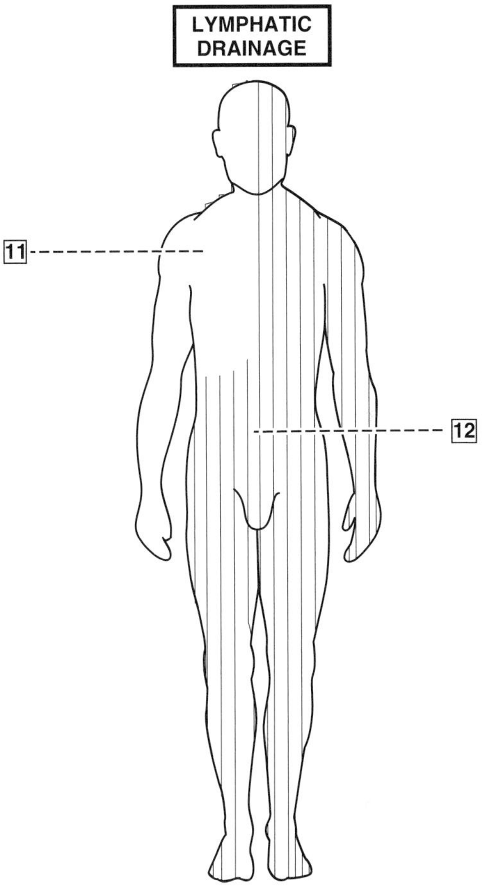

LYMPHATIC DRAINAGE

1 Right lymphatic duct draining into right subclavian vein

2 Axillary nodes

3 Cisterna chyli

4 Inguinal nodes

5 Palatine tonsils

6 Cervical nodes

7 Thoracic duct draining into left subclavian vein

8 Thymus

9 Thoracic duct

10 Spleen

11 Area drained by right lymphatic duct

12 Area drained by thoracic duct

REVIEW QUESTIONS: Major lymphatics

Fill in the blanks by choosing the appropriate terms from the list below.

1. The _____ consists of a network of lymphatic vessels linking lymph nodes throughout most of the body.

2. The lymphatics are a part of the _____ and help fight disease processes such as infection and cancer, while serving other functions in the body; the lymphatics consist of vessels, nodes, ducts, and tonsils.

3. The lymphatic system also includes all the structures dedicated to the circulation and production of the white blood cells, the _____; it is important to note that these structures include the spleen, thymus, bone marrow, and the lymphoid tissue associated with the digestive system.

4. The conducting system carries the clear fluid, the _____, and consists of tubular vessels that include the lymph capillaries, the lymph vessels, and the right and left thoracic ducts.

5. The _____ is the tissue that is primarily involved in the immune response and consists of lymphocytes and other white blood cells enmeshed in connective tissue through which the lymph passes.

6. Both the thymus and the bone marrow constitute the _____ involved in the production and early selection of lymphocytes.

7. The _____ provides the environment for foreign or altered native molecules, immunogens or *antigens*, to interact with lymphocytes; it is exemplified by the lymph nodes and the lymphoid follicles in tonsils, Peyer patches, spleen, adenoids, skin, and any area associated with mucosa-associated lymphoid tissue.

8. The regions of the lymphoid tissue that are densely packed with lymphocytes are the _____; lymphoid tissue can either be structurally well organized as lymph nodes or may consist of loosely organized tissue such as the mucosa-associated lymphoid tissue.

9. The _____ is a lymphoid organ located on the left side of the abdomen posterior to the stomach, lying between the ninth and eleventh ribs on the left side; it is the primary filtering element for the blood as well as a storage site for red blood cells (or erythrocytes) and platelets (or thrombocytes).

10. The _____ consist of masses of lymphoid tissue located in the oral cavity and pharynx and like lymph nodes they contain lymphocytes that remove toxins; they are located near airway and food passages to protect the body against disease processes from toxins.

immune system	lymph	secondary lymphoid tissue
lymphatic system	tonsils	lymphocytes
primary lymphoid tissue	lymphoid follicles	lymphoid tissue
spleen		

References Chapter 10, Lymphatic system. In Fehrenbach MJ, Herring SW: *Illustrated anatomy of the head and neck,* ed 6, St. Louis, 2021, Saunders; Various chapters. In Drake R, Vogl AW, Mitchell AWM: *Gray's anatomy for students,* ed 4, Philadelphia, 2020, Churchill Livingstone.

ANSWER KEY 1. lymphatic system, 2. immune system, 3. lymphocytes, 4. lymph, 5. lymphoid tissue, 6. primary lymphoid tissue, 7. secondary lymphoid tissue, 8. lymphoid follicles, 9. spleen, 10. tonsils

FIGURE 1.32 Lymph node (sagittal section with microanatomic views)

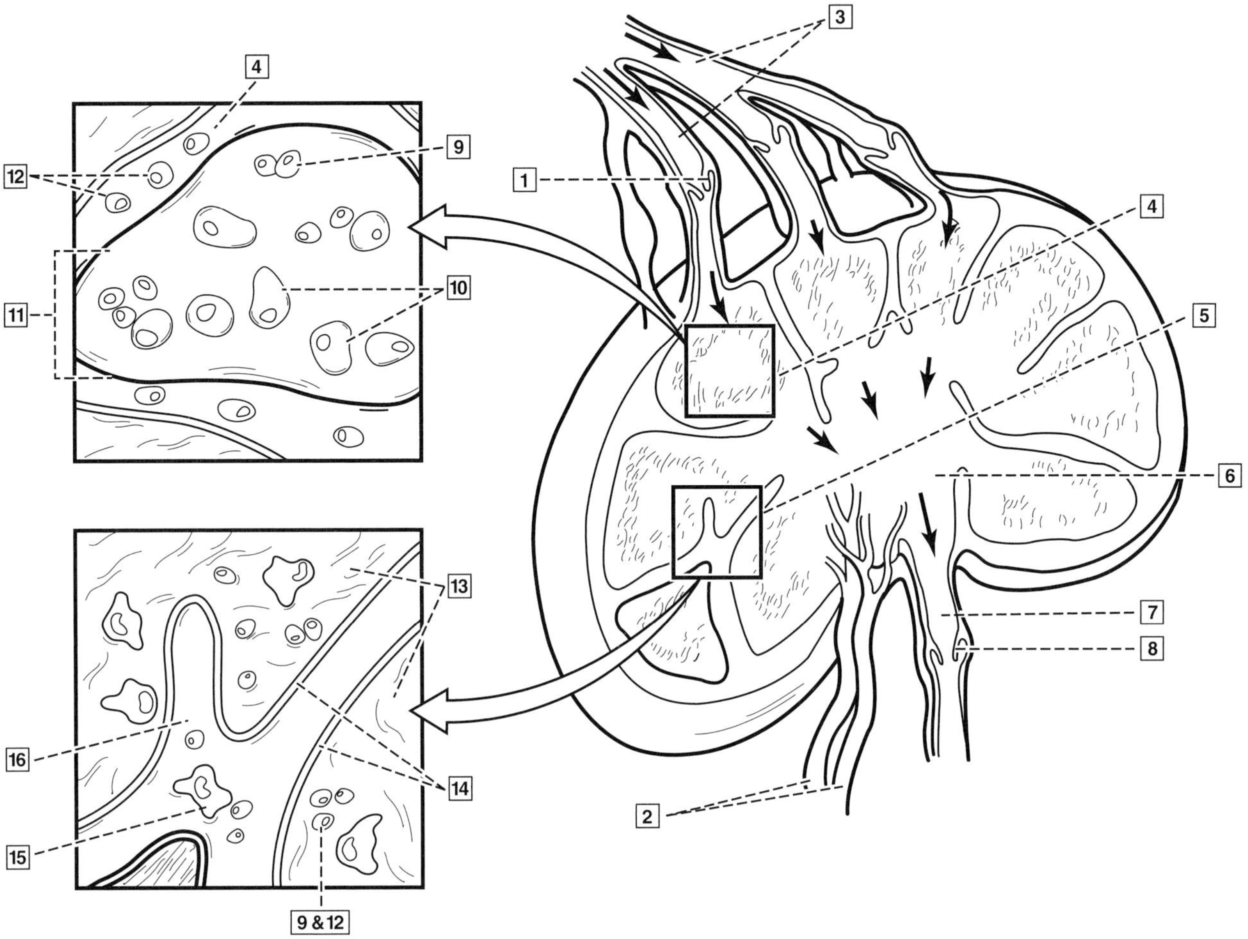

1 Valve	5 Medulla	9 B-cell lymphocytes	13 Medullary cords
2 Blood vessels, vein and artery	6 Hilus	10 Dendritic cells	14 Trabeculae
3 Afferent lymphatic vessels	7 Efferent lymphatic vessel	11 Germinal center	15 Macrophage
4 Lymphatic nodule	8 Valve	12 T-cell lymphocytes	16 Medullary sinus

REVIEW QUESTIONS: Lymph node

Fill in the blanks by choosing the appropriate terms from the list below.

1. The _____ are bean-shaped bodies grouped in clusters along the connecting lymphatic vessels; positioned beside the lymphatic vessels, they filter toxic products from the lymph to prevent their entry into the vascular system.

2. The lymph nodes are composed of organized lymphoid tissue and contain _____, the white blood cells of the immune system that actively remove toxins to help fight disease processes in the body.

3. The lymph nodes can be superficially located with superficial veins or located deep in the tissue with the deeper blood vessels; however, in a healthy patient, they are usually small, soft, and free or mobile in the surrounding tissue and therefore they are not able to be _____ or felt when palpated by the clinician.

4. The _____ are a system of channels that are parallel to the venous blood vessels yet are more numerous; they are larger and thicker than the vascular system's capillaries, but unlike capillaries, they have one-way valves similar to veins to ensure the one-way flow of lymph through the lymphatic vessel.

5. The lymph flows into the lymph node by way of multiple _____.

6. On one side of the node is a depression or hilus where the lymph flows out of the node by way of a single _____.

7. The lymph from a particular tissue region first drains into a(n) _____ (regional node or master node) before the lymph flows to a more distant region.

8. The primary nodes, in turn, drain into a(n) _____ (central node).

9. Within the tissue located in outer regions of the body, smaller lymphatic vessels containing lymph converge into larger _____, which empty into the venous component of the vascular system in the thorax (chest).

10. The final drainage endpoint of the lymphatic vessels into the lymphatic ducts depends on which _____ of the body is involved, which mirrors a similar concept in the vascular system.

lymphatic ducts	primary node	lymphocytes
lymph nodes	secondary node	side
efferent lymphatic vessel	afferent lymphatic vessels	lymphatic vessels
visualized		

Reference   Chapter 10, Lymphatic system. In Fehrenbach MJ, Herring SW: *Illustrated anatomy of the head and neck,* ed 6, St. Louis, 2021, Saunders.

FIGURE 1.33 Central and peripheral nervous systems (section with microanatomic views)

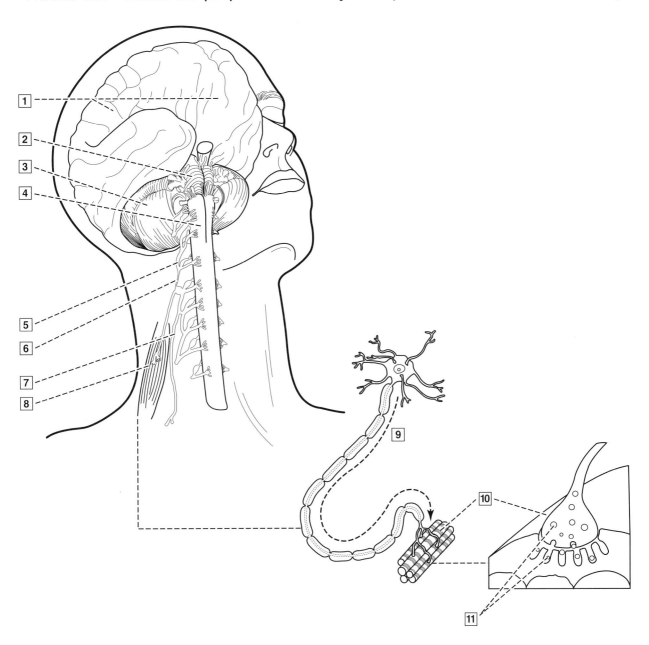

CENTRAL NERVOUS SYSTEM

1 Cerebrum (Cerebral hemispheres)

2 Brainstem

3 Cerebellum

4 Spinal cord

PERIPHERAL NERVOUS SYSTEM

5 Nerve ganglion

6 Nerve

7 Afferent nerve from skin

8 Efferent nerve to muscle

NEURON

9 Action potential (impulse propagation)

10 Muscle fiber

SYNAPSE

10 Muscle fiber

11 Neurotransmitter

REVIEW QUESTIONS: Central and peripheral nervous systems

Fill in the blanks by choosing the appropriate terms from the list below.

1. The _____ is an extensive intricate network of neural structures that activates, coordinates, and controls all functions of the body.

2. One of the major divisions of the nervous system, the _____ includes the brain and spinal cord.

3. The major divisions of the _____ include the cerebrum, cerebellum, brainstem, and diencephalon.

4. The _____ is the largest division of the brain and consists of two cerebral hemispheres; it coordinates sensory data and motor functions and governs many aspects of intelligence and reasoning, learning, and memory.

5. The _____ is the second largest division of the brain after the cerebrum; it functions to produce muscle coordination and maintains the usual muscle tone and posture as well as coordinates balance.

6. The _____ has a number of divisions that include the medulla, pons, and midbrain.

7. A major division of the nervous system, the _____, is composed of all the nerves creating their pathways between the central nervous system and the receptors, muscles, and glands of the body.

8. The peripheral nervous system is further divided into the _____ or *sensory nervous system*, which carries information from receptors to the brain or spinal cord, and the efferent nervous system or *motor nervous system*, which carries information from the brain or spinal cord to muscles or glands.

9. The _____ of the peripheral nervous system is further subdivided into the somatic nervous system and the autonomic nervous system.

10. The _____ includes both afferent and efferent nerves and involves both receptors and effectors; specifically, this includes all nerves controlling the voluntary muscular system.

efferent division	central nervous system	nervous system
peripheral nervous system	cerebrum	brainstem
cerebellum	somatic nervous system	afferent nervous system
brain		

References   Chapter 8, Basic tissue. In Fehrenbach MJ, Popowics T: *Illustrated dental embryology, histology, and anatomy,* ed 5, St. Louis, 2020, Saunders; Chapter 8, Nervous system. In Fehrenbach MJ, Herring SW: *Illustrated anatomy of the head and neck,* ed 6, St. Louis, 2021, Saunders.

FIGURE 1.34 Neurons with muscular involvement

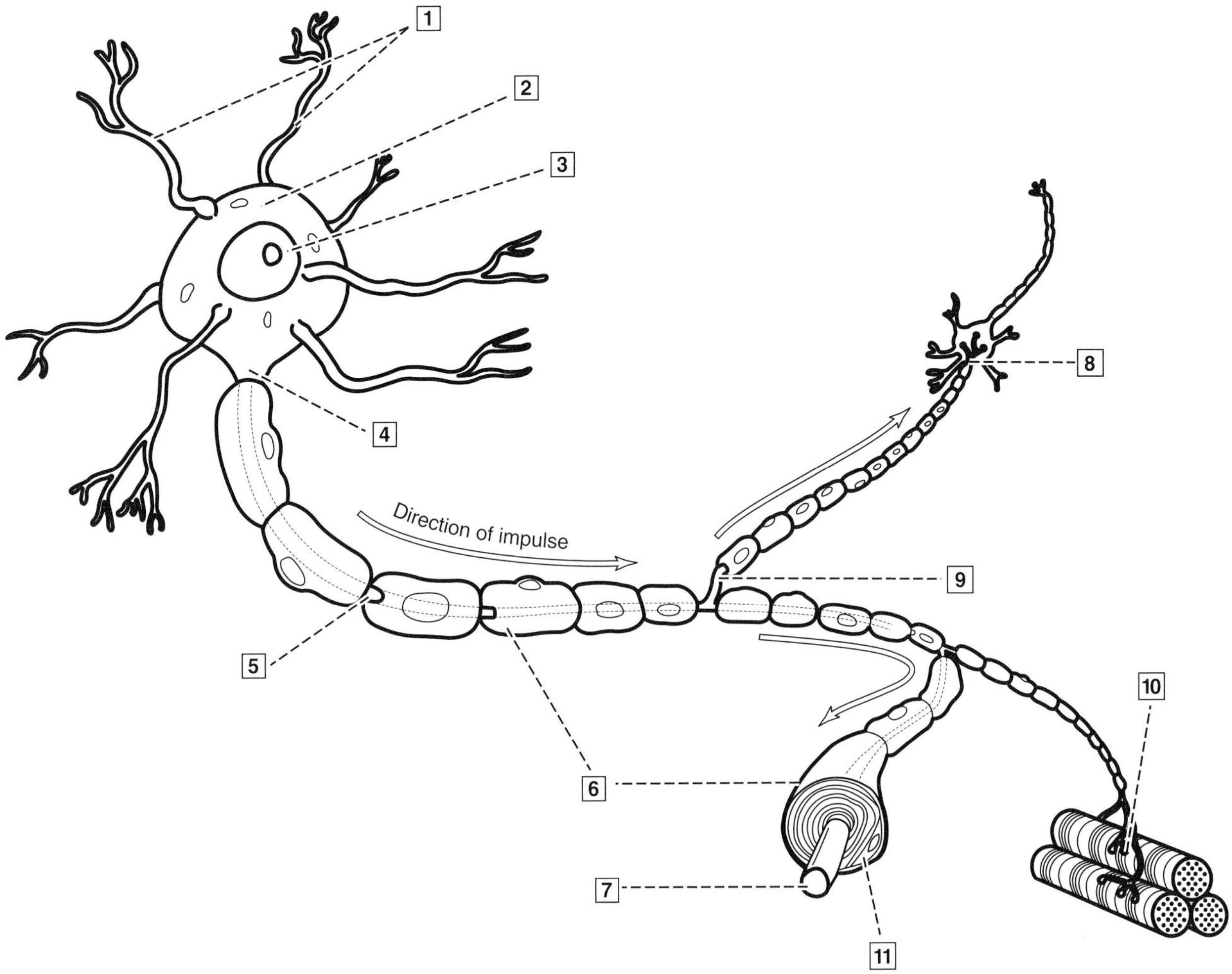

1	Dendrites	7	Axon
2	Cell body	8	Synapse with another neuron
3	Nucleus	9	Collateral branch
4	Axon	10	Synapse with myofibers
5	Node of Ranvier	11	Nucleus of Schwann cell
6	Myelin sheath		

REVIEW QUESTIONS: Neurons with muscular involvement

Fill in the blanks by choosing the appropriate terms from the list below.

1. The _____ is the functional cellular component of the nervous system and is composed of one neural cell body and with two different types of neural cytoplasmic processes; one type is an axon, a cablelike process that conducts impulses away from the cell body, while the other type is the dendrite, which is a threadlike process that usually contains multiple branches and functions to receive and conduct impulses toward the cell body.

2. A(n) _____ is a bundle of neural processes outside the central nervous system and in the peripheral nervous system, while an accumulation of neuron cell bodies outside the central nervous system is a ganglion; there are two functional types of nerves: afferent and efferent.

3. A(n) _____ is the junction between two neurons or between a neuron and an effector organ where neural impulses are transmitted by chemical means (neurotransmitter).

4. A(n) _____ or *sensory nerve* carries information or relays impulses from the periphery of the body to the brain (or spinal cord).

5. A(n) _____ or *motor nerve* carries information away from the brain to the periphery of the body.

6. The cell membrane of a neuron, like all other cells, has an unequal distribution of ions and electric charges between the two sides of the membrane, with the fluid outside of the membrane having a positive charge and the fluid inside having a negative charge; the charge difference is a(n) _____ and is measured in millivolts.

7. The rapid depolarization of the cell membrane results in a(n) _____, which then causes propagation of the nerve impulse along the membrane; this is a temporary reversal of the electric potential along the membrane for a brief period.

8. To have the impulse cross the synapse to another cell requires the actions of chemical agents that are considered the _____, which are discharged with the arrival of the action potential; these released agents diffuse across the synapse and bind to receptors on the membrane of the other cell.

9. The myelin sheath consists of tightly wrapped layers of the phospholipid-rich membrane surrounding the _____ cytoplasm that has formed it; there is very little cytoplasm sandwiched between them.

10. The _____ are gaps between the Schwann cells occurring at regular intervals along the myelinated axon; the insulating properties of the myelin sheath and its uninsulated gaps allow the axon to conduct impulses more quickly.

resting potential	synapse	neurotransmitters
efferent nerve	action potential	nerve
neuron	Schwann cell	afferent nerve
nodes of Ranvier		

References   Chapter 8, Basic tissue. In Fehrenbach MJ, Popowics T: *Illustrated dental embryology, histology, and anatomy,* ed 5, St. Louis, 2020, Saunders; Chapter 8, Nervous system. In Fehrenbach MJ, Herring SW: *Illustrated anatomy of the head and neck,* ed 6, St. Louis, 2021, Saunders.

ANSWER KEY 1. neuron, 2. nerve, 3. synapse, 4. afferent nerve, 5. efferent nerve, 6. resting potential, 7. action potential, 8. neurotransmitters, 9. Schwann cell, 10. nodes of Ranvier

FIGURE 2.1 Anatomic position with head and neck sections and planes

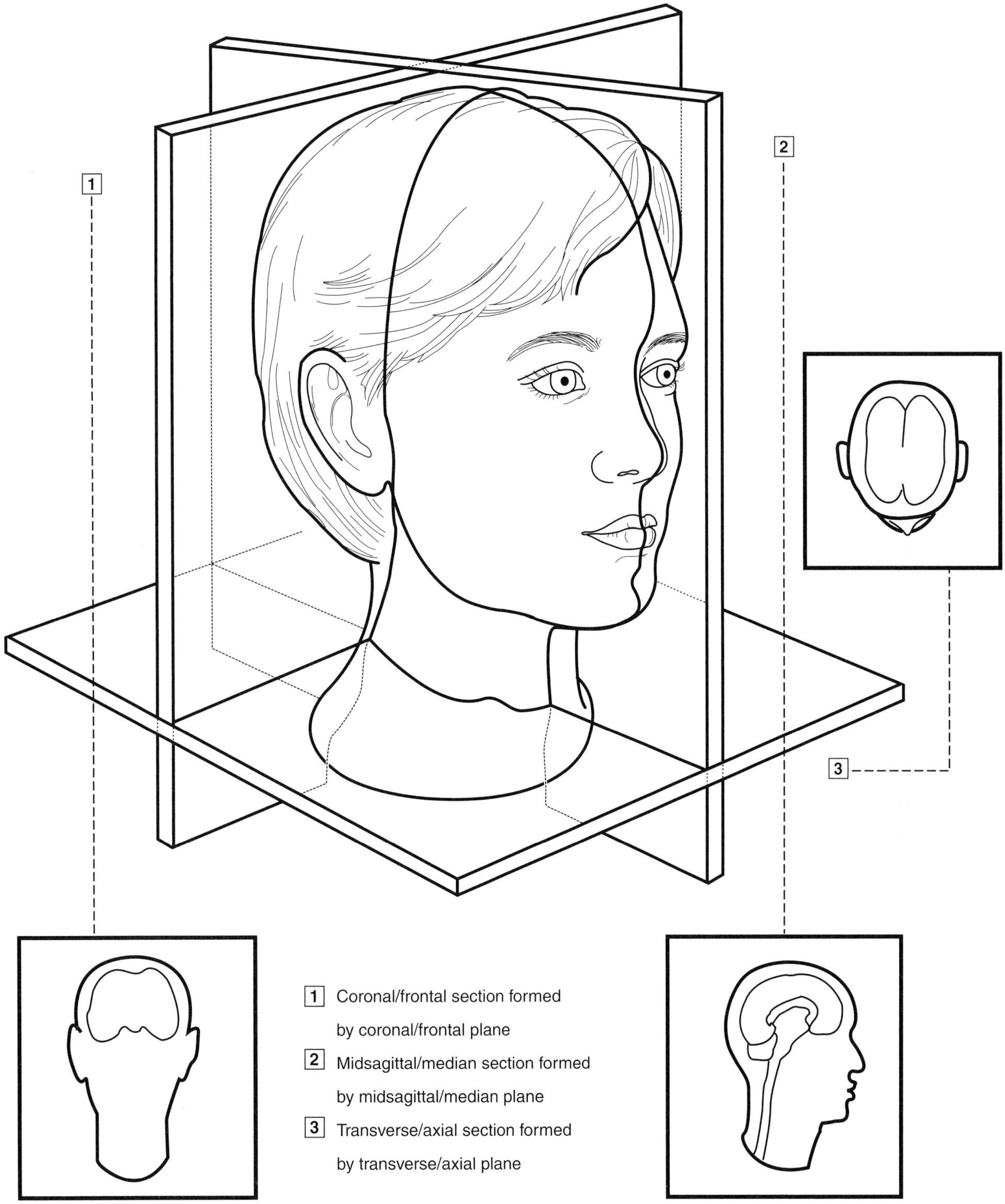
1
2
3
1 Coronal/frontal section formed by coronal/frontal plane
2 Midsagittal/median section formed by midsagittal/median plane
3 Transverse/axial section formed by transverse/axial plane

REVIEW QUESTIONS: Anatomic position with head and neck sections and planes

Fill in the blanks by choosing the appropriate terms from the list below.

1. The _____ is the system of names for anatomic structures.

2. The nomenclature of anatomy is based on the body being in _____.

3. In anatomic position, the body can be standing erect, with the arms at the sides with the palms and toes directed _____ and the eyes looking forward.

4. The midsagittal section or *median section* is a division through the _____.

5. The _____ or *coronal section* is a division through any frontal plane.

6. The _____ or *transverse section* is a division through an axial plane.

7. The _____ or *median plane* divides the body into equal right and left halves.

8. Dividing the body into anterior and posterior parts at any level relates to the _____ or *frontal plane.*

9. An axial plane _____ the body at any level into superior and inferior parts and is perpendicular to the median plane.

10. Any plane related to the median plane is considered the _____.

midsagittal plane	anatomic nomenclature	sagittal plane
forward	median plane	coronal plane
frontal section	divides	axial section
anatomic position		

Reference Chapter 1, Introduction to head and neck anatomy. In Fehrenbach MJ, Herring SW: *Illustrated anatomy of the head and neck,* ed 6, St. Louis, 2021, Saunders.

NOTES

FIGURE 2.2 Facial development within third to fourth week of embryonic period during prenatal development (frontal aspects)

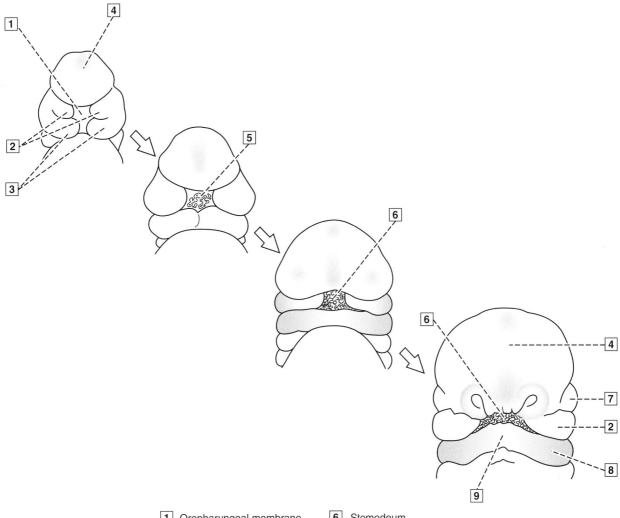

1	Oropharyngeal membrane	6	Stomodeum
2	Maxillary processes	7	Lens placode
3	Mandibular processes	8	Mandibular arch
4	Frontonasal processes	9	Mandibular symphysis
5	Oropharyngeal membrane disintegrating		

REVIEW QUESTIONS: Facial development within third to fourth week of embryonic period during prenatal development

Fill in the blanks by choosing the appropriate terms from the list below.

1. The face and its associated tissue begin to form during the fourth week of prenatal development within the

_____.

2. All three embryonic layers are involved in facial development, the ectoderm, mesoderm, and

_____.

3. At the beginning of the fourth week of prenatal development, the primitive mouth has become the

_____, which initially appeared as a shallow depression in the embryonic surface ectoderm at its cephalic end.

4. At this time, the stomodeum is limited in depth by the _____, which is a temporary membrane consisting of external ectoderm overlying endoderm formed during the third week of prenatal development that also separates the stomodeum from the primitive pharynx.

5. After formation of the stomodeum but still during the fourth week, two bulges of tissue appear inferior to the primitive mouth, the two _____, which consist of a core of mesenchyme formed in part by migrating neural crest cells and are covered externally by ectoderm and internally by endoderm.

6. The paired mandibular processes fuse at the midline to form the _____, the developmental form of the future lower jaw, the mandible.

7. In the midline, on the surface of the mature bony mandible, is the _____ indicating where the mandible is formed by fusion of right and left mandibular processes.

8. During the fourth week, the _____ forms as a bulge of tissue at the most cephalic end of the embryo, which is the cranial boundary of the stomodeum; in the future, this process gives rise to the upper face, which includes the forehead, bridge of the nose, primary palate, nasal septum, and all structures associated with the medial nasal processes.

9. During the fourth week of prenatal development within the embryonic period, a tissue swelling forms from increased growth of the mandibular arch on each side of the stomodeum, the _____, which will each later grow superiorly and anteriorly around the stomodeum.

10. In the future, the maxillary processes will form the midface, which includes the sides of the upper lip, cheeks, secondary palate, and posterior part of the _____ with its canines, certain posterior teeth, and associated tissue, as well as forming the zygomatic bones and parts of the temporal bones.

mandibular processes	mandibular symphysis	stomodeum
maxilla	frontonasal process	embryonic period
mandibular arch	maxillary process	endoderm
oropharyngeal membrane		

Reference   Chapter 4, Face and neck development. In Fehrenbach MJ, Popowics T: *Illustrated dental embryology, histology, and anatomy,* ed 5, St. Louis, 2020, Saunders.

FIGURE 2.3 Facial development within fourth week of embryonic period during prenatal development (frontal and lateral aspects)

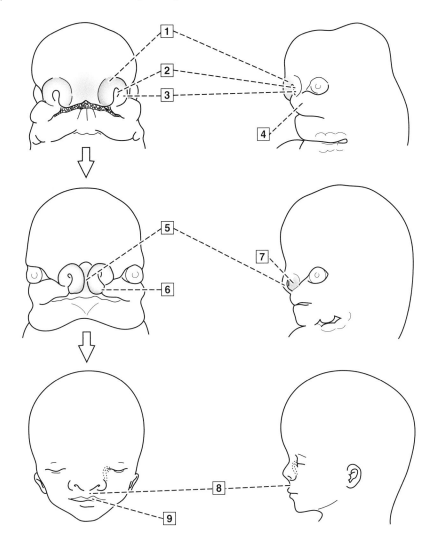

1 Medial nasal process	6 Medial nasal process fusing with maxillary process on each side
2 Nasal pit	7 Lateral nasal process
3 Lateral nasal process	8 Philtrum
4 Maxillary process	9 Upper lip
5 Medial nasal processes fusing with each other	

REVIEW QUESTIONS: Facial development within fourth week of embryonic period during prenatal development

Fill in the blanks by choosing the appropriate terms from the list below.

1. The two _____ form in the anterior part of the frontonasal process just superior to the stomodeum during the fourth week of embryonic period as button-like structures, which are bilateral ectodermal thickenings that later develop into olfactory epithelium located in the mature nose for the sensation of smell.

2. During the fourth week, the tissue around the nasal placodes on the frontonasal process undergoes growth, thus starting the development of the nasal region and the nose; the placodes become submerged forming a depression in the center of each placode, the _____.

3. The middle part of the tissue growing around the nasal placodes appears as two crescent-shaped swellings located between the nasal pits, the _____ .

4. In the future, the medial nasal processes will fuse together externally to form the middle part of the nose from the root of the nose to the apex of the nose as well as the tubercle of the upper lip and

   _____.

5. On the outer part of the nasal pits are two crescent-shaped swellings, the _____.

6. In the future, the lateral nasal processes will form the _____ of the nose.

7. The fusion of the lateral nasal, maxillary, and medial nasal processes forms the _____.

8. The paired medial nasal processes fuse internally and grow inferiorly on the inside of the stomodeum, forming the _____ by the seventh week.

9. The intermaxillary segment is involved in the formation of certain maxillary teeth, incisors, and associated structures, such as the _____ and nasal septum.

10. The facial development that starts during the embryonic period will be completed later in the twelfth week within the _____.

fetal period	nasal pits	nasal placodes
nares	primary palate	medial nasal processes
intermaxillary segment	alae	lateral nasal processes
philtrum		

Reference Chapter 4, Face and neck development. In Fehrenbach MJ, Popowics T: *Illustrated dental embryology, histology, and anatomy,* ed 5, St. Louis, 2020, Saunders.

FIGURE 2.4 **Internal development of head and neck within fourth week of embryonic period**

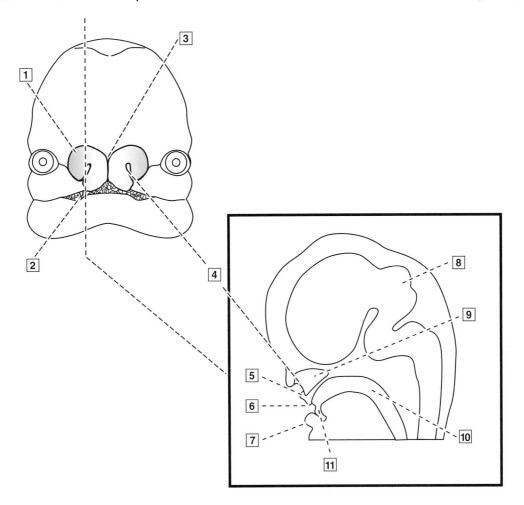

1 Lateral nasal process		**7** Developing lower lip	
2 Stomodeum		**8** Developing brain	
3 Fused medial nasal processes		**9** Developing nasal cavity	
4 Nasal pit		**10** Primitive pharynx	
5 Intermaxillary segment		**11** Primitive mouth	
6 Developing upper lip			

REVIEW QUESTIONS: Internal development of head and neck within fourth week of embryonic period during prenatal development

Fill in the blanks by choosing the appropriate terms from the list below.

1. The first event in the development of the face during the latter part of the fourth week of prenatal development is the disintegration of the oropharyngeal membrane, which allows the primitive mouth to be increased in depth and enlarged across the surface of the midface; access now occurs through the stomodeum between the internal _____ and the outside fluids of the amniotic cavity that surrounds the embryo.

2. During the fourth week, the tissue around the _____ on the frontonasal process undergoes growth, thus starting the development of the nasal region and the nose by forming a depression in the center of each placode, the nasal pits (or olfactory pits).

3. The middle part of the tissue growing around the nasal placodes appears as two crescent-shaped _____ located between the nasal pits and the medial nasal processes.

4. In the future, the medial nasal processes will fuse together externally to form the middle part of the nose from the root of the nose to the apex of the nose as well as the tubercle of the _____ and philtrum.

5. The paired medial nasal processes fuse internally and grow inferiorly on the inside of the_____, forming the intermaxillary segment.

6. The intermaxillary segment is involved in the formation of certain maxillary teeth (incisors) and associated structures, such as the primary palate and _____.

7. On the outer part of the _____ are two crescent-shaped swellings, the lateral nasal processes.

8. In the future, the _____ form the alae of the nose, and the fusion of the lateral nasal, maxillary, and medial nasal processes forms the nares.

9. Deepening of the nasal pits produces a nasal sac that grows internally toward the developing brain, with the nasal sacs initially separated from the stomodeum by the _____.

10. The oronasal membrane disintegrates, bringing the _____ and oral cavity into communication in the area of the primitive choanae, posterior to the developing primary palate; at the same time, the superior, middle, and inferior nasal conchae are forming on the lateral walls of the developing nasal cavities.

nasal pits	upper lip	nasal cavity
stomodeum	primitive pharynx	nasal septum
oronasal membrane	swellings	nasal placodes
lateral nasal processes		

Reference Chapter 4, Face and neck development. In Fehrenbach MJ, Popowics T: *Illustrated dental embryology, histology, and anatomy,* ed 5, St. Louis, 2020, Saunders.

ANSWER KEY 1. primitive pharynx, 2. nasal placodes, 3. swellings, 4. upper lip, 5. stomodeum, 6. nasal septum, 7. nasal pits, 8. lateral nasal processes, 9. oronasal membrane, 10. nasal cavity

FIGURE 2.5 Neck development during prenatal development with branchial apparatus formation (external view and internal sections)

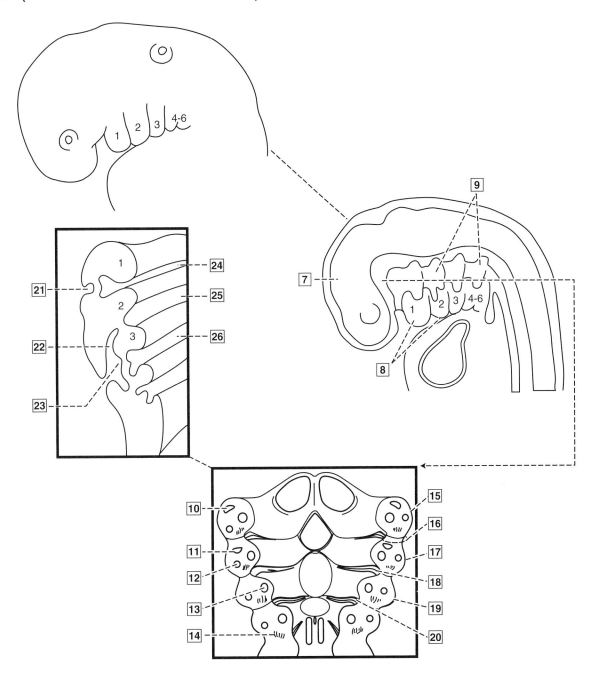

7	Brain	12	Nerve	17	Second branchial arch (hyoid arch)	22	Second branchial groove
8	Branchial arches	13	Vessel	18	Second branchial pouch	23	Third branchial groove
9	Pharyngeal pouches	14	Muscle	19	Third branchial arch	24	First branchial pouch
10	Meckel cartilage	15	First branchial arch (mandibular arch)	20	Third branchial pouch	25	Second branchial pouch
11	Reichert cartilage	16	First branchial membrane	21	First branchial groove	26	Third branchial pouch

REVIEW QUESTIONS: Neck development during prenatal development with branchial apparatus formation

Fill in the blanks by choosing the appropriate terms from the list below.

1. The development of the _____ parallels the development of the face over time, beginning during the fourth week of prenatal development within the embryonic period and completed during the fetal period.

2. During the fourth week of prenatal development, stacked bilateral swellings of tissue forming the brachial arches appear inferior to the stomodeum and include the _____.

3. The pharyngeal or _____ are a total of six pairs of U-shaped bars with a central core of mesenchyme derived from mesoderm invaded by neural crest cells, now referred to as *ectomesenchyme;* they are covered externally by ectoderm, lined internally by endoderm and support the lateral walls of the primitive pharynx.

4. The pharyngeal or _____ consists of arches, grooves and membranes, as well as pouches.

5. The endodermal invaginations from the lateral walls lining the pharynx will form four well-defined pairs of balloon-like structures, the _____.

6. The first branchial arch or pharyngeal arch, also known as the *mandibular arch*, and its associated tissue include _____.

7. Forming within the second branchial arch or pharyngeal arch, also known as the *hyoid arch*, is cartilage similar to that of the mandibular arch, _____, with most of this structure disappearing during development; however, parts of it are responsible in the future for a middle ear bone, a process of the temporal bone, and parts of the hyoid bone.

8. Between neighboring branchial arches, external grooves are noted on each side of the embryo, the pharyngeal or _____.

9. The _____ are derived from the lining of the second pharyngeal pouches and also from the pharyngeal walls.

10. The parathyroid glands and _____ are derived from the lining of the third and fourth pharyngeal pouches; additionally, the latter has a part that is of ectodermal origin.

mandibular arch	branchial arches	branchial grooves
thymus gland	neck	branchial apparatus
pharyngeal pouches	palatine tonsils	Reichert cartilage
Meckel cartilage		

Reference Chapter 4, Face and neck development. In Fehrenbach MJ, Popowics T: *Illustrated dental embryology, histology, and anatomy,* ed 5, St. Louis, 2020, Saunders.

FIGURE 2.6   **Regions of head**

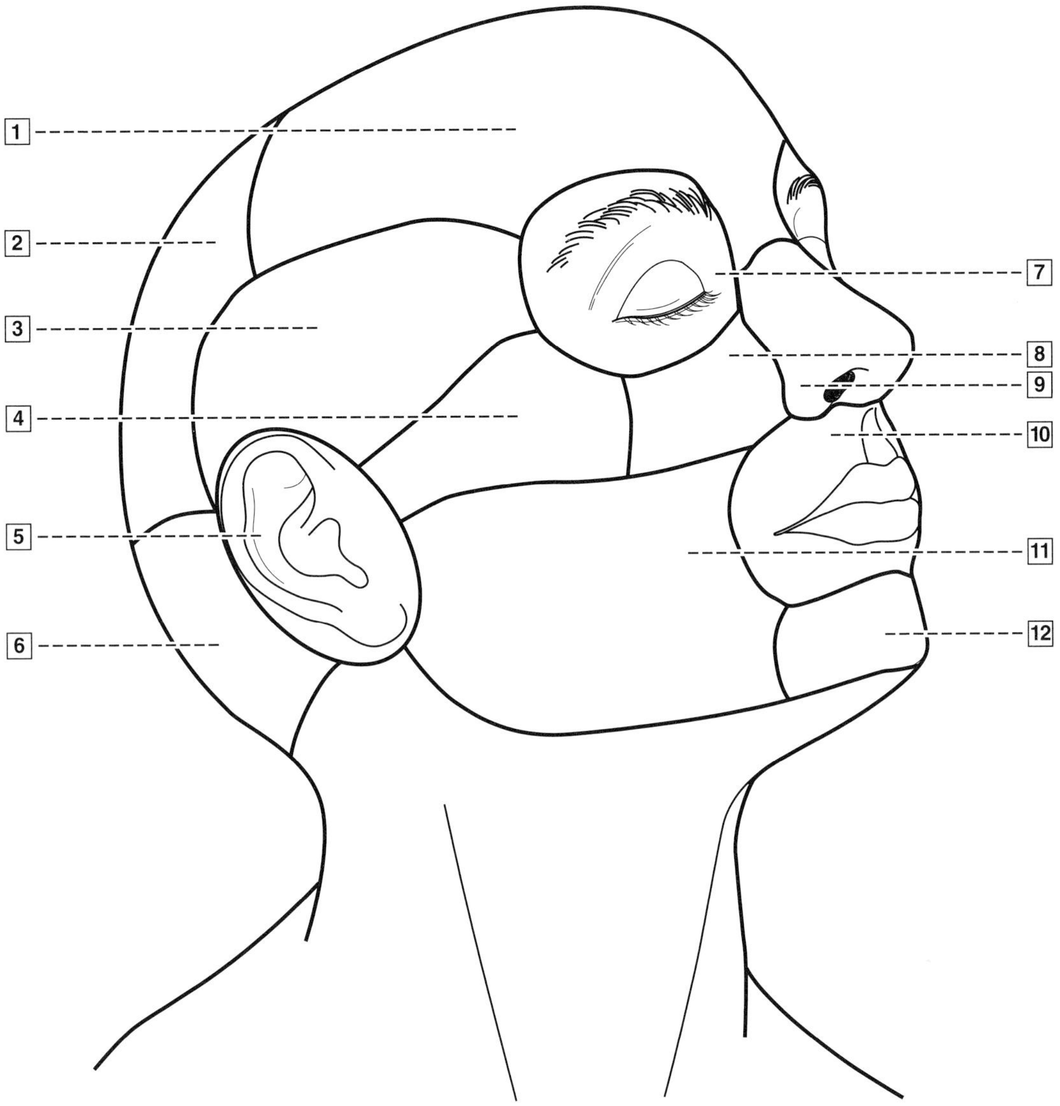

1	Frontal region	**7**	Orbital region
2	Parietal region	**8**	Infraorbital region
3	Temporal region	**9**	Nasal region
4	Zygomatic region	**10**	Oral region
5	Auricular region	**11**	Buccal region
6	Occipital region	**12**	Mental region

REVIEW QUESTIONS: Regions of head

Fill in the blanks by choosing the appropriate terms from the list below.

1. The _____ is the study of the structural relationships of the external features of the body to the internal organs and parts.

2. The _____ include the frontal, parietal, occipital, temporal, auricular, orbital, nasal, infra-orbital, zygomatic, buccal, oral, and mental regions.

3. The _____ as a region of the head includes the forehead and the area superior to the eyes and is defined by the deeper skull bone.

4. The scalp covers both the parietal region and the _____ of the head, which consists of layers of soft tissue overlying the bones of the braincase.

5. Within the _____ is the region of the head that has the temple, which is located on the superficial side of the head posterior to each eye and is defined by the deeper skull bone.

6. The _____ is a region of each side of the head that has the external ear as a prominent feature.

7. In the _____ is a region of each side of the head with the eyeball and all its supporting structures contained within the bony socket or orbit, which is formed by various skull bones.

8. The main feature of the _____ as a region of the head is the external nose; the root of the nose is located between the eyes, and the tip is the apex of the nose, with the naris or nostril on each side.

9. The infraorbital region, zygomatic region, and _____ on each side of the head are all located on the facial aspect.

10. The _____ is a region of the head that has many structures within it such as the lips, oral cavity, palate, tongue, floor of the mouth, and parts of the pharynx.

auricular region	oral region	regions of the head
buccal region	temporal region	nasal region
orbital region	surface anatomy	occipital region
frontal region		

References Chapter 2, Surface anatomy. In Fehrenbach MJ, Herring SW: *Illustrated anatomy of the head and neck,* ed 6, St. Louis, 2021, Saunders; Chapter 1, Face and neck regions. In Fehrenbach MJ, Popowics T: *Illustrated dental embryology, histology, and anatomy,* ed 5, St. Louis, 2020, Saunders.

ANSWER KEY 1. surface anatomy, 2. regions of the head, 3. frontal region, 4. occipital region, 5. temporal region, 6. auricular region, 7. orbital region, 8. nasal region, 9. buccal region, 10. oral region

FIGURE 2.7 Frontal region with skin region noted (microanatomic view)

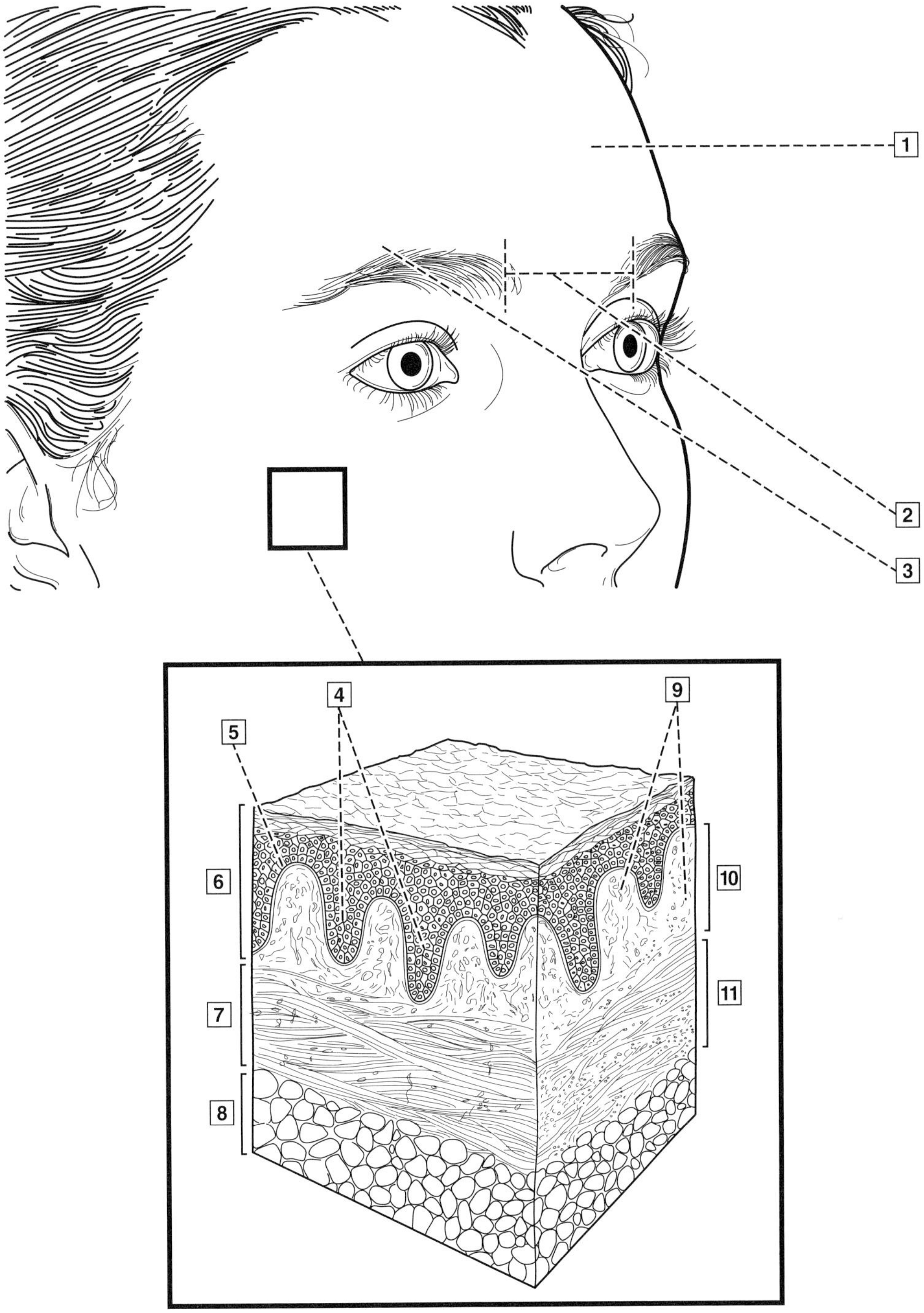

1	Frontal eminence	7	Dermis (connective tissue proper)
2	Glabella	8	Hypodermis
3	Supraorbital ridge	9	Connective tissue papillae
4	Rete ridges	10	Loose connective tissue or papillary layer
5	Basement membrane	11	Dense connective tissue or dense layer
6	Epidermis (epithelium)		

REVIEW QUESTIONS: Frontal region with skin region noted

Fill in the blanks by choosing the appropriate terms from the list below.

1. The _____ of the head includes the forehead and the area superior to the eyes.

2. Directly inferior to each eyebrow is the _____.

3. The smooth elevated area between the eyebrows is the _____.

4. The prominence of the forehead is the _____.

5. The _____ is the tissue type that covers and lines both the external and internal body surfaces, including vessels and small cavities; it not only serves as a protective covering or lining but is also involved in tissue absorption, secretion, sensory, and other specialized functions.

6. Depending on individual classification, epithelial tissue can be derived from any of the _____ embryonic cell layers based on the location when developing.

7. Most epithelium in the body is composed of _____, which includes the superficial layer of both the skin and oral mucosa.

8. An example of keratinized stratified squamous epithelium is the _____, which is the superficial layer of the skin that overlies a basement membrane and adjoins the deeper layers of connective tissue.

9. The connective tissue proper in the skin is the _____ and is found deep to the epidermis.

10. Even deeper into the dermis within the skin is the _____, which is composed of loose connective tissue and adipose connective tissue with large blood vessels and nerves; the adipose tissue is a specialized connective tissue as well as glandular tissue.

epidermis	stratified squamous epithelium	hypodermis
three	epithelium	frontal region
glabella	dermis	supraorbital ridge
frontal eminence		

References Chapter 2, Surface anatomy. In Fehrenbach MJ, Herring SW: *Illustrated anatomy of the head and neck,* ed 6, St. Louis, 2021, Saunders; Chapter 8, Basic tissue. In Fehrenbach MJ, Popowics T: *Illustrated dental embryology, histology, and anatomy,* ed 5, St. Louis, 2020, Saunders.

NOTES

FIGURE 2.8 Interface between epithelium and connective tissue: Skin example (microanatomic views)

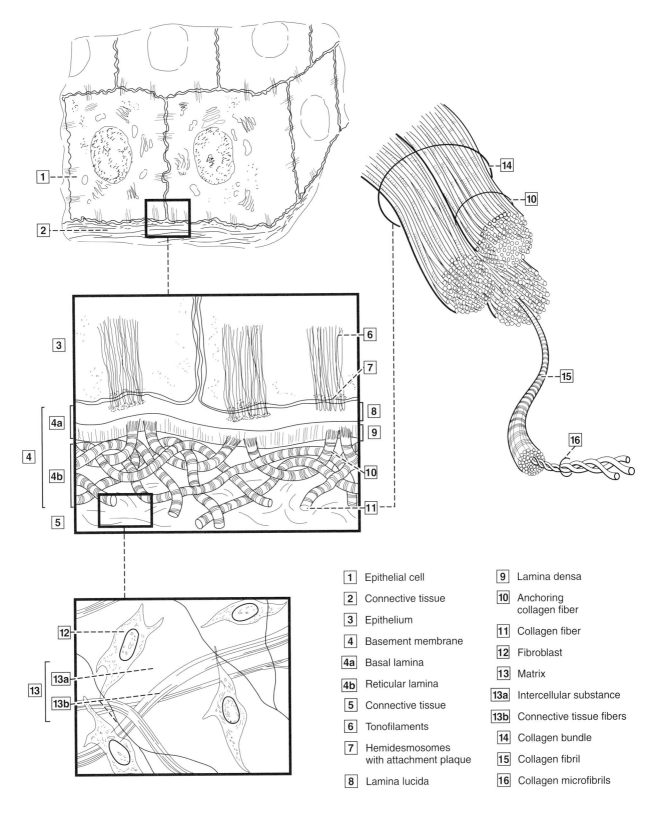

1	Epithelial cell	**9**	Lamina densa
2	Connective tissue	**10**	Anchoring collagen fiber
3	Epithelium	**11**	Collagen fiber
4	Basement membrane	**12**	Fibroblast
4a	Basal lamina	**13**	Matrix
4b	Reticular lamina	**13a**	Intercellular substance
5	Connective tissue	**13b**	Connective tissue fibers
6	Tonofilaments	**14**	Collagen bundle
7	Hemidesmosomes with attachment plaque	**15**	Collagen fibril
8	Lamina lucida	**16**	Collagen microfibrils

REVIEW QUESTIONS: Interface between epithelium and connective tissue: Skin example

Fill in the blanks by choosing the appropriate terms from the list below.

1. The _____ is a thin acellular structure located between any form of epithelium and the underlying connective tissue as noted in both the skin and oral mucosa; this type of structure is even present between the components of the tooth germ during tooth development.

2. The basement membrane consists of two layers, _____ and reticular lamina.

3. The superficial layer of the basement membrane is the basal lamina and is produced by the _____.

4. The basal lamina consists of two sublayers, the lamina lucida, which is a clear layer closer to the epithelium and the _____, which is a dense layer closer to the connective tissue.

5. The deeper layer of the basement membrane is usually the reticular lamina, which consists of collagen fibers and reticular fibers produced and secreted by the underlying _____.

6. Attachment mechanisms are part of the basement membrane and involve hemidesmosomes with the attachment plaque as well as tonofilaments from the epithelium and the _____ from the connective tissue.

7. The _____ from the epithelium loop through the attachment plaque, whereas the collagen fibers of the reticular lamina loop into the lamina densa of the basal lamina, forming a flexible attachment between the two tissue types.

8. The _____ are the main connective tissue fiber type found in the body and are composed of the protein collagen, including distinct types that have been shown by immunologic studies to have great tensile strength.

9. The most common distinct type of collagen protein is _____ collagen, which is found in the teeth, lamina propria of the oral mucosa, dermis of the skin, bone, tendons, and virtually all other types of connective tissue.

10. Cells responsible for the synthesis of Type I collagen protein include _____ that produce fibers and intercellular substance, and osteoblasts that produce bone as well as odontoblasts that produce dentin.

anchoring collagen fibers	tonofilaments	basal lamina
fibroblasts	lamina densa	collagen fibers
Type I	epithelium	basement membrane
connective tissue		

Reference Chapter 8, Basic tissue. In Fehrenbach MJ, Popowics T: *Illustrated dental embryology, histology, and anatomy,* ed 5, St. Louis, 2020, Saunders.

FIGURE 2.9 Auricular region: External ear (lateral view)

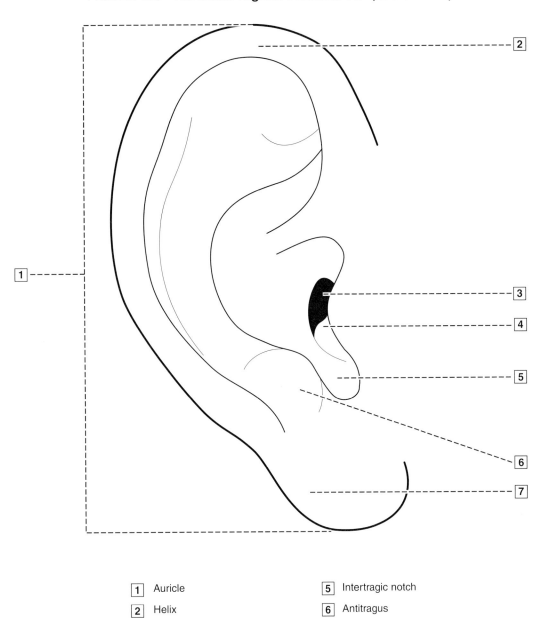

1	Auricle	**5**	Intertragic notch
2	Helix	**6**	Antitragus
3	External acoustic meatus	**7**	Lobule
4	Tragus		

REVIEW QUESTIONS: Auricular region: External ear

Fill in the blanks by choosing the appropriate terms from the list below.

1. The _____ is a region on each side of the head that has the external ear as a prominent feature.

2. The first part of the ear consists of the external ear that is attached to the lateral aspect of the head and a canal leading inward to the eardrum or _____.

3. The _____ is composed of an oval flap or *auricle* and the external acoustic meatus.

4. As the visible part of the external ear, the _____ collects sound waves.

5. The _____ is a centrally located tube through which sound waves are transmitted to the middle ear within the skull; it is an important landmark when taking certain radiographs and administering certain local anesthetic nerve blocks.

6. The superior and posterior free margin of the auricle is the _____.

7. The helix ends inferiorly at the _____, the fleshy protuberance of the earlobe.

8. The _____ is the smaller flap of tissue of the auricle anterior to the external acoustic meatus.

9. The other flap of tissue opposite the tragus is the _____, which is a landmark when taking radiographs and administering local anesthetic nerve blocks.

10. Between the tragus and antitragus is a small groove, the _____.

intertragic notch	tympanic membrane	external ear
helix	auricular region	antitragus
auricle	external acoustic meatus	lobule
tragus		

References Chapter 2, Surface anatomy. In Fehrenbach MJ, Herring SW: *Illustrated anatomy of the head and neck,* ed 6, St. Louis, 2021, Saunders; Chapter 1, Face and neck regions. In Fehrenbach MJ, Popowics T: *Illustrated dental embryology, histology, and anatomy,* ed 5, St. Louis, 2020, Saunders; Chapter 8, Head and neck. In Drake R, Vogel AW, Mitchell AWM: *Gray's anatomy for students,* ed 4, Philadelphia, 2020, Churchill Livingstone.

NOTES

FIGURE 2.10 Auricular region: Middle and internal ear (sagittal sections)

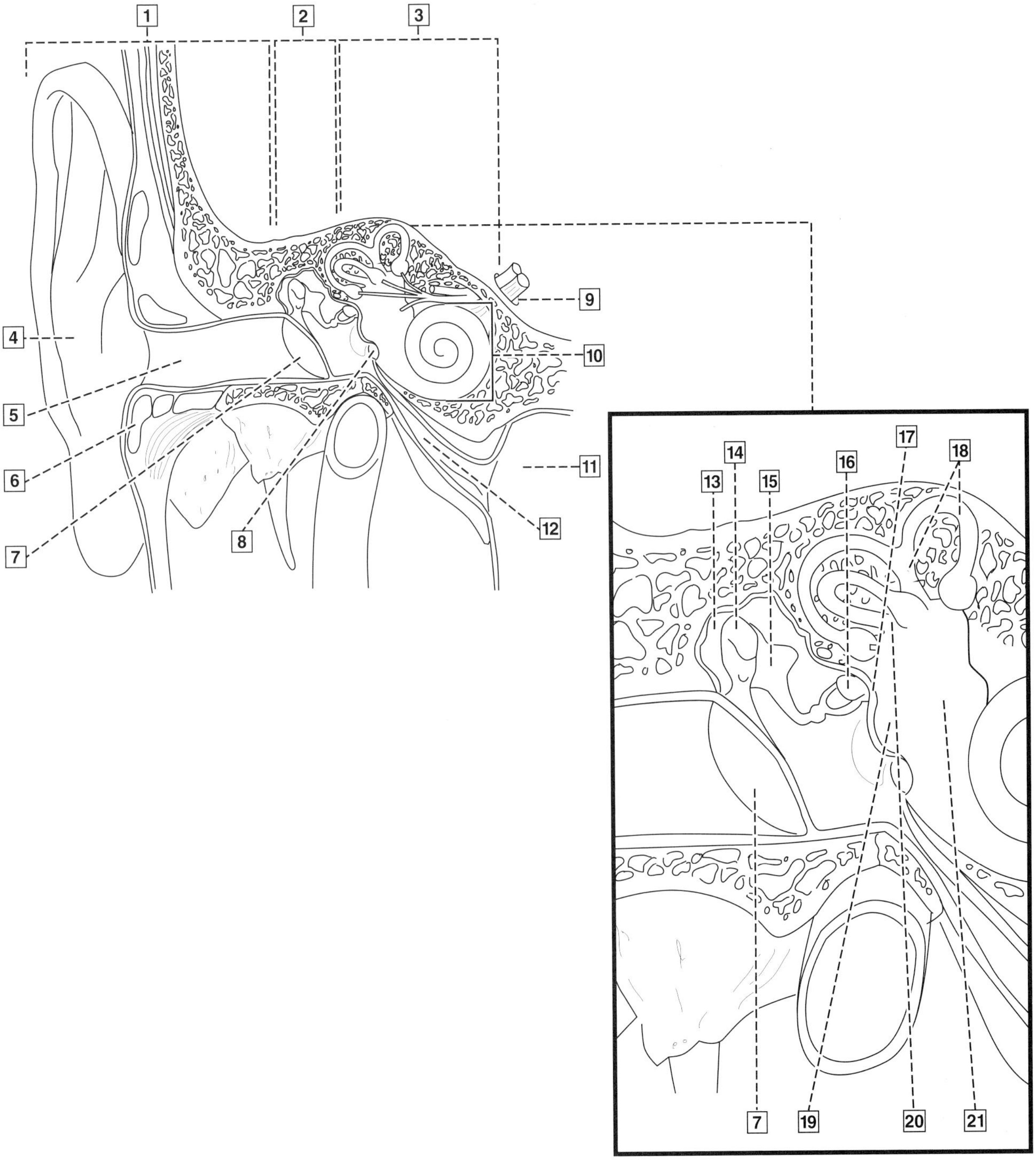

1 External ear	**7** Tympanic membrane	**13** Epitympanic recess	**19** Vestibule
2 Middle ear	**8** Round window	**14** Malleus	**20** Utricle
3 Internal ear	**9** Internal acoustic meatus	**15** Incus	**21** Saccule
4 Auricle	**10** Cochlea	**16** Stapes	
5 External acoustic meatus	**11** Pharynx	**17** Oval window	
6 Cartilage	**12** Pharyngotympanic tube	**18** Semicircular canals	

REVIEW QUESTIONS: Auricular region: Middle and internal ear

Fill in the blanks by choosing the appropriate terms from the list below.

1. The second part of the ear is the _____, which is a cavity in the petrous part of the temporal bone bounded laterally and separated from the external canal by a membrane and connected internally to the pharynx by a narrow tube.

2. The _____ separates the external acoustic meatus from the middle ear and consists of a connective tissue core lined with skin on the outer part and mucous membrane on the inner part.

3. The function of the middle ear is to transmit _____ of the tympanic membrane across the cavity of the middle ear to the internal ear, which is accomplished through three interconnected but movable bones that bridge the space between the tympanic membrane and the internal ear.

4. The bones of the middle ear include the _____ (connected to the tympanic membrane), the incus (connected to the malleus by a synovial joint), and the stapes (connected to the incus by a synovial joint and attached to the lateral wall of the internal ear at the oval window).

5. The third part of the ear is the _____, which consists of a series of cavities within the petrous part of the temporal bone between the laterally located middle ear and the medially located internal acoustic meatus.

6. The internal ear consists of the _____, which is a series of bony cavities and the membranous labyrinth with its membranous ducts and sacs within these cavities.

7. The bony labyrinth consists of the _____, three semicircular canals, and cochlea that contain a clear fluid, the perilymph.

8. Suspended within the perilymph but not filling all spaces of the bony labyrinth is the _____, which consists of the semicircular ducts, cochlear duct, and two sacs filled with endolymph, the utricle and the saccule.

9. The vestibule contains the _____ in its lateral wall, which is the central part of the bony labyrinth that communicates anteriorly with the cochlea and posterosuperiorly with the semicircular canals.

10. Projecting in an anterior direction from the vestibule is the _____, which is a bony structure that twists on itself around a central column of bone.

internal ear	middle ear	tympanic membrane
oval window	malleus	vibrations
vestibule	cochlea	bony labyrinth
membranous labyrinth		

Reference Chapter 8, Head and neck. In Drake R, Vogl AW, Mitchell AWM: *Gray's anatomy for students,* ed 4, Philadelphia, 2020, Churchill Livingstone.

8. membranous labyrinth, 9. oval window, 10. cochlea
ANSWER KEY 1. middle ear, 2. tympanic membrane, 3. vibrations, 4. malleus, 5. internal ear, 6. bony labyrinth, 7. vestibule,

88 Copyright © 2023 Elsevier Inc. All Rights Reserved.

FIGURE 2.11 Orbital region (frontal view with internal view)

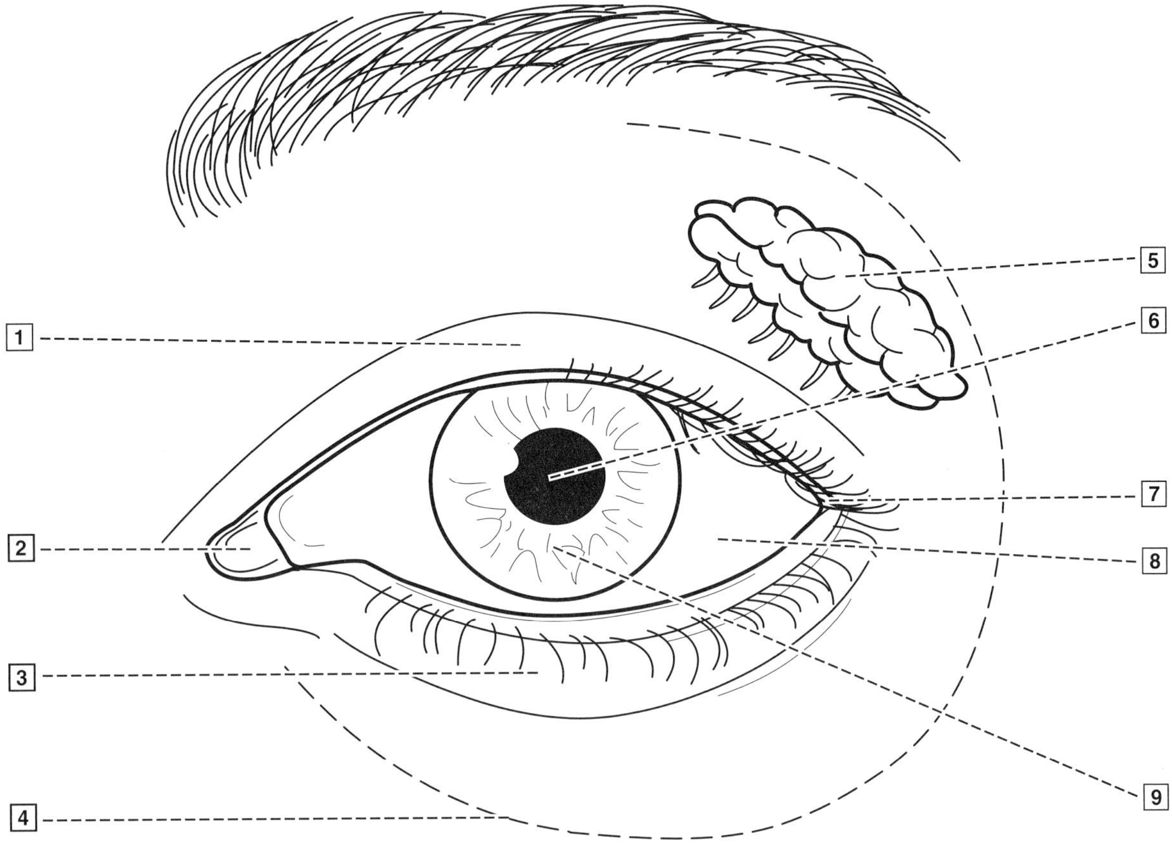

1	Upper eyelid	7	Lateral canthus
2	Medial canthus	8	Sclera (covered by conjunctiva)
3	Lower eyelid	9	Iris
4	Orbit (outlined)		
5	Lacrimal gland (deep)		
6	Pupil		

REVIEW QUESTIONS: Orbital region

Fill in the blanks by choosing the appropriate terms from the list below.

1. In the orbital region of each side of the head, the eyeball and all its supporting structures are contained within the _____, a bony socket of the skull.

2. The orbits are a pair of conical or four-sided pyramidal cavities, which open into the midline of the face and point posteriorly into the head, with each having a(n) _____, an orbital apex and four orbital walls.

3. On the eyeball is the _____, the white area of the eye.

4. The sclera has a central area of coloration, the circular _____.

5. The opening in the center of the iris is the _____, which appears black and changes size as the iris responds to changing light conditions.

6. Two movable eyelids, upper and lower, cover and protect each _____.

7. Behind each upper eyelid and deep within the orbit are the _____, which produce lacrimal fluid or *tears* from its ducts.

8. The _____ is the delicate and thin membrane lining the inside of the eyelids and the front of the eyeball.

9. The outer corner where the upper and lower eyelids meet is the _____ or *outer canthus;* the canthi are landmarks when taking certain extraoral radiographs.

10. The inner angle of the eye is the _____ or *inner canthus;* the canthi are landmarks when taking certain extraoral radiographs.

eyeball	Conjunctiva	orbit
pupil	lateral canthus	medial canthus
lacrimal glands	base	sclera
iris		

References   Chapter 2, Surface anatomy. In Fehrenbach MJ, Herring SW: *Illustrated anatomy of the head and neck,* ed 6, St. Louis, 2021, Saunders; Chapter 1, Face and neck regions. In Fehrenbach MJ, Popowics T: *Illustrated dental embryology, histology, and anatomy,* ed 5, St. Louis, 2020, Saunders; Chapter 3, Skeletal system. In Fehrenbach MJ, Popowics T: *Illustrated dental embryology, histology, and anatomy,* ed 5, St. Louis, 2020, Saunders.

NOTES

ANSWER KEY   1. orbit, 2. base, 3. sclera, 4. iris, 5. pupil, 6. eyeball, 7. lacrimal glands, 8. conjunctiva, 9. lateral canthus, 10. medial canthus

FIGURE 2.12 Orbital region: Eye (sagittal section)

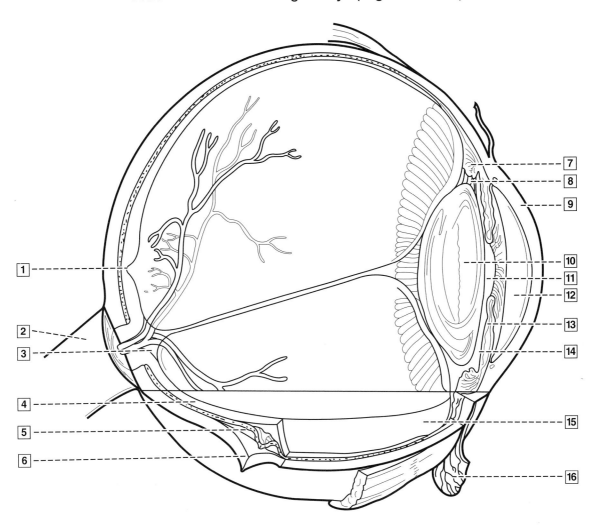

1	Fovea centralis	6	Sclera	11	Pupil
2	Optic nerve	7	Ciliary body	12	Anterior chamber filled with aqueous humor
3	Optic disk	8	Suspensory ligament	13	Iris
4	Retina	9	Cornea	14	Posterior chamber
5	Choroid	10	Lens	15	Postremal chamber filled with vitreous humor
				16	Conjunctiva

REVIEW QUESTIONS: Orbital region: Eye

Fill in the blanks by choosing the appropriate terms from the list below.

1. The _____ is the area directly posterior to the cornea and anterior to the colored part of the eye, the iris; the central opening in the iris is the pupil and posterior to the iris but anterior to the lens is the smaller posterior chamber.

2. Both the anterior and posterior chambers are continuous with each other through the pupillary opening and filled with a fluid, _____, which is secreted into the posterior chamber and flows into the anterior chamber through the pupil.

3. The _____ is a transparent biconvex elastic disc attached circumferentially to muscles associated with the outer wall of the eyeball, and whose lateral attachment provides it with the ability to change its refractive ability to maintain visual acuity.

4. The posterior part of the eyeball from the lens to the retina is filled with a gelatinous substance, the _____.

5. The _____ is an opaque layer of dense connective tissue that can be noted anteriorly through its covering of conjunctiva; it is pierced by numerous vessels and nerves, including the optic nerve posteriorly, and provides attachment for the various muscles involved in eyeball movements.

6. Continuous with the sclera anteriorly is the transparent _____, which covers the anterior surface of the eyeball and allows light to enter the eyeball.

7. The _____ is a posterior part of the eyeball and consists of a thin highly vascular pigmented layer with smaller vessels adjacent to the retina and larger vessels more peripherally; it is firmly attached to the retina internally and loosely attached to the sclera externally.

8. Extending from the anterior border of the choroid is the _____, which is a triangular-shaped structure located between the choroid and the iris, forming a complete ring around the eyeball.

9. The inner layer of the eyeball is the _____, which consists of two parts that include posteriorly and laterally the optic part, which is sensitive to light, and anteriorly the nonvisual part, which covers the internal surface of the ciliary body and the iris.

10. The optic disc is where the optic nerve leaves the retina (its "blind spot"); lateral to the optic disc is a small area with a hint of yellowish coloration, the macula lutea with its central depression, the _____, which is the thinnest and most sensitive part.

sclera	aqueous humor	anterior chamber
choroid	lens	vitreous humor
retina	cornea	fovea centralis
ciliary body		

Reference   Chapter 8, Head and neck. In Drake R, Vogl AW, Mitchell AWM: *Gray's anatomy for students,* ed 4, Philadelphia, 2020, Churchill Livingstone.

ANSWER KEY   1. anterior chamber, 2. aqueous humor, 3. lens, 4. vitreous humor, 5. sclera, 6. cornea, 7. choroid, 8. ciliary body, 9. retina, 10. fovea centralis

FIGURE 2.13 Nasal region: External nose (frontal view)

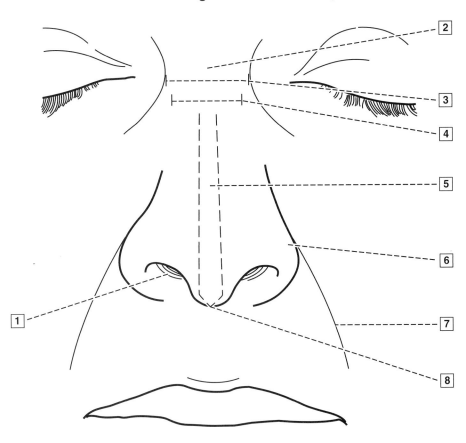

1 Naris
2 Position of nasion
3 Root of nose
4 Bridge of nose
5 Nasal septum (outlined)
6 Ala
7 Nasolabial sulcus
8 Apex of nose

REVIEW QUESTIONS: Nasal region: External nose

Fill in the blanks by choosing the appropriate terms from the list below.

1. The main feature of the nasal region of the head is the _____.

2. The _____ is located between the eyes in the nasal region.

3. Inferior to the glabella is a midpoint cephalometric landmark of the nasal region that corresponds with the junction between the underlying bones, the _____, which is a landmark when taking certain extraoral radiographs.

4. Inferior to the nasion is the bony structure of the skull that forms the _____.

5. The _____ or *tip* is flexible when palpated because it is formed from cartilage.

6. Inferior to the apex on each side of the nose is a(n) _____ or *nostril.*

7. The nares are separated by the midline _____.

8. The nares are bounded laterally on each side by a winglike cartilaginous structure, the _____ of the nose, which is a landmark when taking certain extraoral radiographs.

9. The nose is a structure on the face that admits and expels air for respiration in conjunction with the _____.

10. Deep to the nose are _____ and the paranasal sinuses.

oral cavity	bridge of the nose	ala
olfactory mucosa	nasion	root of the nose
naris	external nose	nasal septum
apex of the nose		

References Chapter 2, Surface anatomy. In Fehrenbach MJ, Herring SW: *Illustrated anatomy of the head and neck,* ed 6, St. Louis, 2021, Saunders; Chapter 1, Face and neck regions. In Fehrenbach MJ, Popowics T: *Illustrated dental embryology, histology, and anatomy,* ed 5, St. Louis, 2020, Saunders.

NOTES

FIGURE 2.14   Nasal region: Nasal cavity (sagittal section with microanatomic view)

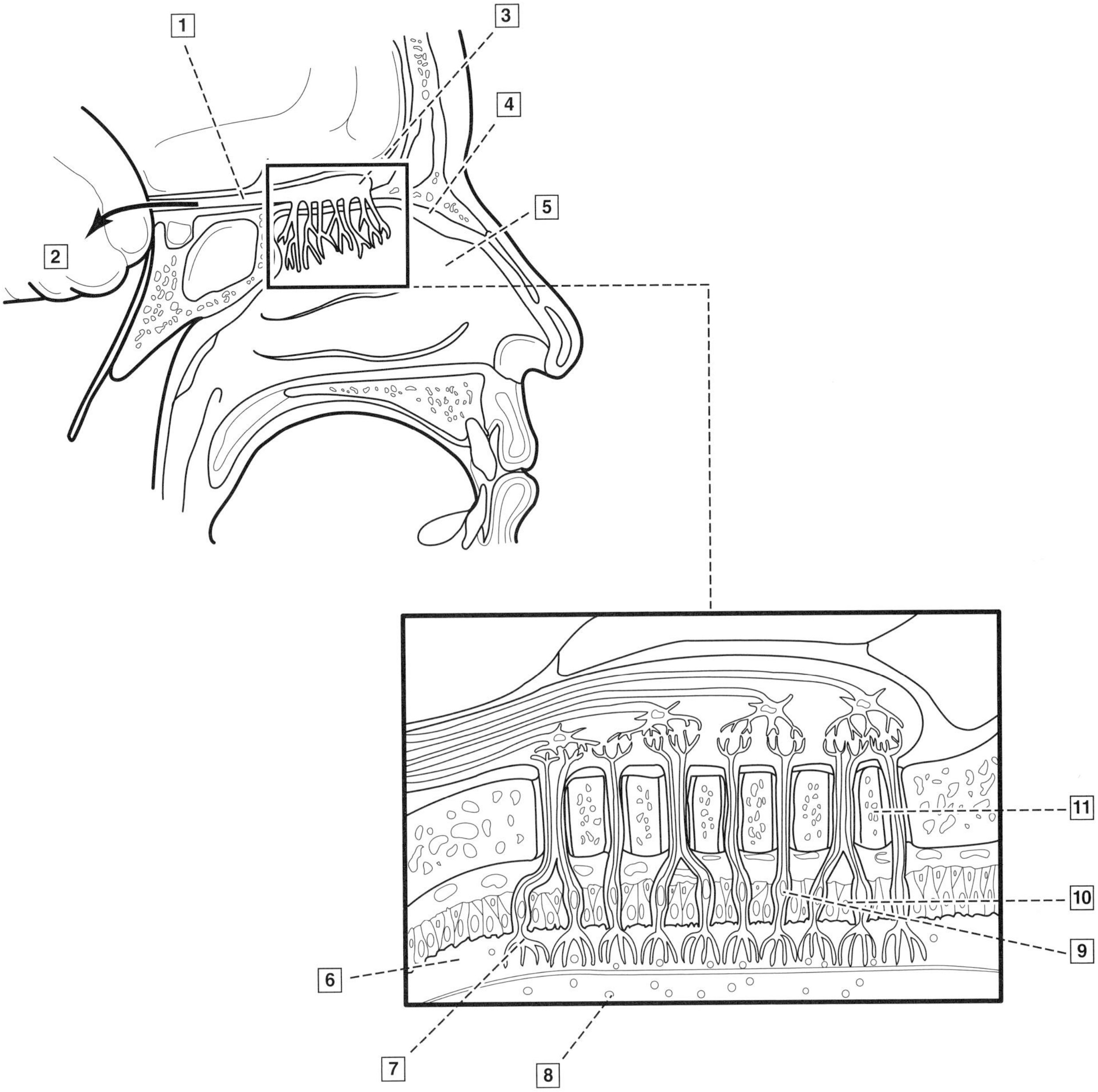

1	Olfactory tract	**6**	Mucous layer
2	Olfactory cortex	**7**	Cilia of receptor cell
3	Olfactory bulb	**8**	Odor molecule
4	Olfactory epithelium	**9**	Cell body of olfactory neuron
5	Nasal cavity	**10**	Supporting cells
		11	Cribriform plate of ethmoid bone

REVIEW QUESTIONS: Nasal region: Nasal cavity

Fill in the blanks by choosing the appropriate terms from the list below.

1. Each _____ consists of three general regions that include the nasal vestibule, respiratory region, and olfactory region, with each having a floor, roof, medial wall, and lateral wall.

2. The nasal vestibule is just internal to each _____ of the nasal cavity and is lined by skin that contains hair follicles.

3. The _____ is the largest general region of the nasal cavity and is lined by respiratory epithelium composed mainly of ciliated and mucous cells.

4. The olfactory region at the apex of each nasal cavity is lined by _____ and contains the olfactory receptors.

5. In addition to functioning for the sense of smell, the nasal cavities adjust the temperature and humidity; these cavities also filter the air through the hair in the vestibule and capture foreign material in the _____, which is moved posteriorly by cilia on epithelial cells in the nasal cavities into the digestive tract.

6. The lateral wall is characterized by three curved shelves of bone, the _____, which are superior to each other and project medially and inferiorly across the nasal cavity, dividing each nasal cavity into four air channels to also increase the surface area.

7. The openings of the _____, the air-filled spaces in the bones of the skull, are located on the lateral wall and roof of the nasal cavities.

8. The lateral wall of the nasal cavity contains the opening of the _____, which drains lacrimal fluid or *tears* from the lacrimal gland of the eye into the nasal cavity.

9. The _____ of the ethmoid bone is at the apex of the nasal cavities and separates the nasal cavities located inferiorly from the cranial cavity located superiorly; there are small perforations in the bone that allow the fibers of the first cranial nerve or the olfactory nerve to pass between the two regions.

10. The _____, which transmits the sense of smell from the nose to the brain, is supported and protected by the cribriform plate of the ethmoid bone that separates it from the olfactory epithelium and is perforated by olfactory nerve axons.

naris	mucus	respiratory region
nasolacrimal duct	conchae	olfactory epithelium
paranasal sinuses	nasal cavity	cribriform plate
olfactory bulb		

Reference Chapter 8, Head and neck. In Drake R, Vogl AW, Mitchell AWM: *Gray's anatomy for students,* ed 4, Philadelphia, 2020, Churchill Livingstone.

ANSWER KEY 1. nasal cavity, 2. naris, 3. respiratory region, 4. olfactory epithelium, 5. mucus, 6. conchae, 7. paranasal sinuses, 8. nasolacrimal duct, 9. cribriform plate, 10. olfactory bulb

FIGURE 2.15 Zygomatic, infraorbital, buccal, oral, and mental regions (anterolateral and frontal views with internal notations)

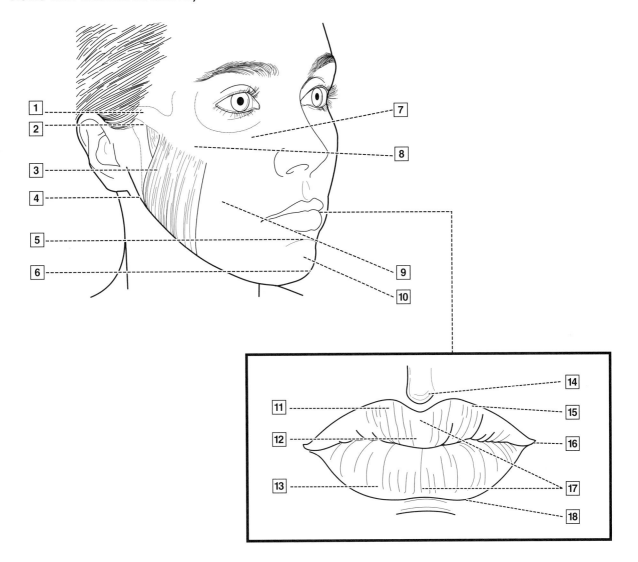

1	Zygomatic arch (deep)	11	Upper lip
2	Temporomandibular joint	12	Tubercle of the upper lip
3	Masseter muscle (deep)	13	Lower lip
4	Angle of mandible	14	Philtrum
5	Labiomental groove	15	Mucocutaneous junction at the vermilion border
6	Mental protuberance	16	Labial commissure
7	Infraorbital region	17	Vermilion zone
8	Zygomatic region	18	Mucocutaneous junction at the vermilion border
9	Buccal region		
10	Mental region		

REVIEW QUESTIONS: Zygomatic, infraorbital, buccal, oral, and mental regions

Fill in the blanks by choosing the appropriate terms from the list below.

1. The _____ of the head is a region located inferior to the orbital region and lateral to the nasal region.

2. Further laterally to the infraorbital region is the _____, which is a region that overlies the zygomatic arch or *cheekbone.*

3. Within the zygomatic region is the _____, which is formed from various skull bones and extends from just inferior to the lateral margin of the eye toward the middle part of the ear.

4. Inferior to the zygomatic arch and just anterior to the ear is the _____, a location where the upper skull forms a joint with the lower jaw.

5. The _____ of the head is a region composed of the soft tissue of the cheek.

6. One of the muscles within the cheek is the strong _____, which is felt or palpated when a patient clenches the teeth together.

7. The sharp angle of the lower jaw inferior to the lobule of the ear is the _____.

8. The lips are the gateway of the oral region and each lip begins as a(n) _____, having a darker appearance than the surrounding skin.

9. Superior to the midline of the upper lip, extending downward from the nasal septum, is a vertical groove on the skin, the _____; inferior to this the midline of the upper lip terminates in a thicker area or tubercle of the upper lip.

10. The _____ is the prominence of the chin, which is inferior to the labiomental groove, a horizontal groove between the lower lip and the chin.

zygomatic arch	temporomandibular joint	masseter muscle
buccal region	mental protuberance	vermilion border
infraorbital region	angle of the mandible	philtrum
zygomatic region		

References Chapter 2, Surface anatomy. In Fehrenbach MJ, Herring SW: *Illustrated anatomy of the head and neck,* ed 6, St. Louis, 2021, Saunders; Chapter 2, Oral cavity and pharynx. In Fehrenbach MJ, Popowics T: *Illustrated dental embryology, histology, and anatomy,* ed 5, St. Louis, 2020, Saunders.

NOTES

FIGURE 2.16 Oral region: Oral cavity (oral view with microanatomic view)

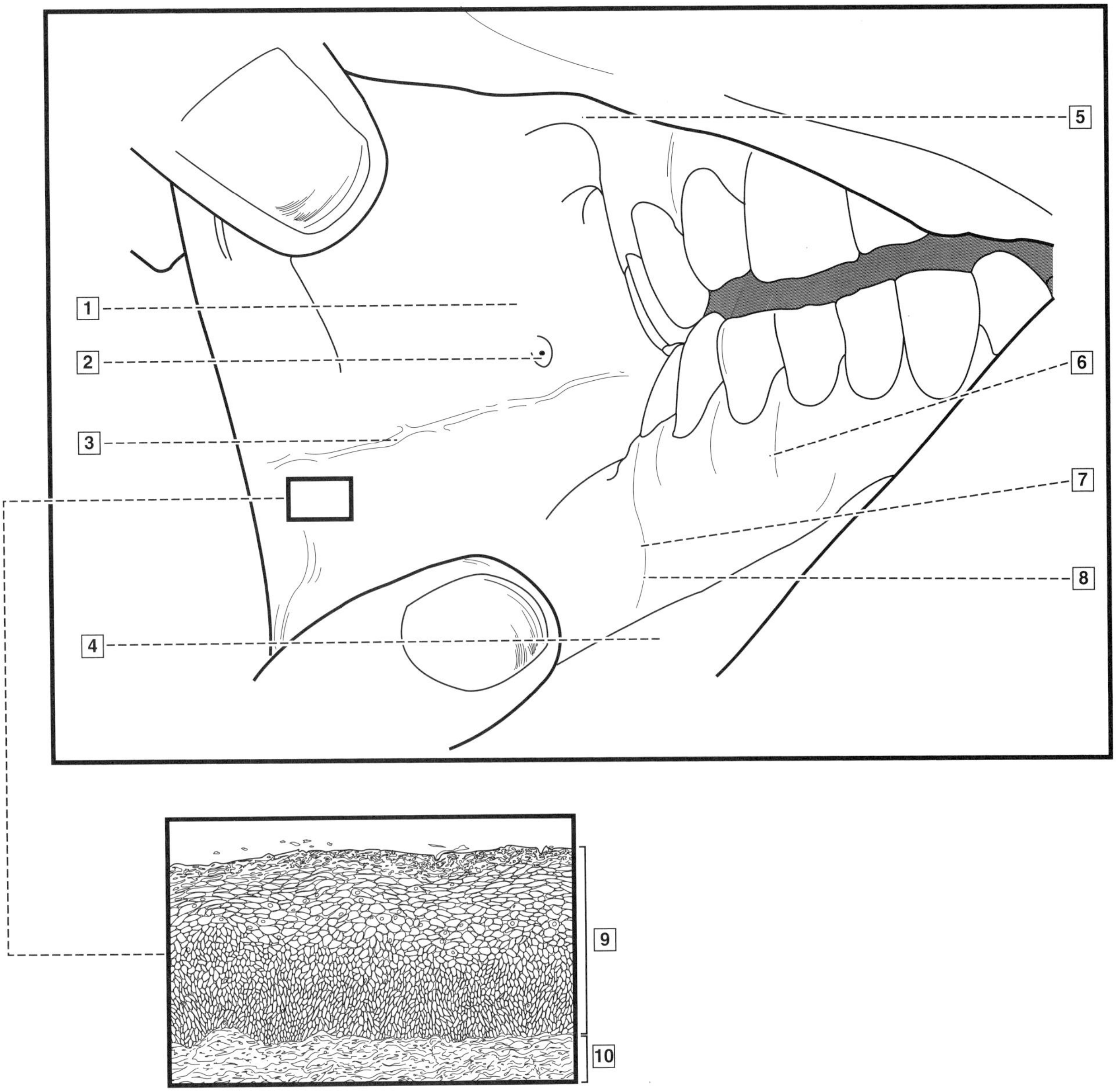

1 Buccal mucosa	**6** Alveolar mucosa
2 Parotid papilla	**7** Mucobuccal fold
3 Linea alba	**8** Mandibular vestibule
4 Labial mucosa	**9** Epithelium
5 Maxillary vestibule	**10** Lamina propria

REVIEW QUESTIONS: Oral region: Oral cavity

Fill in the blanks by choosing the appropriate terms from the list below.

1. The inside of the mouth is known as the _____.

2. Underlying the upper lip is the bony _____ or *upper jaw.*

3. The bone underlying the lower lip is the bony _____ or *lower jaw.*

4. The oral cavity is lined by a mucous membrane or _____.

5. The inner parts of the lips are lined by a thick _____.

6. The labial mucosa is continuous with the equally thick _____ that lines the inner cheek.

7. The upper and lower horseshoe-shaped spaces in the oral cavity between the lips anteriorly or cheeks laterally and the teeth with their soft tissue medially and posteriorly are considered the maxillary and mandibular _____.

8. Deep within each vestibule is the vestibular fornix, where the thicker labial or buccal mucosa meets the thinner _____ at the mucobuccal fold.

9. On the inner part of the buccal mucosa, just opposite the maxillary second molar, is the _____, a small elevation of tissue that protects the duct opening of the parotid salivary gland.

10. The _____ is a fold of tissue located at the midline between the labial mucosa and the alveolar mucosa on both the maxilla and mandible.

alveolar mucosa	vestibules	oral cavity
labial mucosa	parotid papilla	maxillae
buccal mucosa	mandible	labial frenum
oral mucosa		

References   Chapter 2, Surface anatomy. In Fehrenbach MJ, Herring SW: *Illustrated anatomy of the head and neck,* ed 6, St. Louis, 2021, Saunders; Chapter 2, Oral cavity and pharynx. In Fehrenbach MJ, Popowics T: *Illustrated dental embryology, histology, and anatomy,* ed 5, St. Louis, 2020, Saunders.

NOTES

FIGURE 2.17 Oral region: Gingiva (frontal views)

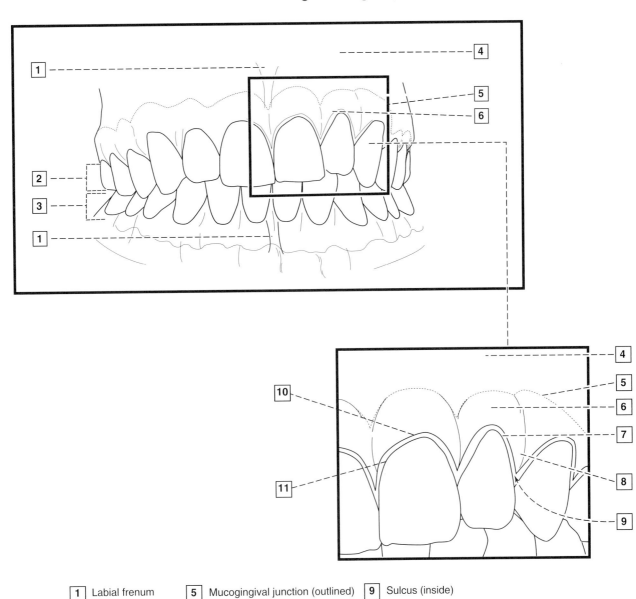

1 Labial frenum	**5** Mucogingival junction (outlined)	**9** Sulcus (inside)
2 Maxillary teeth	**6** Attached gingiva	**10** Free gingival groove
3 Mandibular teeth	**7** Marginal gingiva	**11** Free gingival crest
4 Alveolar mucosa	**8** Interdental gingiva (with papilla)	

REVIEW QUESTIONS: Oral region: Gingiva

Fill in the blanks by choosing the appropriate terms from the list below.

1. The teeth in the maxillary arch are the _____ and the teeth in the mandibular arch are the mandibular teeth.

2. Surrounding the maxillary and mandibular teeth in the alveoli or *tooth sockets* and covering the alveolar processes or *alveolar bone* are the soft tissue gums or _____.

3. The gingival tissue that tightly adheres to the alveolar process surrounding the roots of the teeth is the _____ and it may have areas of melanin pigmentation.

4. The line of demarcation between the firmer attached gingiva and the movable alveolar mucosa is the scallop-shaped _____.

5. At the gingival margin of each tooth is the _____ or *free gingiva*, which forms a cuff above the neck of the tooth.

6. The circular inner surface of the marginal gingiva of each tooth faces an equally rounded space(s) or _____.

7. The _____ is the gingival tissue between adjacent teeth adjoining attached gingiva, with each individual extension being an interdental papilla.

8. The labial frenum is a fold(s) of tissue located at the _____ between the labial mucosa and the alveolar mucosa on the upper and lower dental arches.

9. The _____ separates the marginal gingiva from the attached gingiva; at the most coronal part of the marginal gingiva is the free gingival crest.

10. Both dental arches in the adult have _____ that include the incisors, canines, premolars, and molars.

permanent teeth	attached gingiva	gingiva
free gingival groove	maxillary teeth	mucogingival junction
gingival sulcus	interdental gingiva	midline
marginal		

References Chapter 2, Surface anatomy. In Fehrenbach MJ, Herring SW: *Illustrated anatomy of the head and neck,* ed 6, St. Louis, 2021, Saunders; Chapter 2, Oral cavity and pharynx. In Fehrenbach MJ, Popowics T: *Illustrated dental embryology, histology, and anatomy,* ed 5, St. Louis, 2020, Saunders.

NOTES

FIGURE 2.18 Oral region: Oral vestibule and gingiva (frontal view with microanatomic view)

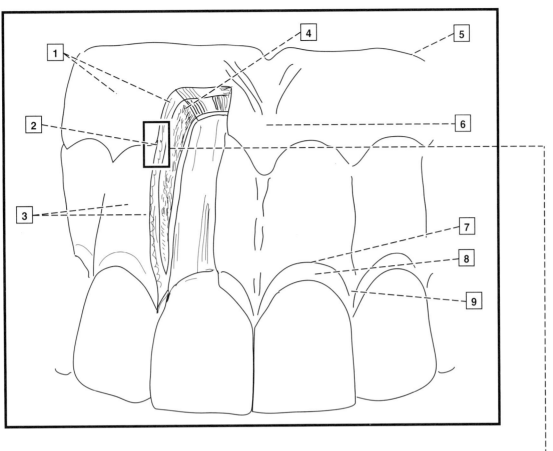

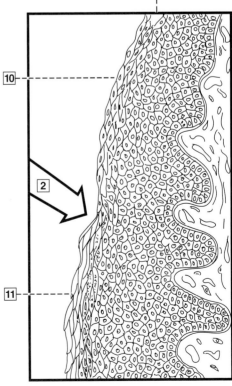

1 Alveolar mucosa (nonkeratinized epithelium)	**6** Labial frenum
2 Mucogingival junction	**7** Free gingival groove
3 Attached gingiva (keratinized epithelium)	**8** Marginal gingiva
4 Alveolar process	**9** Interdental papilla
5 Height of mucobuccal fold	**10** Lining mucosa (nonkeratinized)
	11 Masticatory mucosa (keratinized)

REVIEW QUESTIONS: Oral region: Oral vestibule and gingiva

Fill in the blanks by choosing the appropriate terms from the list below.

1. The _____ is a shiny, moist, and extremely mobile region as it lines the vestibules of the oral cavity.

2. Alveolar mucosa is classified as a(n) _____, a type of oral mucosa noted for its softer surface texture, moist surface, and ability to stretch and be compressed, acting as a cushion for the underlying structures.

3. The epithelium of the alveolar mucosa is extremely thin _____ stratified squamous epithelium that overlies but does not obscure an extensive vascular supply in the lamina propria.

4. The connective tissue papillae in the alveolar mucosa are sometimes absent and numerous elastic fibers are present in the _____, thus allowing mobility of the tissue.

5. The _____ is a sharply defined scalloped junction between the attached gingiva and the alveolar mucosa.

6. The _____ has a thick layer of mainly parakeratinized stratified squamous epithelium that obscures the extensive vascular supply in the lamina propria, making the tissue appear opaque as it covers the alveolar process of the dental arches.

7. The lamina propria of the attached gingiva has tall and narrow _____.

8. The attached gingiva that covers the bony _____ of each of the dental arches is classified as a masticatory mucosa, which is a type of oral mucosa noted for its rubbery texture and consistency.

9. The attached gingiva as a mucous membrane when combined with the periosteum of the underlying bony jaws is termed a(n) _____ since it attaches directly to the underlying alveolar process of each of jaw without the usual intervening submucosa, providing a firm inelastic attachment.

10. The mucogingival junction can be seen as a dividing zone between the keratinized attached gingiva and the nonkeratinized alveolar mucosa, and thus is also considered a junction between a(n) _____ and a lining mucosa.

masticatory mucosa	nonkeratinized	lamina propria
mucoperiosteum	alveolar process	attached gingiva
connective tissue papillae	alveolar mucosa	lining mucosa
mucogingival junction		

References Chapter 9, Oral mucosa. In Fehrenbach MJ, Popowics T: *Illustrated dental embryology, histology, and anatomy,* ed 5, St. Louis, 2020, Saunders; Chapter 10, Gingival and dentogingival junctional tissue. In Fehrenbach MJ, Popowics T: *Illustrated dental embryology, histology, and anatomy,* ed 5, St. Louis, 2020, Saunders.

ANSWER KEY 1. alveolar mucosa, 2. lining mucosa, 3. nonkeratinized, 4. lamina propria, 5. mucogingival junction, 6. attached gingiva, 7. connective tissue papillae, 8. alveolar process, 9. mucoperiosteum, 10. masticatory mucosa

FIGURE 2.19 Oral region: Oral mucosa with (ortho)keratinized and nonkeratinized types (microanatomic views)

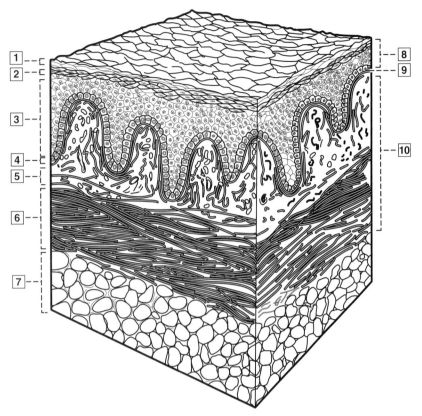

Keratinized Oral Mucosa (and underlying tissue)

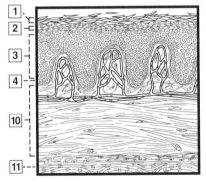

Orthokeratinized Stratified
Squamous Epithelium (and
deeper tissue)

Nonkeratinized Stratified
Squamous Epithelium (and
deeper tissue)

1	Keratin layer	7	Submucosa
2	Granular layer	8	Oral epithelium
3	Prickle layer	9	Basement membrane
4	Basal layer	10	Lamina propria
5	Papillary layer	11	Bone
6	Dense fibrous layer	12	Muscle

REVIEW QUESTIONS: Oral region: Oral mucosa with (ortho)keratinized and nonkeratinized types

Fill in the blanks by choosing the appropriate terms from the list below.

1. The _____ almost continuously lines the oral cavity.

2. Microscopically the oral mucosa is composed of _____ overlying a connective tissue proper or lamina propria, with possibly a deeper submucosa.

3. A(n) _____ lies between the epithelium and connective tissue in the oral mucosa; it serves not as a separation between the two tissue types but as a continuous structure linking the two.

4. There are _____ main types of oral mucosa found in the oral cavity that include lining, masticatory, and specialized mucosa; the classification of mucosa is based on the general histologic features of the tissue.

5. The lining mucosa is a type of oral mucosa that is associated with _____ stratified squamous epithelium and includes the buccal mucosa, labial mucosa, and alveolar mucosa, as well as the mucosa lining the ventral surface of the tongue, floor of the mouth, and soft palate.

6. The _____ is a type of oral mucosa associated with orthokeratinized stratified squamous epithelium as well as parakeratinized stratified squamous epithelium, and includes the hard palate, attached gingiva, and dorsal surface of the tongue.

7. The _____ or *stratum basale* is the deepest layer of the oral mucosa and consists of a single layer of cuboidal epithelial cells overlying the basement membrane, which in turn is located superior to the lamina propria.

8. Superficial to the basal layer in keratinized oral mucosa is the _____, or *stratum spinosum,* in which a spiky look results when the individual dehydrated epithelial cells are shrinking when fixed for prolonged microscopic study but still joined at their outer edges by desmosomes.

9. In keratinized oral mucosa, superficial to the prickle layer is the _____ or *stratum granulosum,* with each of its epithelial cells having prominent keratohyaline granules, which appear microscopically as dark spots.

10. In keratinized oral mucosa, the most superficial layer is the _____ or *stratum corneum,* which has keratin-filled epithelial cells.

basal layer	nonkeratinized	basement membrane
prickle layer	keratin layer	stratified squamous epithelium
granular layer	three	oral mucosa
masticatory mucosa		

Reference   Chapter 9, Oral mucosa. In Fehrenbach MJ, Popowics T: *Illustrated dental embryology, histology, and anatomy,* ed 5, St. Louis, 2020, Saunders.

FIGURE 2.20 Oral region: Gingival tissue (microanatomic views)

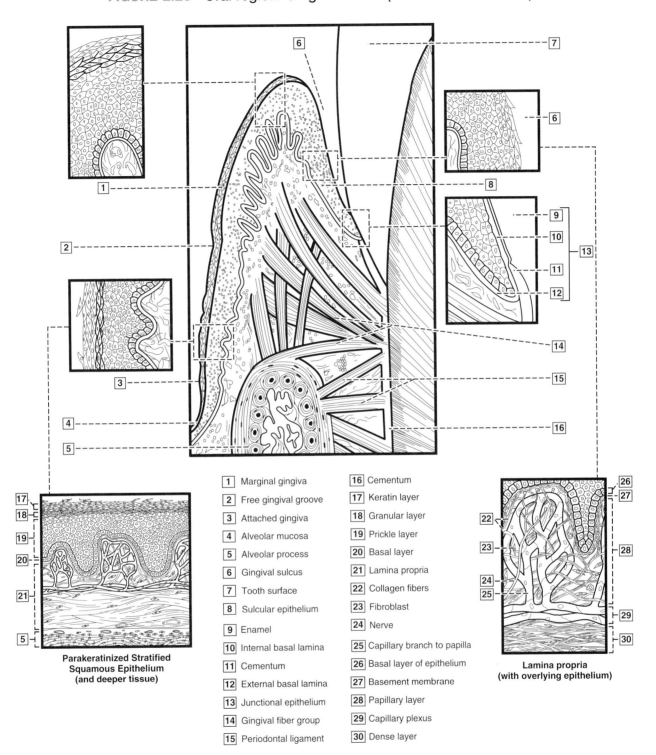

1 Marginal gingiva	16 Cementum
2 Free gingival groove	17 Keratin layer
3 Attached gingiva	18 Granular layer
4 Alveolar mucosa	19 Prickle layer
5 Alveolar process	20 Basal layer
6 Gingival sulcus	21 Lamina propria
7 Tooth surface	22 Collagen fibers
8 Sulcular epithelium	23 Fibroblast
9 Enamel	24 Nerve
10 Internal basal lamina	25 Capillary branch to papilla
11 Cementum	26 Basal layer of epithelium
12 External basal lamina	27 Basement membrane
13 Junctional epithelium	28 Papillary layer
14 Gingival fiber group	29 Capillary plexus
15 Periodontal ligament	30 Dense layer

Parakeratinized Stratified
Squamous Epithelium
(and deeper tissue)

Lamina propria
(with overlying epithelium)

REVIEW QUESTIONS: Oral region: Gingival tissue

Fill in the blanks by choosing the appropriate terms from the list below.

1. Surrounding the maxillary and mandibular teeth in the alveoli and covering the alveolar processes is the _____ or *gums.*

2. The gingival tissue that tightly adheres to the bone around the roots of the teeth is the

   _____.

3. At the gingival margin of each tooth is the _____ or *free gingiva,* which is continuous with the attached gingiva.

4. The _____ or *gingival margin* is at the most superficial part of the marginal gingiva.

5. The _____ separates the attached gingiva from the marginal gingiva on the superficial surface of gingival tissue.

6. Together the sulcular epithelium and junctional epithelium form the _____.

7. The _____ or *crevicular epithelium* stands away from the tooth, creating a gingival sulcus that is filled with gingival crevicular fluid from the adjacent blood supply in the lamina propria.

8. A deeper extension of the sulcular epithelium is the _____, which lines the floor of the gingival sulcus and is attached to the tooth surface.

9. The junctional epithelium is attached to the tooth surface by way of a(n) _____, which attaches this tissue to the tooth surface of either enamel, cementum, or dentin; the suprabasal cells that make up the most superficial layer of the junctional epithelium serve as part of the epithelial attachment of the gingiva to the tooth surface.

10. The deeper interface between the thin junctional epithelium and the underlying _____ is relatively smooth, without rete ridges or connective tissue papillae; its epithelial cells are loosely packed, with fewer intercellular junctions using desmosomes between cells and more intercellular spaces compared with other types of gingival tissue.

sulcular epithelium	epithelial attachment	free gingival crest
free gingival groove	attached gingiva	junctional epithelium
dentogingival junctional tissue	gingival tissue	lamina propria
marginal gingiva		

References Chapter 9, Oral mucosa. In Fehrenbach MJ, Popowics T: *Illustrated dental embryology, histology, and anatomy,* ed 5, St. Louis, 2020, Saunders; Chapter 10, Gingival and dentogingival junctional tissue. In Fehrenbach MJ, Popowics T: *Illustrated dental embryology, histology, and anatomy,* ed 5, St. Louis, 2020, Saunders.

FIGURE 2.21 Oral region: Dentogingival junction including junctional epithelium with epithelial attachment (microanatomic views)

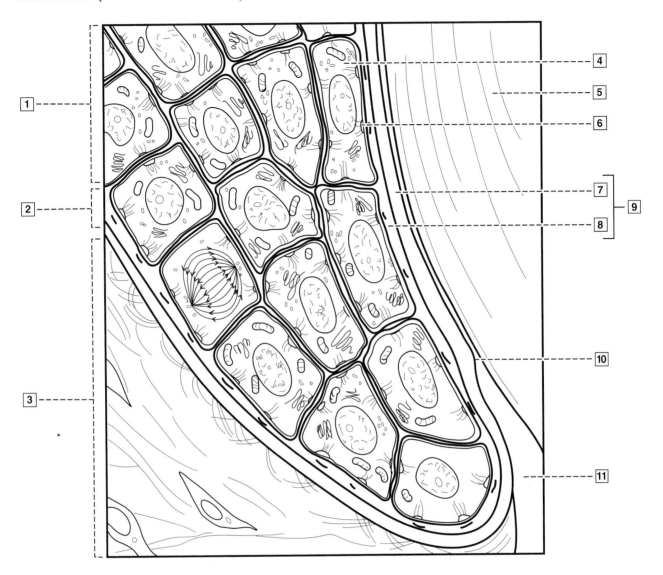

1 Basal layer	**7** Lamina densa
2 External basal lamina	**8** Lamina lucida
3 Lamina propria	**9** Internal basal lamina
4 Suprabasal epithelial cell	**10** Cementoenamel junction
5 Enamel	**11** Cementum
6 Hemidesmosome	

REVIEW QUESTIONS: Oral region: Dentogingival junction including junctional epithelium with epithelial attachment

Fill in the blanks by choosing the appropriate terms from the list below.

1. The more suprabasal cells of the junctional epithelium provide the hemidesmosomes and an internal basal lamina that create the _____, a cell-to-noncellular type of intercellular junction.

2. The structure of the epithelial attachment is similar to that of the junction between the epithelium and sub-adjacent connective tissue because the internal basal lamina also consists of a(n) _____ and lamina densa.

3. The internal basal lamina of the epithelial attachment is also continuous with the external basal lamina between the junctional epithelium and the _____ at the apical extent of the junctional epithelium.

4. The deepest layer of the _____ or basal layer undergoes constant and rapid cell division or mitosis, a process that allows a constant coronal migration as the cells die and are shed into the gingival sulcus at the coronal end of it.

5. The junctional epithelium cells do not _____ like keratinized tissue and thus do not show any change in cellular structure related to that process such as the marginal gingiva or attached gingiva, which both fills its matured superficial cells with keratin, forming into either a granular layer or intermediate layer.

6. Before the eruption of the tooth and after enamel maturation, the enamel-producing _____ secrete a basal lamina on the tooth surface that serves as a part of the primary epithelial attachment.

7. As the tooth actively erupts, the coronal part of the fused tissue consisting of the _____ and surrounding epithelium peel back off the crown serving as the primary epithelial attachment, which is later replaced by a definitive junctional epithelium as the root is formed.

8. The position of the epithelial attachment on the tooth surface is initially on the cervical half of the _____ when the tooth first becomes functional after eruption.

9. The _____ seeps between epithelial cells and into the gingival sulcus, allowing the components of the blood to reach the tooth surface through the junctional epithelium from the blood vessels of the adjacent lamina propria.

10. A calibrated periodontal probe measures the probing depth of the healthy _____; after the probe is gently inserted, it slides by the sulcular epithelium, and is stopped by the epithelial attachment of the junctional epithelium.

gingival sulcus	epithelial attachment	reduced enamel epithelium
gingival crevicular fluid	lamina lucida	junctional epithelium
anatomic crown	lamina propria	ameloblasts
mature		

References Chapter 9, Oral mucosa. In Fehrenbach MJ, Popowics T: *Illustrated dental embryology, histology, and anatomy,* ed 5, St. Louis, 2020, Saunders; Chapter 10, Gingival and dentogingival junctional tissue. In Fehrenbach MJ, Popowics T: *Illustrated dental embryology, histology, and anatomy,* ed 5, St. Louis, 2020, Saunders.

ANSWER KEY 1. epithelial attachment, 2. lamina lucida, 3. lamina propria, 4. junctional epithelium, 5. mature, 6. ameloblasts, 7. reduced enamel epithelium, 8. anatomic crown, 9. gingival crevicular fluid, 10. gingival sulcus

FIGURE 2.22 Palate: Hard palate and soft palate (inferior view with microanatomic views)

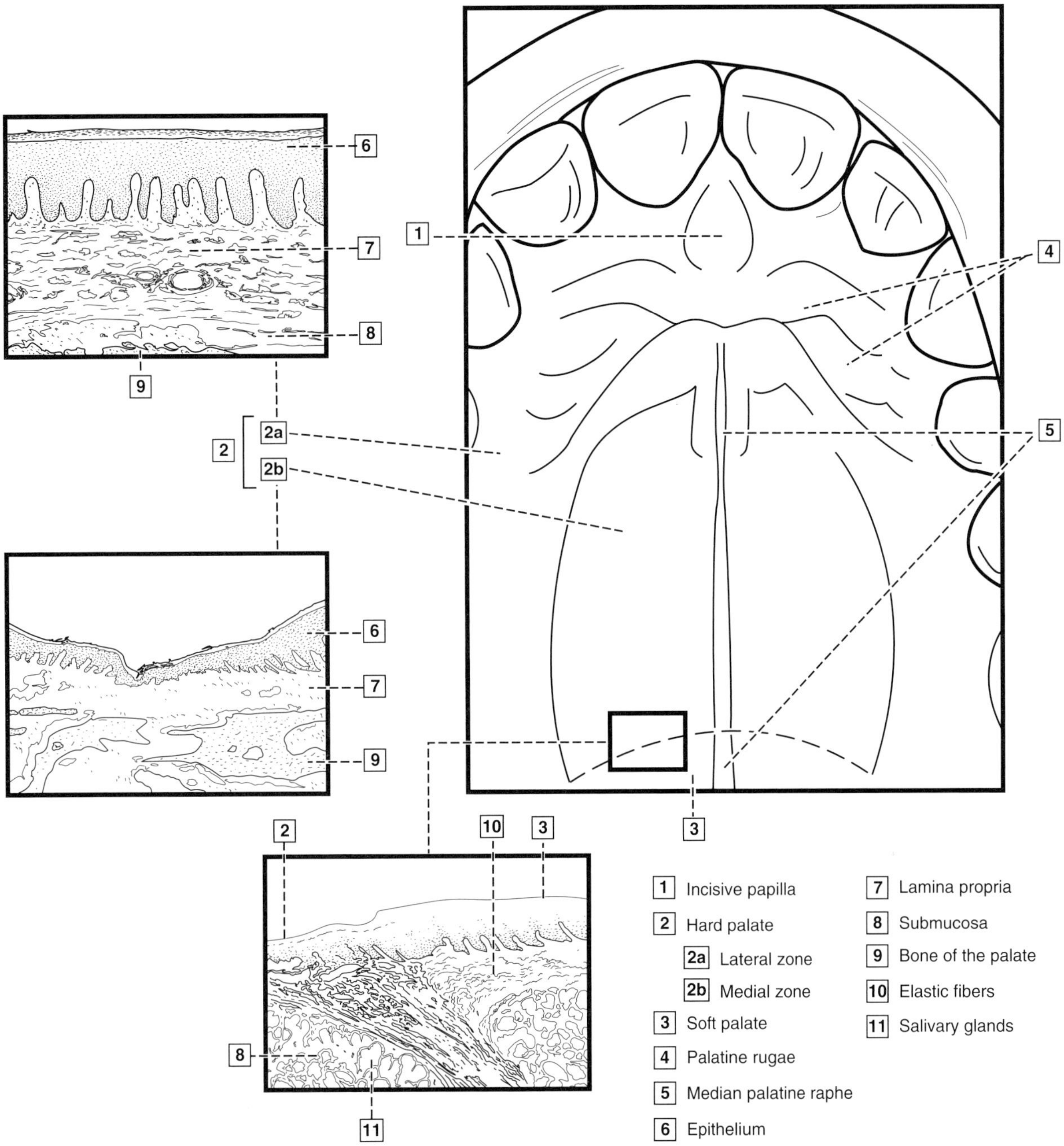

1	Incisive papilla	**7**	Lamina propria
2	Hard palate	**8**	Submucosa
2a	Lateral zone	**9**	Bone of the palate
2b	Medial zone	**10**	Elastic fibers
3	Soft palate	**11**	Salivary glands
4	Palatine rugae		
5	Median palatine raphe		
6	Epithelium		

REVIEW QUESTIONS: Palate: Hard palate and soft inferior view (with microanatomic views)

Fill in the blanks by choosing the appropriate terms from the list below.

1. At the anterior part of the inferior surface of the skull is the _____, which is bordered by the alveolar process of the maxilla that usually contains the roots of the maxillary teeth within the alveoli; a cushioned feeling is noted when it is palpated in the posterior lateral zones (has submucosa present) and a firmer feeling in the adjacent medial zone (no submucosa present).

2. The hard palate located anterior to the soft palate is formed by two separate bones, the two palatine processes of the maxillae anteriorly and the two horizontal plates of the _____ posteriorly; the junction of the soft palate and hard palate is also a junction between a lining mucosa and a masticatory mucosa as well as a junction between nonkeratinized epithelium and keratinized epithelium.

3. The articulation between the maxillae and palatine bones on the hard palate is noted by the prominent _____.

4. The median palatine suture underlies the _____ .

5. The nearby transverse palatine suture is an articulation located between the two palatine processes of the _____ and the two horizontal plates of the palatine bones.

6. The hard palate forms the floor of the _____ as well as the roof of the mouth; during an intraoral examination, tilt the head back slightly and extend the tongue to visually inspect the soft palate and throat (or pharynx).

7. The posterior edge of the hard palate forms the inferior border of two funnel-shaped cavities, the _____ or *choanae,* which serve as posterior openings of the nasal cavity.

8. Each posterior nasal aperture is bordered medially by the vomer, inferiorly by the horizontal plate of the palatine bone, laterally by the medial pterygoid plate of the _____, and superiorly by the body of the sphenoid bone.

9. The posterior nasal apertures are located between the nasal cavity and the _____, allowing for communication between the two spaces.

10. Near the superior border of each posterior nasal aperture is the _____, which runs anteriorly by the pterygoid process of the sphenoid bone to open into the pterygopalatine fossa and carries the nerve of the structure and associated blood vessels.

palatine bones	posterior nasal apertures	maxillae
pterygoid canal	hard palate	nasal cavity
nasopharynx	median palatine raphe	sphenoid bone
median palatine suture		

References Chapter 3, Skeletal system. In Fehrenbach MJ, Herring SW: *Illustrated anatomy of the head and neck,* ed 6, St. Louis, 2021, Saunders; Chapter 9, Oral mucosa. In Fehrenbach MJ, Popowics T: *Illustrated dental embryology, histology, and anatomy,* ed 5, St. Louis, 2020, Saunders.

ANSWER KEY 1. hard palate, 2. palatine bones, 3. median palatine suture, 4. median palatine raphe, 5. maxillae, 6. nasal cavity, 7. posterior nasal apertures, 8. sphenoid bone, 9. nasopharynx, 10. pterygoid canal

FIGURE 2.23 Palatal and nasal cavity development during prenatal development (sagittal sections)

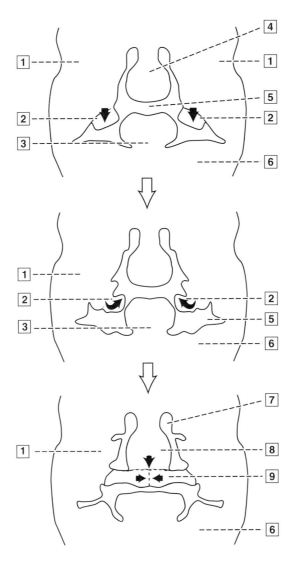

1 Maxillary process   6 Developing mandible

2 Palatal shelf   7 Developing nasal cavity

3 Developing tongue   8 Nasal septum

4 Developing nasal septum   9 Fusing palate

5 Stomodeum

REVIEW QUESTIONS: Palatal and nasal cavity development during prenatal development

Fill in the blanks by choosing the appropriate terms from the list below.

1. The formation of the palate, initially in the embryo and later in the fetus, takes place over several weeks of _____.

2. During the _____ week of prenatal development and still within the embryonic period, the intermaxillary segment forms.

3. The intermaxillary segment arises as a result of fusion of the two _____ internally within the embryo.

4. The _____ is an internal wedge-shaped mass that extends inferiorly and deep to the nasal pits on the inside of the stomodeum.

5. The intermaxillary segment initially serves as a partial floor of the _____ and the nasal septum.

6. The intermaxillary segment also gives rise to the _____ (or primitive palate).

7. At this time, the primary palate serves only as a partial separation between the developing _____ and nasal cavity.

8. In the future, the primary palate will form the premaxillary part of the _____, which is the anterior one-third of the hard palate.

9. The premaxillary part of the maxilla is a smaller part of the _____, which is located anterior to the incisive foramen and will contain certain maxillary teeth (incisors).

10. The formation of the primary palate completes the _____ stage of palate development.

oral cavity proper	prenatal development	primary palate
fifth	intermaxillary segment	first
nasal cavity	medial nasal processes	hard palate
maxilla		

Reference Chapter 5, Orofacial development. In Fehrenbach MJ, Popowics T: *Illustrated dental embryology, histology, and anatomy,* ed 5, St. Louis, 2020, Saunders.

NOTES

FIGURE 2.24 Palatal and nasal cavity development during prenatal development (inferior views)

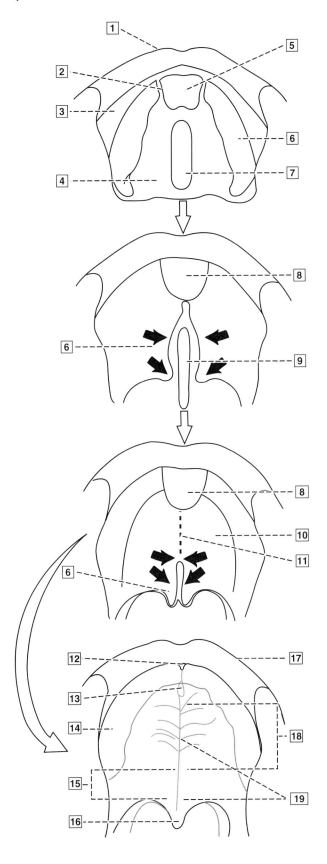

1 Developing upper lip

2 Site of future fusion

3 Developing maxillary alveolar process

4 Developing nasal cavity

5 Intermaxillary segment

6 Palatal shelf

7 Developing nasal septum

8 Primary palate

9 Nasal septum

10 Secondary palate

11 Median palatine suture

12 Labial frenum

13 Incisive papilla

14 Gingiva covering maxillary process

15 Soft palate

16 Uvula

17 Upper lip

18 Hard palate

19 Median palatine raphe

REVIEW QUESTIONS: Palatal and nasal cavity development during prenatal development

Fill in the blanks by choosing the appropriate terms from the list below.

1. During the sixth week of prenatal development within the embryonic period, the bilateral maxillary processes give rise to two _____ (or lateral palatine processes).

2. The palatal shelves grow inferiorly and deep on the inside of the stomodeum in a vertical direction along both sides of the developing _____, which will later contract and move anteriorly and inferiorly out of the way of the developing palatal shelves.

3. The palatal shelves will later move into a horizontal position, which is now superior to the developing tongue; the two palatal shelves elongate and move medially toward each other meeting to join and then fusing to form the _____; the formation of this structure is completed during the second stage of palatal development.

4. The secondary palate will give rise to the posterior two-thirds of the hard palate, which contains certain _____ anterior teeth (canines) and posterior teeth, all located posterior to the incisive foramen; it also gives rise to the soft palate and its uvula.

5. The _____ within the mucosa lining and the associated deeper median palatine suture on the adult bone of the hard palate indicate the fusion of the palatal shelves.

6. The completion of the final palate involves the _____ of swellings, which involve tissue from different surfaces of the embryo meeting and joining, similar to that of the neural tube and the components of the upper lip.

7. To complete the final stage of palatal development, the posterior part of the primary palate meets the secondary palate due to increased growth, and these structures gradually fuse in an anterior to posterior direction; the three processes completely fuse, forming the final palate including the hard and soft palates during the _____ of prenatal development.

8. The future nasal septum of the nasal cavity is also developing when the palate is forming from a growth from the fused _____, similar to the primary palate.

9. The tissue types that form the nasal septum will grow inferiorly and deep to the medial nasal processes and superior to the _____.

10. The vertical nasal septum then fuses with the horizontally oriented final palate after it forms; this fusion begins in the _____ week and is completed by the twelfth week, resulting in the paired nasal cavity and the single oral cavity in the fetus becoming completely separate.

median palatine raphe	stomodeum	tongue
maxillary	fusion	medial nasal processes
secondary palate	twelfth week	ninth
palatal shelves		

Reference Chapter 5, Orofacial development. In Fehrenbach MJ, Popowics T: *Illustrated dental embryology, histology, and anatomy,* ed 5, St. Louis, 2020, Saunders.

ANSWER KEY 1. palatal shelves, 2. tongue, 3. secondary palate, 4. maxillary, 5. median palatine raphe, 6. fusion, 7. twelfth week, 8. medial nasal processes, 9. stomodeum, 10. ninth

FIGURE 2.25   Oral region: Tongue (lateral view with microanatomic views)

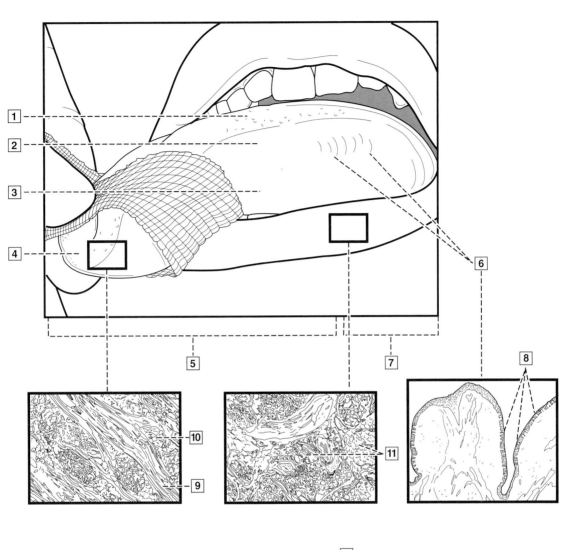

1 Dorsal surface	**5** Body of the tongue	**9** Striated muscle bundles
2 Lateral surface	**6** Foliate lingual papillae	**10** Adipose connective tissue
3 Ventral surface	**7** Base of the tongue	**11** Salivary glands
4 Apex of the tongue	**8** Taste buds	

REVIEW QUESTIONS: Oral region: Tongue

Fill in the blanks by choosing the appropriate terms from the list below.

1. The tongue is a prominent feature of the oral region, with its _____ considered its *pharyngeal part* or base of the tongue.

2. The _____ attaches to the floor of the mouth.

3. The base of the tongue does not lie within the oral cavity but within the oral part of the _____.

4. The anterior two-thirds of the tongue is termed the _____; in the mobile anterior tongue, the striated muscle bundles are tightly packed with relatively little intervening adipose connective tissue, unlike the less mobile posterior where collections of salivary glands are numerous in the submucosa and muscular core.

5. The body of the tongue is considered its *oral part* since it lies within the _____ .

6. The tip of the tongue is the _____.

7. Certain surfaces of the tongue have small elevated structures of specialized mucosa, the _____, some of which are associated with taste buds; they consist of small discrete structures or appendages of keratinized epithelium, with both orthokeratinized and parakeratinized epithelium present overlying a lamina propria.

8. The side or lateral surface of the tongue is noted for its vertical ridges parallel to one another, the _____, which consist of leaf-shaped structures with a layer of orthokeratinized or parakeratinized epithelium that contains taste buds overlying a lamina propria core.

9. The top surface of the tongue is considered the _____; to examine this surface as well as the lateral surface, slightly extend the tongue and wrap gauze around its body or anterior two-thirds of the tongue in order to obtain a firm grasp.

10. The underside of the tongue is considered the _____.

oral cavity	base of the tongue	apex of the tongue
pharynx	posterior one-third	lingual papillae
ventral surface	body of the tongue	dorsal surface
foliate lingual papillae		

References Chapter 2, Surface anatomy. In Fehrenbach MJ, Herring SW: *Illustrated anatomy of the head and neck,* ed 6, 2021; Chapter 2, Oral cavity and pharynx. In Fehrenbach MJ, Popowics T: *Illustrated dental embryology, histology, and anatomy,* ed 5, St. Louis, 2020, Saunders; Chapter 9, Oral mucosa. In Fehrenbach MJ, Popowics T: *Illustrated dental embryology, histology, and anatomy,* ed 5, St. Louis, 2020, Saunders.

ANSWER KEY 1. posterior one-third, 2. base of the tongue, 3. pharynx, 4. body of the tongue, 5. oral cavity, 6. apex of the tongue, 7. lingual papillae, 8. foliate lingual papillae, 9. dorsal surface, 10. ventral surface

FIGURE 2.26 Oral region: Tongue (dorsal surface and microanatomic views)

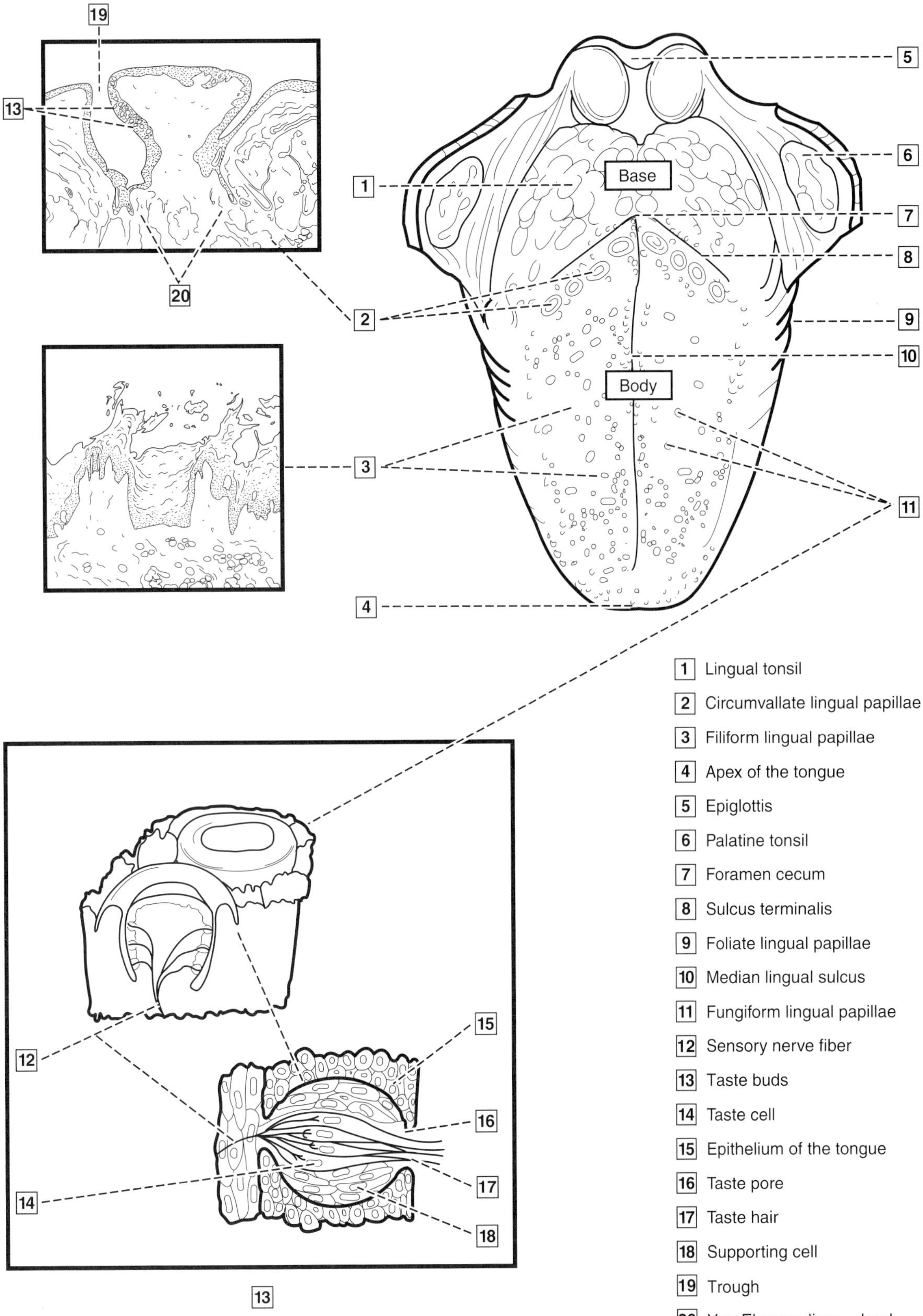

1 Lingual tonsil
2 Circumvallate lingual papillae
3 Filiform lingual papillae
4 Apex of the tongue
5 Epiglottis
6 Palatine tonsil
7 Foramen cecum
8 Sulcus terminalis
9 Foliate lingual papillae
10 Median lingual sulcus
11 Fungiform lingual papillae
12 Sensory nerve fiber
13 Taste buds
14 Taste cell
15 Epithelium of the tongue
16 Taste pore
17 Taste hair
18 Supporting cell
19 Trough
20 Von Ebner salivary gland

REVIEW QUESTIONS: Oral region: Tongue

Fill in the blanks by choosing the appropriate terms from the list below.

1. The top or dorsal surface of the tongue has a midline depression, the _____, corresponding with the position of a midline fibrous structure deeper within the tongue from fusion tissue of the area, the median septum.

2. The lingual papillae shaped like fine-pointed cones are the _____, which give the dorsal surface of the tongue its velvety texture; they consist of a thick layer of orthokeratinized or parakeratinized epithelium overlying a lamina core, with an increased amount of keratin on the surface of each cone.

3. The slightly raised mushroom-shaped dots are the _____, which are not found near the sulcus terminalis; they consist of a thin layer of orthokeratinized or parakeratinized epithelium with taste buds in the superficial part overlying a highly vascularized lamina propria core.

4. Posteriorly on the dorsal surface of the tongue is a V-shaped groove, the _____, which separates the base of the tongue from the body of the tongue, and where a small pit-like depression, the foramen cecum, is located.

5. The _____ line up along just anterior to the sulcus terminalis; these larger mushroom-shaped structures consist of orthokeratinized or parakeratinized epithelium with hundreds of taste buds surrounding the base overlying a lamina propria core and are surrounded by a circular trough lined by the surrounding tongue surface tissue.

6. The _____ are present in the submucosa deep to the lamina propria of the circumvallate lingual papillae; with ducts that open into the trough, these minor serous salivary glands flush the area near the taste pores so as to introduce new taste sensations from several sequential food molecules.

7. The _____ is a barrel-shaped organ of taste derived from the epithelium and composed of spindle-shaped cells that extend from the basement membrane of the oral mucosa to the epithelial surface of the lingual papilla.

8. The supporting cells maintain the taste bud and are usually located on the outer part of the taste bud and in contrast, the _____ are usually located in the central part of the taste bud; taste hairs are hair-like projections of gustatory cells of taste buds and electron micrographs show them to be clusters of microvilli.

9. The taste cells have taste receptors that are responsible for making contact with dissolved molecules of food at the _____, which is an opening in the most superficial part of the taste bud; this process produces a taste sensation by way of the messages being sent by the sensory neurons processes to the central nervous system.

10. At the most posterior surface of the tongue base on each side is an irregular mass of lymphoid tissue, the _____.

fungiform lingual papillae	circumvallate lingual papillae	taste bud
lingual tonsil	median lingual sulcus	taste cells
sulcus terminalis	filiform lingual papillae	taste pore
von Ebner salivary glands		

References Chapter 2, Surface anatomy. In Fehrenbach MJ, Herring SW: *Illustrated anatomy of the head and neck,* ed 6, 2021; Chapter 2, Oral cavity and pharynx. In Fehrenbach MJ, Popowics T: *Illustrated dental embryology, histology, and anatomy,* ed 5, St. Louis, 2020, Saunders; Chapter 9, Oral mucosa. In Fehrenbach MJ, Popowics T: *Illustrated dental embryology, histology, and anatomy,* ed 5, St. Louis, 2020, Saunders.

ANSWER KEY 1. median lingual sulcus, 2. filiform lingual papillae, 3. fungiform lingual papillae, 4. sulcus terminalis, 5. circumvallate lingual papillae, 6. von Ebner salivary glands, 7. taste bud, 8. taste cells, 9. taste pore, 10. lingual tonsil

FIGURE 2.27   Tongue development during prenatal development

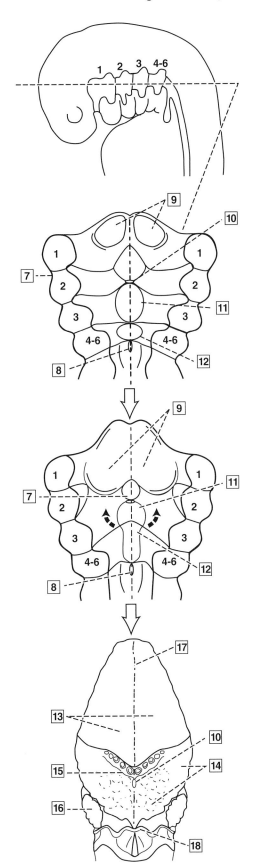

7	Tuberculum impar
8	Laryngeal orifice
9	Lateral lingual swellings
10	Foramen cecum
11	Copula
12	Epiglottic swelling
13	Body of the tongue
14	Base of the tongue
15	Sulcus terminalis
16	Palatine tonsil
17	Median lingual sulcus
18	Epiglottis

REVIEW QUESTIONS: Tongue development during prenatal development

Fill in the blanks by choosing the appropriate terms from the list below.

1. The tongue develops during the fourth to eighth weeks of prenatal development from independent swellings located internally on the floor of the primitive pharynx, formed by the first four pharyngeal or _____.

2. The _____ develops from the first pharyngeal or branchial arch, and the base of the tongue originates later from the second, third, and fourth pharyngeal or branchial arches.

3. During the fourth week of prenatal development within the embryonic period, the tongue begins its development as a triangular median swelling, the _____ (or median tongue bud), which is located in the midline on the mandibular arch at the floor of the primitive pharynx within the conjoined embryo's nasal and oral cavities.

4. Later, two oval _____ (or distal tongue buds) develop and merge with each other on each side of the tuberculum impar, which are from the further growth of the mesenchyme of the first pharyngeal or branchial arch or *mandibular arch.*

5. Later the two fused lateral lingual swellings overgrow and encompass the disappearing tuberculum impar to form the anterior two-thirds or body of the mature tongue, which lies within the oral cavity proper; the _____ is a superficial demarcation of the fusion of lateral lingual swellings as well as of a deeper fibrous structure.

6. Around the lingual swellings, the cells degenerate, forming a sulcus, which frees the body of the tongue from the floor of the mouth, except for the attachment of the midline _____.

7. Immediately posterior to these fused anterior swellings, the single midline _____ is mostly formed from the fusion of the mesenchyme of the third and parts of the fourth pharyngeal or branchial arch; it gradually overgrows the second pharyngeal or branchial arch or *hyoid arch* to form the posterior one-third or base of the mature tongue.

8. Even farther posterior to the copula is the projection of a third median swelling, the _____, which develops from the mesenchyme of the posterior parts of the fourth pharyngeal or branchial arches.

9. As the tongue develops further, the copula of the tongue base after overgrowing the second arch, merges with the anterior swellings of the first arch of the tongue body during the eighth week of prenatal development, which has its fusion superficially demarcated by the _____.

10. The sulcus terminalis points backward toward the oropharynx at a small pit-like depression, the _____, which is the beginning of the thyroglossal duct that is the origin of the thyroid gland; this duct shows the origin of the thyroid gland and migration pathway into the neck region.

copula	sulcus terminalis	branchial arches
median lingual sulcus	tuberculum impar	epiglottic swelling
lingual frenum	lateral lingual swellings	foramen cecum
body of the tongue		

Reference Chapter 5, Orofacial development. In Fehrenbach MJ, Popowics T: *Illustrated dental embryology, histology, and anatomy,* ed 5, St. Louis, 2020, Saunders.

FIGURE 2.28 Oral region: Tongue (ventral surface with microanatomic view)

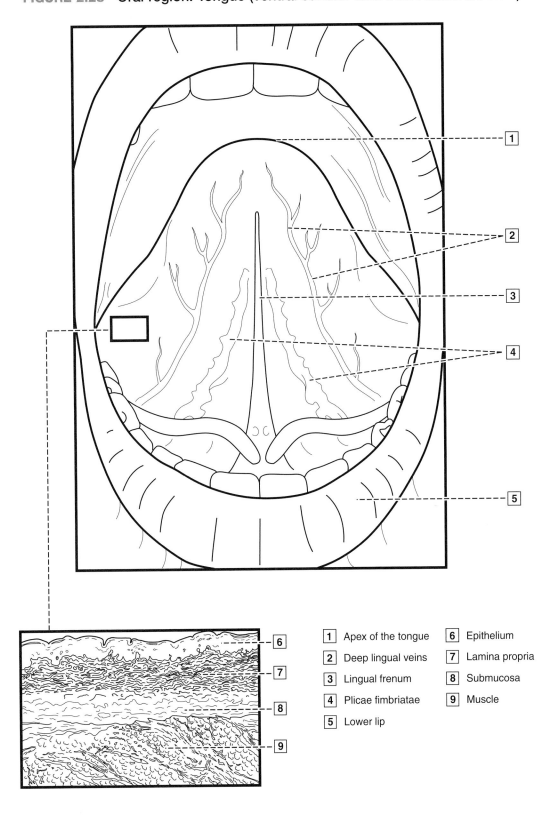

1	Apex of the tongue	6	Epithelium
2	Deep lingual veins	7	Lamina propria
3	Lingual frenum	8	Submucosa
4	Plicae fimbriatae	9	Muscle
5	Lower lip		

REVIEW QUESTIONS: Oral region: Tongue

Fill in the blanks by choosing the appropriate terms from the list below.

1. The underside of the tongue is considered the _____.

2. The ventral surface of the tongue has large visible blood vessels, the _____, which pass close to the surface.

3. Lateral to each deep lingual vein on each side of the tongue is the _____, a fold with its fringelike projections.

4. Having the patient slightly lift the _____ to visually inspect and digitally palpate its surface.

5. The patient should gently touch the surface of the _____ with the apex of the tongue to fully visualize the underside of the tongue.

6. One excellent example of the venous variability involves the lingual veins; these include the dorsal lingual veins that drain the dorsal surface of the tongue, the highly visible branching blue deep lingual vein noted during an intraoral examination that drains the ventral surface of the tongue, and the _____ that drains the floor of the mouth.

7. The lingual veins may join to form a single vessel or may empty into larger vessels separately; they also may drain indirectly into the facial vein or directly into the _____.

8. The internal jugular vein drains most of the structures of the head and neck after it originates in the _____ and leaves the skull through the jugular foramen; it receives many tributaries including the veins from the lingual, sublingual, and pharyngeal areas as well as the facial vein.

9. The lining of the ventral surface of the tongue is _____.

10. The ventral surface of the tongue has an extremely thin epithelium overlying, but not obscuring, a lamina propria with an extensive _____, thus making the veins (such as the deep lingual veins) more apparent.

sublingual veins	internal jugular vein	nonkeratinized stratified squamous epithelium
hard palate	deep lingual veins	vascular supply
apex of the tongue	ventral surface of the tongue	
plica fimbriata	cranial cavity	

References   Chapter 2, Surface anatomy. In Fehrenbach MJ, Herring SW: *Illustrated anatomy of the head and neck,* ed 6, St. Louis, 2021, Saunders; Chapter 7, Vascular system. In Fehrenbach MJ, Herring SW: *Illustrated anatomy of the head and neck,* ed 6, St. Louis, 2021, Saunders; Chapter 2, Oral cavity and pharynx. In Fehrenbach MJ, Popowics T: *Illustrated dental embryology, histology, and anatomy,* ed 5, St. Louis, 2020, Saunders; Chapter 9, Oral mucosa. In Fehrenbach MJ, Popowics T: *Illustrated dental embryology, histology, and anatomy,* ed 5, St. Louis, 2020, Saunders.

ANSWER KEY   1. ventral surface of the tongue, 2. deep lingual veins, 3. plica fimbriata, 4. apex of the tongue, 5. hard palate, 6. sublingual veins, 7. internal jugular vein, 8. cranial cavity, 9. nonkeratinized stratified squamous epithelium, 10. vascular supply

FIGURE 2.29 Oral region: Floor of the mouth (superior view)

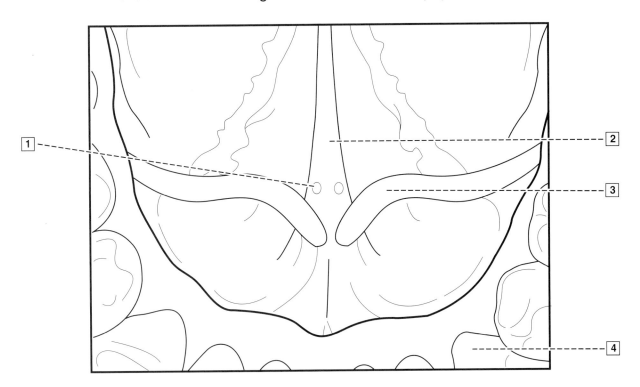

1 Sublingual caruncle

2 Lingual frenum

3 Sublingual fold

4 Mandibular teeth

REVIEW QUESTIONS: Oral region: Floor of the mouth

Fill in the blanks by choosing the appropriate terms from the list below.

1. The _____ is located in the oral cavity proper, inferior to the ventral surface of the tongue.

2. The _____ is a midline fold of tissue between the ventral surface of the tongue and the floor of the mouth.

3. A ridge of tissue exists on each side of the floor of the mouth, the _____, which represents the sublingual salivary gland and also contains openings of the sublingual duct.

4. Together the sublingual folds are arranged in a V-shaped configuration extending from the lingual frenum to the _____.

5. The small papilla or _____ at the anterior end of each sublingual fold contains the duct openings of the submandibular duct and sublingual duct from both the submandibular and sublingual salivary glands.

6. The roof of the mouth or palate marks the superior border, while the floor of the mouth is the _____ of the oral cavity.

7. The _____ supplies the mylohyoid muscle, sublingual salivary gland, and oral mucosa of the floor of the mouth as well as the lingual periodontium and gingiva of the mandibular teeth in most cases.

8. During tongue development, the cells degenerate around the lingual swellings, forming a sulcus, which frees the _____ from the floor of the mouth, except for the attachment of the midline lingual frenum.

9. The _____ comprises the lining of the floor of the mouth.

10. The floor of the mouth has an extremely thin epithelium overlying, but not obscuring, a(n) _____ with an extensive vascular supply, thus making the veins more apparent.

inferior border	body of the tongue	nonkeratinized stratified squamous epithelium
base of the tongue	lingual frenum	lamina propria
sublingual caruncle	floor of the mouth	
sublingual fold	sublingual artery	

References Chapter 2, Surface anatomy. In Fehrenbach MJ, Herring SW: *Illustrated anatomy of the head and neck,* ed 6, St. Louis, 2021, Saunders; Chapter 6, Vascular system. In Fehrenbach MJ, Herring SW: *Illustrated anatomy of the head and neck,* ed 6, St. Louis, 2021, Saunders; Chapter 2, Oral cavity and pharynx. In Fehrenbach MJ, Popowics T: *Illustrated dental embryology, histology, and anatomy,* ed 5, St. Louis, 2020, Saunders; Chapter 5, Orofacial development. In Fehrenbach MJ, Popowics T: *Illustrated dental embryology, histology, and anatomy,* ed 5, St. Louis, 2020, Saunders; Chapter 9, Oral mucosa. In Fehrenbach MJ, Popowics T: *Illustrated dental embryology, histology, and anatomy,* ed 5, St. Louis, 2020, Saunders.

FIGURE 2.30 Pharynx with landmarks (midsagittal section)

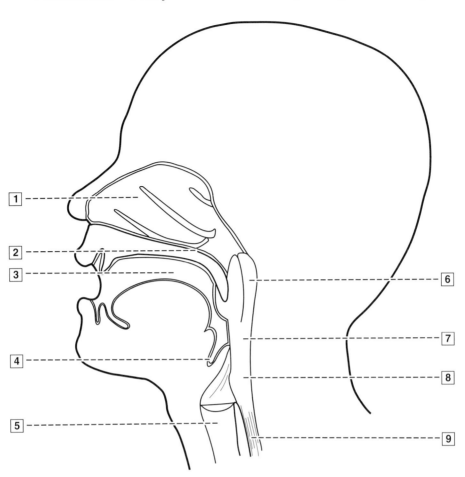

1	Nasal cavity	**6**	Nasopharynx
2	Soft palate	**7**	Oropharynx
3	Oral cavity	**8**	Laryngopharynx
4	Epiglottis	**9**	Esophagus
5	Larynx		

REVIEW QUESTIONS: Pharynx with landmarks

Fill in the blanks by choosing the appropriate terms from the list below.

1. The oral cavity also provides the entrance into the deeper structure of the _____ or *throat.*

2. The pharynx is a muscular tube that serves both the respiratory and digestive systems; it consists of _____ parts, which includes the nasopharynx, oropharynx, and laryngopharynx.

3. The _____ is the part of the pharynx that is located more inferiorly than the other parts as well as close to the laryngeal opening.

4. The part of the pharynx that is superior to the level of the soft palate is the _____, which is continuous with the nasal cavity.

5. The part of the pharynx that is between the soft palate and the opening of the larynx is the _____.

6. The lips of the face mark the anterior boundary of the oral cavity, and the throat or pharynx is the _____.

7. During the fourth week of prenatal development after the embryonic folding, there is the formation of a long hollow tube; the anterior part is the _____, which forms the primitive pharynx or primitive throat and includes a part of the primitive yolk sac as it becomes enclosed with folding.

8. The two more posterior parts of the tube formed during the fourth week of prenatal development are the _____ and the hindgut, which will form the rest of the mature pharynx as well as the remainder of the digestive tract.

9. During development of the digestive tract, four pairs of _____ will form from evaginations on the lateral walls lining the pharynx.

10. The primitive pharynx widens cranially during prenatal development where it joins the primitive mouth and later the stomodeum, and also narrows caudally as it joins the esophagus; the _____ of the pharynx lines the internal parts of the pharyngeal or branchial arches and passes into balloon-like areas of the pharyngeal pouches.

midgut	posterior boundary	foregut
nasopharynx	oropharynx	pharyngeal pouches
laryngopharynx	pharynx	endoderm
three		

References Chapter 2, Surface anatomy. In Fehrenbach MJ, Herring SW: *Illustrated anatomy of the head and neck,* ed 6, St. Louis, 2021, Saunders; Chapter 2, Oral cavity and pharynx. In Fehrenbach MJ, Popowics T: *Illustrated dental embryology, histology, and anatomy,* ed 5, St. Louis, 2020, Saunders; Chapter 4, Face and neck development. In Fehrenbach MJ, Popowics T: *Illustrated dental embryology, histology, and anatomy,* ed 5, St. Louis, 2020, Saunders; Chapter 8, Head and neck. In Drake R, Vogl AW, Mitchell AWM: *Gray's anatomy for students,* ed 4, Philadelphia, 2020, Churchill Livingstone.

ANSWER KEY 1. pharynx, 2. three, 3. laryngopharynx, 4. nasopharynx, 5. oropharynx, 6. posterior boundary, 7. foregut, 8. midgut, 9. pharyngeal pouches, 10. endoderm

FIGURE 2.31 Oropharynx with landmarks (frontal view)

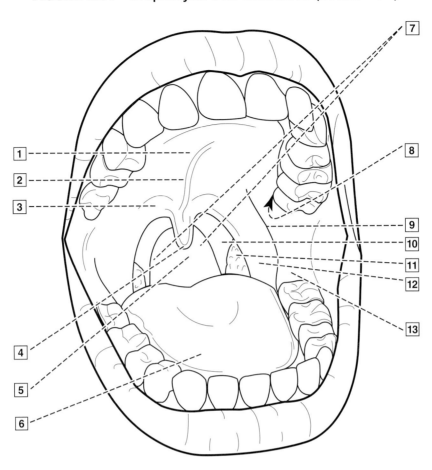

1 Hard palate		**7** Fauces	
2 Median palatine raphe		**8** Maxillary tuberosity	
3 Soft palate		**9** Pterygomandibular fold	
4 Uvula		**10** Posterior faucial pillar	
5 Posterior wall of pharynx		**11** Palatine tonsil	
6 Dorsal surface of the tongue		**12** Anterior faucial pillar	
		13 Retromolar pad	

REVIEW QUESTIONS: Oropharynx with landmarks

Fill in the blanks by choosing the appropriate terms from the list below.

1. The part of the pharynx that is between the _____ and the opening of the larynx is the oropharynx.

2. Behind the base of the tongue and in front of the oropharynx is the _____, a flap of cartilage, which at rest is upright and allows air to pass through the larynx and into the rest of the respiratory system; during swallowing, it folds back to cover the entrance to the larynx, preventing food and liquid from entering the deeper still trachea and then entering the lungs.

3. The opening from the oral region into the oropharynx is the _____ or *faucial isthmus*.

4. The fauces are formed laterally on each side of the oral cavity by both the _____ and the posterior faucial pillar.

5. The tonsillar tissue, the _____, is located between the faucial pillars or folds of tissue created by underlying muscles.

6. The _____ forms the posterior faucial pillar in the oral cavity, a vertical fold posterior to each palatine tonsil.

7. The _____ forms the anterior faucial pillar in the oral cavity, a vertical fold anterior to each palatine tonsil.

8. Each mass of intraoral tonsillar tissue contains fused-together lymphatic nodules that generally have _____; each tonsil also has 10 to 20 epithelial invaginations or grooves, which penetrate deeply into the tonsil to form tonsillar crypts.

9. Tonsils, like lymph nodes, contain lymphocytes that remove toxic products and then move to the epithelial surface as they mature; unlike lymph nodes, tonsillar tissue is not located along lymphatic vessels but is situated near _____ and food passages to protect the body against disease processes from the related toxins.

10. The palatine tonsils are derived from the lining of the _____ and also from the pharyngeal walls.

airways	palatopharyngeus muscle	second pharyngeal pouches
soft palate	fauces	palatoglossus muscle
anterior faucial pillar	epiglottis	germinal centers
palatine tonsils		

References Chapter 2, Surface anatomy. In Fehrenbach MJ, Herring SW: *Illustrated anatomy of the head and neck,* ed 6, St. Louis, 2021, Saunders; Chapter 7, Muscular system. In Fehrenbach MJ, Herring SW: *Illustrated anatomy of the head and neck,* ed 6, St. Louis, 2021, Saunders; Chapter 2, Oral cavity and pharynx. In Fehrenbach MJ, Popowics T: *Illustrated dental embryology, histology, and anatomy,* ed 5, St. Louis, 2020, Saunders; Chapter 4, Face and neck development. In Fehrenbach MJ, Popowics T: *Illustrated dental embryology, histology, and anatomy,* ed 5, St. Louis, 2020, Saunders; Chapter 11, Head and neck structures. In Fehrenbach MJ, Popowics T: *Illustrated dental embryology, histology, and anatomy,* ed 5, St. Louis, 2020, Saunders.

FIGURE 2.32 Regions of neck: Cervical triangles with landmarks

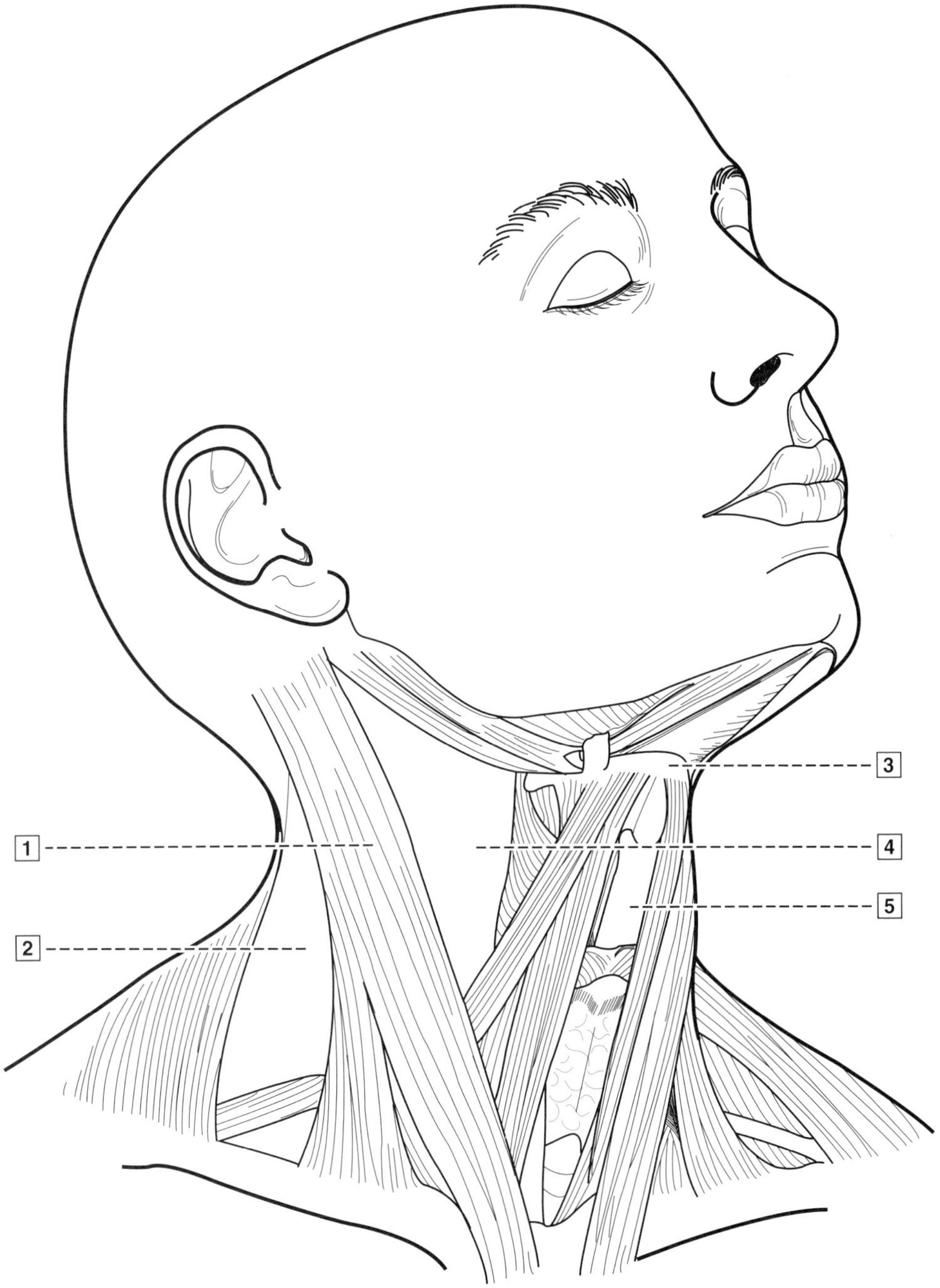

1 Sternocleidomastoid muscle	**4** Anterior cervical triangle
2 Posterior cervical triangle	**5** Thyroid cartilage
3 Hyoid bone	

REVIEW QUESTIONS: Regions of neck: Cervical triangles with landmarks

Fill in the blanks by choosing the appropriate terms from the list below.

1. The _____ extends from the skull and mandible inferiorly to the clavicles and sternum.

2. The large strap muscle, the _____, divides each side of the neck diagonally into a larger anterior cervical triangle and smaller posterior cervical triangle.

3. The anterior region of the neck corresponds with the two _____, which are separated by a midline.

4. The lateral region of the neck that is posterior to the sternocleidomastoid muscle is considered the _____ on each side.

5. At the anterior midline, the largest of the larynx's cartilages, the _____, is visible as the laryngeal prominence or what is called the "Adam's apple"

6. The thyroid cartilage is superior to the _____.

7. The _____ of the thyroid cartilage is just superior to the laryngeal prominence.

8. The vocal cords or ligaments of the _____ or *voice box,* are attached to the posterior surface of the thyroid cartilage.

9. The _____ is located in the anterior midline superior to the thyroid cartilage; it is suspended in the neck without any bony articulations.

10. Instead of bony articulation, _____ are attached to the hyoid bone that controls the tongue and pharynx to assist the muscles of mastication, as well as those muscles involved in swallowing.

larynx	hyoid bone	posterior cervical triangle
thyroid cartilage	superior thyroid notch	neck
anterior cervical triangles	thyroid gland	muscles
sternocleidomastoid muscle		

References   Chapter 2, Surface anatomy. In Fehrenbach MJ, Herring SW: *Illustrated anatomy of the head and neck,* ed 6, St. Louis, 2021, Saunders; Chapter 1, Face and neck regions. In Fehrenbach MJ, Popowics T: *Illustrated dental embryology, histology, and anatomy,* ed 5, St. Louis, 2020, Saunders.

NOTES

FIGURE 2.33 Regions of neck: Anterior cervical triangle with landmarks

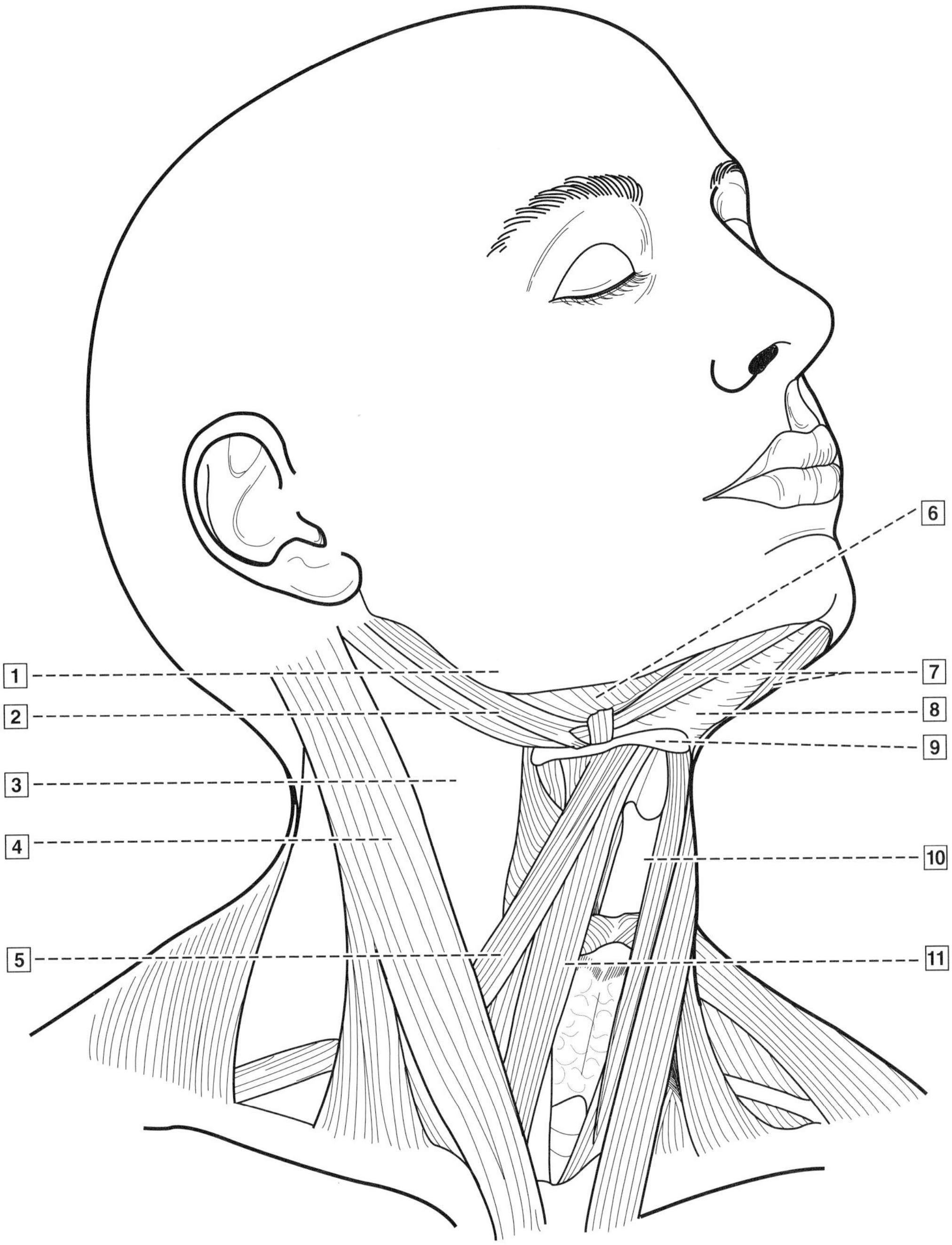

1	Mandible	7	Digastric muscles (anterior bellies)
2	Digastric muscle (posterior belly)	8	Submental triangle
3	Carotid triangle	9	Hyoid bone
4	Sternocleidomastoid muscle	10	Thyroid cartilage
5	Omohyoid muscle (superior belly)	11	Muscular triangle
6	Submandibular triangle		

REVIEW QUESTIONS: Regions of neck: Anterior cervical triangle with landmarks

Fill in the blanks by choosing the appropriate terms from the list below.

1. The _____ is a region of the neck on each side, which can be further subdivided into smaller triangular regions by area muscles that are not as prominent as those of the sternocleidomastoid muscle.

2. The superior part of each anterior cervical triangle is demarcated by the two parts of both the anterior and posterior bellies of the digastric muscle, with the superior mandible forming the _____ on each side as a region of the neck.

3. The inferior part of each anterior cervical triangle is further subdivided by the omohyoid muscle's superior belly into the _____, a region of the neck that is superior to the muscle.

4. The inferior part of each anterior cervical triangle is further subdivided by the omohyoid muscle's superior belly into the _____, a region of the neck that is inferior to the muscle.

5. A single midline _____ is a region of the neck that is formed by the two parts of the digastric muscle, both its right and left anterior bellies as well as the hyoid bone.

6. Passing through the anterior cervical triangle are the _____ and their branches, the external and internal carotid arteries; these blood vessels supply all structures of the head and neck.

7. The superior part of each common carotid artery and its division into _____ occurs in the carotid triangle, which is a subdivision of the anterior cervical triangle.

8. As the _____ passes through the area of the anterior cervical triangle, it innervates the stylopharyngeus muscle, sends a branch to the carotid sinus, and supplies sensory branches to the pharynx.

9. The branches of the _____ as it passes through the anterior cervical triangle include a motor branch to the pharynx, a branch to the carotid body, the superior laryngeal nerve (which divides into external and internal laryngeal branches), and possibly a cardiac branch.

10. The _____ is a muscle of facial expression that runs from the mouth all the way to the neck superficial to the anterior cervical triangle and external jugular vein.

vagus nerve	carotid triangle	external and internal carotid arteries
submandibular triangle	muscular triangle	glossopharyngeal nerve
anterior cervical triangle	common carotid arteries	platysma
submental triangle		

References Chapter 2, Surface anatomy. In Fehrenbach MJ, Herring SW: *Illustrated anatomy of the head and neck,* ed 6, St. Louis, 2021, Saunders; Chapter 6, Vascular system. In Fehrenbach MJ, Herring SW: *Illustrated anatomy of the head and neck,* ed 6, St. Louis, 2021, Saunders; Chapter 8, Nervous system. In Fehrenbach MJ, Herring SW: *Illustrated anatomy of the head and neck,* ed 6, St. Louis, 2021, Saunders; Chapter 1, Face and neck regions. In Fehrenbach MJ, Popowics T: *Illustrated dental embryology, histology, and anatomy,* ed 5, St. Louis, 2020, Saunders; Chapter 8, Head and neck. In Drake R, Vogl AW, Mitchell AWM: *Gray's anatomy for students,* ed 4, Philadelphia, 2020, Churchill Livingstone.

FIGURE 2.34 Regions of neck: Posterior cervical triangle with landmarks

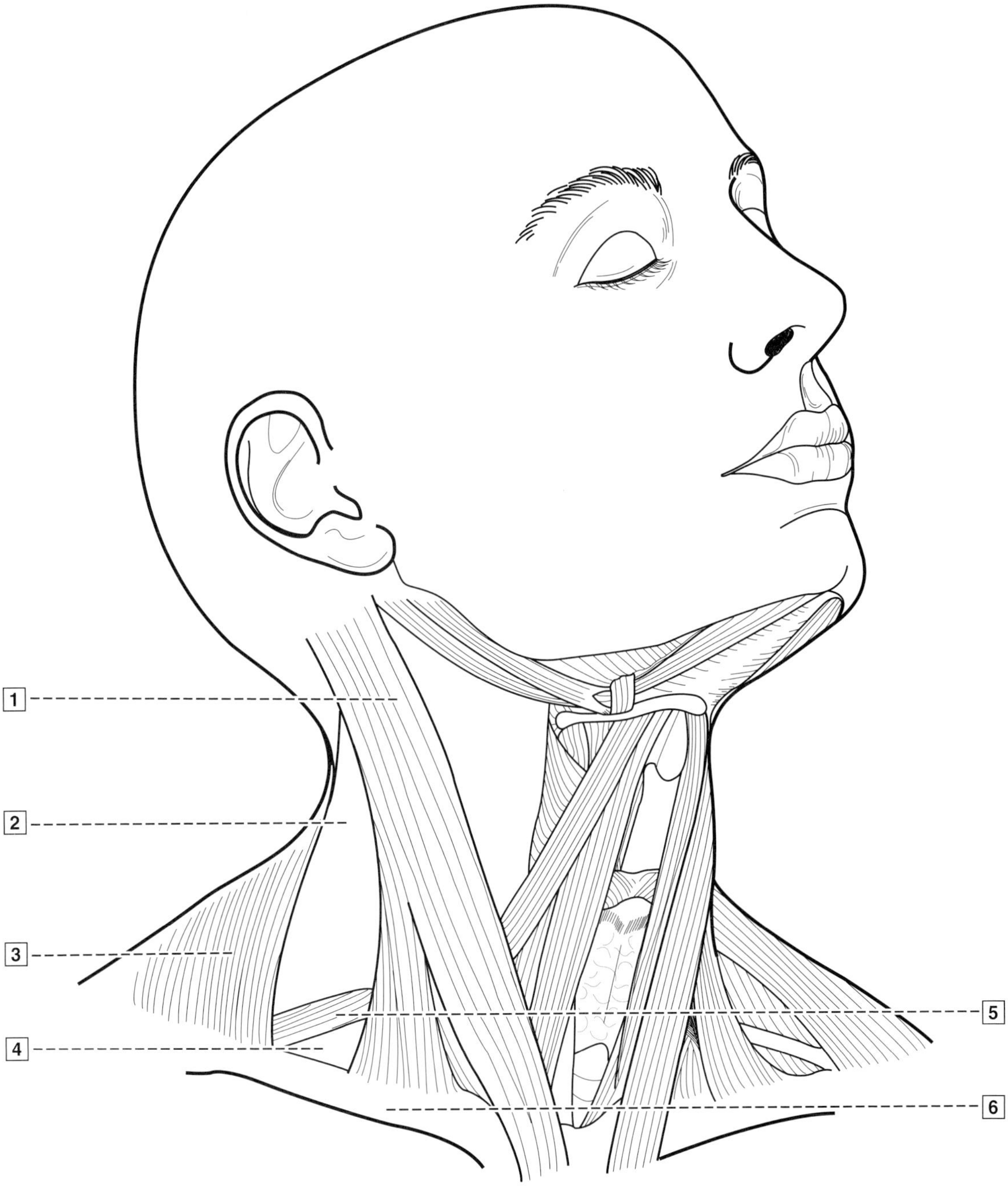

1 Sternocleidomastoid muscle	**3** Trapezius muscle	**5** Omohyoid muscle (inferior belly)
2 Occipital triangle	**4** Subclavian triangle	**6** Clavicle

REVIEW QUESTIONS: Regions of neck: Posterior cervical triangle with landmarks

Fill in the blanks by choosing the appropriate terms from the list below.

1. Each _____ is a region of the neck that can be further subdivided into smaller triangular regions on each side by area muscles.

2. The omohyoid muscle's inferior belly divides the posterior cervical triangle into the larger _____, a region of the neck that is superior to the muscle on each side.

3. The omohyoid muscle's inferior belly divides the posterior cervical triangle into the smaller _____, a region of the neck that is inferior to the muscle on each side but superior to the clavicle.

4. The _____ is a structure of the neck that adjoins the medial aspect of the occipital triangle.

5. The _____ is a structure of the neck that adjoins the lateral aspect of the occipital triangle.

6. The roof of the posterior cervical triangle consists of an investing layer of cervical fascia that surrounds the _____ as it passes through the region.

7. The muscular floor of the posterior cervical triangle is covered by the prevertebral layer of _____; from superior to inferior it consists of the splenius capitis and levator scapulae as well as the posterior, middle, and anterior scalene muscles.

8. One of the most superficial structures passing through the posterior cervical triangle is the _____; after crossing the sternocleidomastoid muscle, the blood vessel then enters the posterior triangle and continues its vertical descent.

9. The borders of the posterior cervical triangle specifically are the middle one-third of the _____, the anterior margin of the trapezius muscle, and the posterior margin of the sternocleidomastoid muscle.

10. The posterior cervical triangle in part lies over the _____, which is the apex of the axillary region and is associated with structures (nerves and blood vessels) that allow passage.

external jugular vein	sternocleidomastoid and trapezius muscles	Clavicle
occipital triangle	posterior cervical triangle	axillary inlet
sternocleidomastoid muscle	subclavian triangle	cervical fascia
trapezius muscle		

References Chapter 2, Surface anatomy. In Fehrenbach MJ, Herring SW: *Illustrated anatomy of the head and neck,* ed 5, St. Louis, 2021, Saunders; Chapter 4, Muscular system. In Fehrenbach MJ, Herring SW: *Illustrated anatomy of the head and neck,* ed 5, St. Louis, 2021, Saunders; Chapter 6, Vascular system. In Fehrenbach MJ, Herring SW: *Illustrated anatomy of the head and neck,* ed 5, St. Louis, 2021, Saunders; Chapter 1, Face and neck regions. In Fehrenbach MJ, Popowics T: *Illustrated dental embryology, histology, and anatomy,* ed 5, St. Louis, 2020, Saunders; Chapter 8, Head and neck. In Drake R, Vogl AW, Mitchell AWM: *Gray's anatomy for students,* ed 4, Philadelphia, 2020, Churchill Livingstone.

ANSWER KEY 1. posterior cervical triangle, 2. occipital triangle, 3. subclavian triangle, 4. sternocleidomastoid muscle, 5. trapezius muscle, 6. sternocleidomastoid and trapezius muscles, 7. cervical fascia, 8. external jugular vein, 9. clavicle, 10. axillary inlet

FIGURE 3.1 Tooth development stages (or odontogenesis)

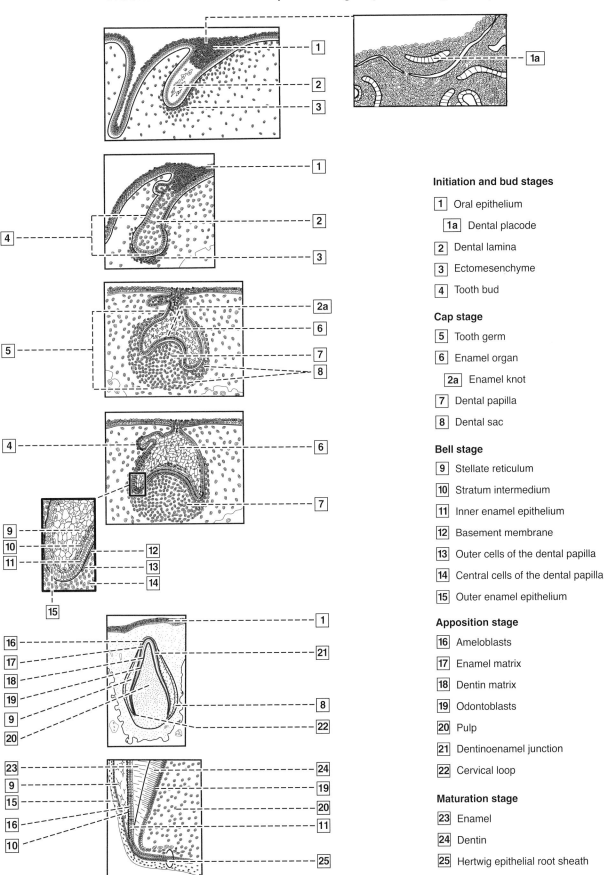

Initiation and bud stages

1 Oral epithelium

1a Dental placode

2 Dental lamina

3 Ectomesenchyme

4 Tooth bud

Cap stage

5 Tooth germ

6 Enamel organ

2a Enamel knot

7 Dental papilla

8 Dental sac

Bell stage

9 Stellate reticulum

10 Stratum intermedium

11 Inner enamel epithelium

12 Basement membrane

13 Outer cells of the dental papilla

14 Central cells of the dental papilla

15 Outer enamel epithelium

Apposition stage

16 Ameloblasts

17 Enamel matrix

18 Dentin matrix

19 Odontoblasts

20 Pulp

21 Dentinoenamel junction

22 Cervical loop

Maturation stage

23 Enamel

24 Dentin

25 Hertwig epithelial root sheath

137

Fill in the blanks by choosing the appropriate terms from the list below.

1. The first stage of tooth development is the _____ stage, which involves the physiologic process of induction, which is an active interaction between the embryologic tissue types.

2. During the second stage of tooth development that occurs at the beginning of the eighth week of prenatal development for the primary dentition, there is an extensive proliferation of the dental placodes within the dental lamina, resulting in both the future maxillary arch and the future mandibular arch each having 10 _____.

3. During the third stage of tooth development that occurs during the ninth and tenth week of prenatal development for the primary dentition and during the fetal period, a depression results in the deepest part of each tooth bud of a dental placode within the dental lamina, with the enamel organ creating a(n) _____ shape.

4. The _____ stage of tooth development occurs between the eleventh and twelfth week of prenatal development for the primary dentition.

5. During the fourth stage of tooth development, the enamel organ differentiates into four different types of cells, one of which is the _____ that will later become enamel-secreting cells or ameloblasts.

6. Within the concavity of the differentiating enamel organ, the _____ undergoes extensive differentiation during the fourth week of prenatal development to later become dentin-secreting cells or odontoblasts.

7. Each hard dental tissue of the mature tooth is initially secreted as a partially mineralized _____ during the stage of appositional growth, thus serving as a framework that will later undergo full maturation when each tissue type is mineralized to its expected level.

8. The first cells to undergo repolarization near the basement membrane in the developing tooth germ are the _____, which then will induce the outer cells of the dental papilla to become odontoblasts.

9. The first cells to begin their synthetic and secretory activity near the basement membrane after repolarization to produce _____ are the odontoblasts, thus obtaining a thicker layer in a developing tooth than any corresponding layer of enamel matrix.

10. The cervical loop, composed only of inner and outer enamel epithelium, begins to grow deeper into the surrounding ectomesenchyme of the dental sac, elongating and moving away from the newly completed crown to enclose more of the dental papilla to form the _____, which functions to shape the root(s) by inducing dentin formation in the root so that it is continuous with coronal dentin.

matrix	bell	cap
inner enamel epithelium	Hertwig epithelial root sheath	preameloblasts
initiation	outer cells of the dental papilla	buds
predentin		

Reference Chapter 6, Tooth development and eruption. In Fehrenbach MJ, Popowics T: *Illustrated dental embryology, histology, and anatomy,* ed 5, St. Louis, 2020, Saunders.

FIGURE 3.2 Primary and permanent teeth comparison (anterior teeth: labial view; posterior teeth: mesial view)

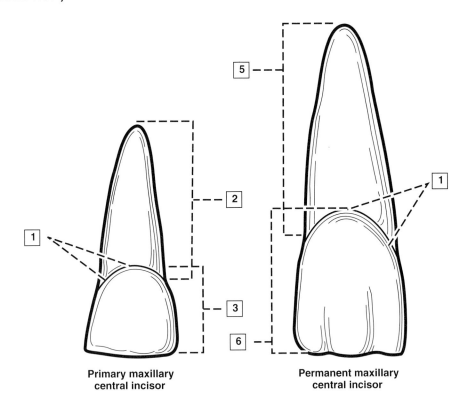

Primary maxillary
central incisor

Permanent maxillary
central incisor

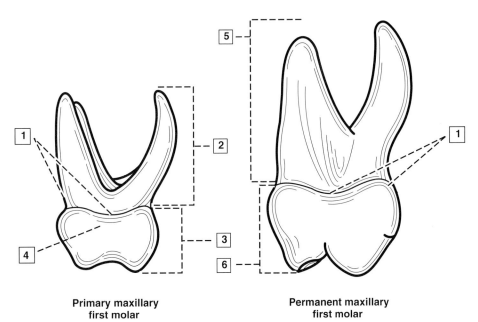

Primary maxillary
first molar

Permanent maxillary
first molar

1 Cementoenamel junction (CEJ)
2 Narrower root(s)
3 Whiter tone crown
4 Prominent cervical ridge
5 Wider root(s)
6 Yellower crown color

REVIEW QUESTIONS: Primary and permanent teeth comparison

Fill in the blanks by choosing the appropriate terms from the list below.

1. Primary teeth have a whiter tone of the _____ of enamel on their crowns than permanent teeth because of increased opacity of the enamel that covers the underlying yellow dentin.

2. Primary teeth have an overall smaller _____, with permanent teeth being larger; however, there are important differences that occur in the structure as well as the size of primary teeth compared with that of permanent teeth.

3. The crowns of primary teeth are more constricted or narrower at the _____, making them appear bulbous in comparison to the thinner necks of the teeth; the crown of any primary tooth is also short in relation to its total length.

4. Primary teeth have a prominent _____ that is present on both the labial and lingual surfaces of anterior teeth and on the buccal surfaces of molars, more than any similar structure on the even larger permanent molars.

5. The _____ of primary teeth are narrower and longer than the crown length, with partial resorption possibly noted radiographically as the teeth begin to shed or exfoliate.

6. Each crown-to-root _____ of primary teeth is smaller than those of their permanent dentition counterparts.

7. The pulp cavity on primary teeth shows that the chambers and horns are relatively large in proportion to those of the permanent teeth, especially the mesial pulpal horns of the _____.

8. Overall, the dentin of the primary dentition is thinner than that of the permanent counterparts; however, the thickness of the _____ between the pulp chambers and the enamel can be in primary teeth, especially in the primary mandibular second molar.

9. The _____ is relatively thin in primary teeth in comparison to the permanent counterparts, but it still has a consistent thickness overlying the dentin of the crown.

10. Within the primary dentition, _____ are present in the dentition of most children because it is necessary for the proper alignment of the larger future permanent dentition; the largest ones are considered primate spaces, mostly involving spaces between the primary maxillary lateral incisor and canine and also between the primary mandibular canine and first molar.

ratio	cementoenamel junction	crown
interproximal spaces	enamel	size
dentin	molars	cervical ridge
roots		

Reference Chapter 18, Primary dentition. In Fehrenbach MJ, Popowics T: *Illustrated dental embryology, histology, and anatomy,* ed 5, St. Louis, 2020, Saunders.

FIGURE 3.3   Primary dentition eruption and shedding timeline

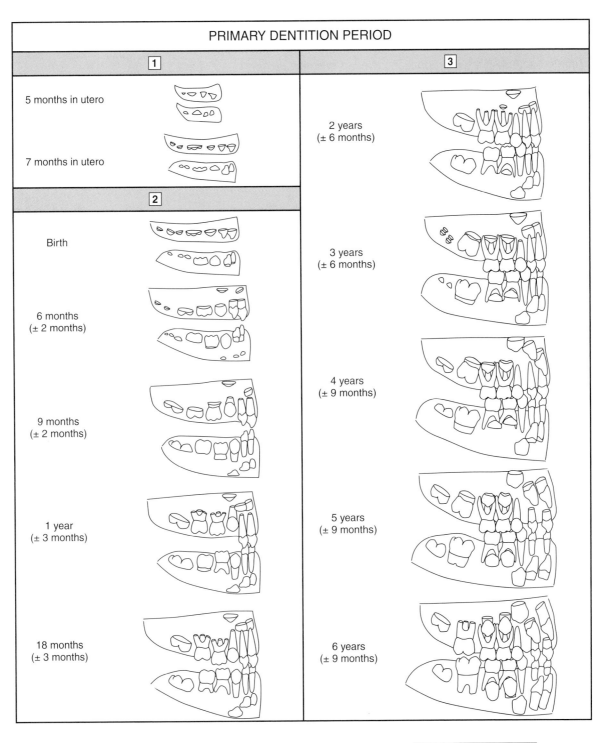

PRIMARY DENTITION PERIOD	
1	**3**
5 months in utero	2 years (± 6 months)
7 months in utero	3 years (± 6 months)
2	4 years (± 9 months)
Birth	5 years (± 9 months)
6 months (± 2 months)	6 years (± 9 months)
9 months (± 2 months)	
1 year (± 3 months)	
18 months (± 3 months)	

1 Prenatal

2 Infancy

3 Early childhood (preschool age)

Primary teeth: white

Permanent teeth: yellow

REVIEW QUESTIONS: Primary dentition eruption and shedding timeline

Fill in the blanks by choosing the appropriate terms from the list below.

1. Although there are only two dentitions, there are three _____ throughout a person's lifetime because the tooth dentitions overlap in time.

2. Each oral cavity should be assigned a dentition period to allow for the most effective dental treatment for that period; this specificity is especially important with the consideration of orthodontic therapy because growth during certain dentition periods is maximized to allow expansion of both the _____ and movement of the teeth.

3. The first dentition period is the _____.

4. The primary dentition period begins with the eruption of the primary _____, which occurs between approximately 6 months and 6 years of age.

5. Only _____ are present in the dentition during the primary dentition period.

6. The primary dentition has its full _____ completed at 30 months.

7. The eruption of the primary teeth is usually completed when the primary _____ are in occlusion.

8. The jaws begin to grow further during the primary dentition period to accommodate the coming larger and more numerous _____.

9. The primary dentition period is a period that usually ends when the first permanent tooth erupts, the permanent _____.

10. The primary dentition period is followed by the _____.

jaws	mixed dentition period	permanent teeth
dentition periods	eruption	mandibular central incisor
primary teeth	primary dentition period	second molars
mandibular first molar		

References Chapter 6, Tooth development and eruption. In Fehrenbach MJ, Popowics T: *Illustrated dental embryology, histology, and anatomy,* ed 5, St. Louis, 2020, Saunders; Chapter 15, Overview of dentitions. In Fehrenbach MJ, Popowics T: *Illustrated dental embryology, histology, and anatomy,* ed 5, St. Louis, 2020, Saunders.

NOTES

FIGURE 3.4   Permanent dentition eruption timeline

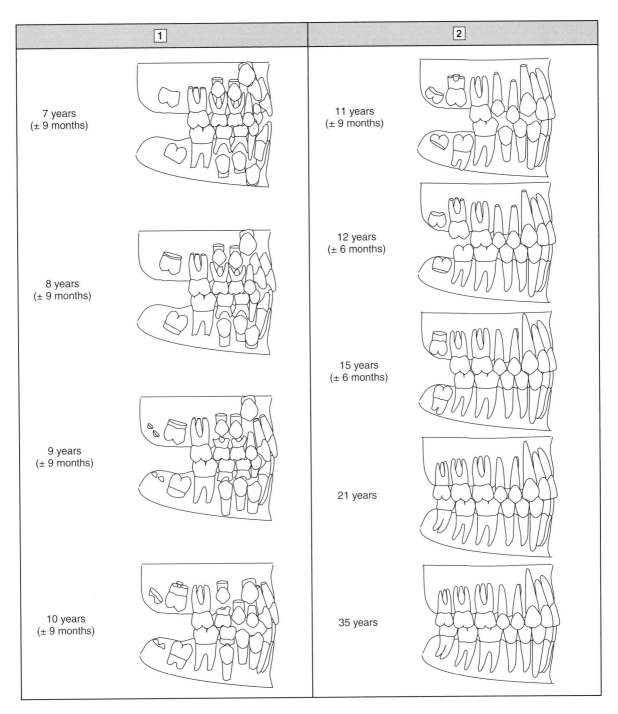

7 years (± 9 months)	11 years (± 9 months)
8 years (± 9 months)	12 years (± 6 months)
9 years (± 9 months)	15 years (± 6 months)
10 years (± 9 months)	21 years
	35 years

1 MIXED DENTITION PERIOD—Late childhood (school age)

2 PERMANENT DENTITION PERIOD—Adolescence and adulthood

Primary teeth: white

Permanent teeth: yellow

REVIEW QUESTIONS: Permanent dentition eruption timeline

Fill in the blanks by choosing the appropriate terms from the list below.

1. The _____ is a period that occurs between approximately 6 and 12 years of age with both primary and permanent teeth present, giving a possible "ugly duckling" appearance.

2. During the mixed dentition period, there is _____ or *exfoliation* of the primary dentition, allowing for the tooth fairy (or helper) to visit.

3. The mixed dentition period begins with the eruption of the first permanent tooth, a permanent mandibular first molar, which is guided by the distal surface of the primary _____.

4. During the mixed dentition period, there is _____ of the permanent teeth after their crowns are completed.

5. Both _____ and permanent teeth are present during the transitional stage of the mixed dentition period.

6. The color differences between the primary and permanent teeth become apparent clinically during the mixed dentition period because the permanent teeth have less overlying opaque _____ and thus the underlying yellow dentin is more visible.

7. The _____ is a period that begins with the shedding of the last primary tooth, which is approximately after 12 years of age, cutting off most of the tooth fairy visits.

8. During the permanent dentition period, there is little growth of the _____ overall given that puberty has passed, which contrasts with the mixed dentition period that has the fastest and most noticeable growth, consistent with the onset of puberty.

9. When an oral cavity is unusually early or late regarding the usual sequential eruption of teeth, the _____ of the biologic family should be reviewed for developmental anomalies.

10. Tooth types tend to erupt in pairs so that if any change in this _____ exists in a patient, a radiograph of the area may be required.

shedding	permanent dentition period	pattern of symmetry
primary teeth	mixed dentition period	mandibular second molar
enamel	eruption	jaws
dental history		

References Chapter 6, Tooth development and eruption. In Fehrenbach MJ, Popowics T: *Illustrated dental embryology, histology, and anatomy,* ed 5, St. Louis, 2020, Saunders; Chapter 15, Overview of dentitions. In Fehrenbach MJ, Popowics T: *Illustrated dental embryology, histology, and anatomy,* ed 5, St. Louis, 2020, Saunders.

ANSWER KEY 1. mixed dentition period, 2. shedding, 3. mandibular second molar, 4. eruption, 5. primary teeth, 6. enamel, 7. permanent dentition period, 8. jaws, 9. dental history, 10. pattern of symmetry

FIGURE 3.5 Dental tissue with crown designations (anterior tooth: labiolingual section; posterior tooth: mesiodistal section)

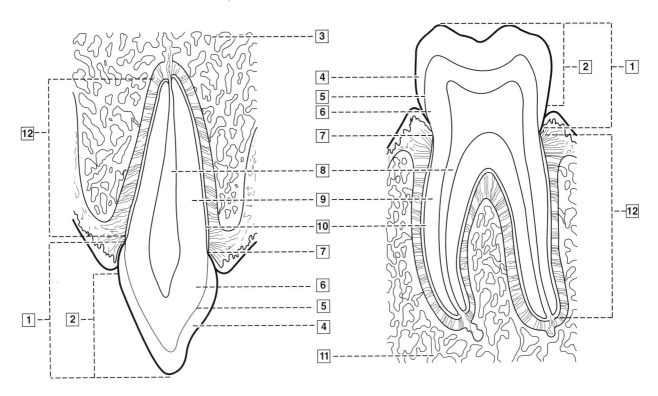

1	Anatomic crown	**7**	Cementoenamel junction (CEJ)
2	Clinical crown	**8**	Pulp cavity
3	Alveolar process of the maxilla	**9**	Dentin
4	Enamel	**10**	Cementum
5	Dentinoenamel junction (DEJ)	**11**	Alveolar process of the mandible
6	Dentin	**12**	Anatomic root

REVIEW QUESTIONS: Dental tissue with crown designations

Fill in the blanks by choosing the appropriate terms from the list below.

1. Each tooth consists of a(n) _____, which is the part covered by enamel that remains mostly constant throughout the life of the tooth, except for the presence of attrition and other physical wear.

2. Each root of a tooth within the jaw has dentin covered by _____.

3. The inner part of the _____ of both the crown and root of the tooth covers the innermost pulp cavity.

4. The _____ has a chamber and canal(s) with an apical foramen.

5. The _____ of the crown and cementum of the root usually meet close to the cementoenamel junction with three interfaces possibly present.

6. The _____ is an external line at the neck or cervix of the tooth and usually feels smooth or evenly grainy or possibly has a slight groove when explored.

7. The _____ of the upper jaw contains the roots of the maxillary teeth.

8. The alveolar process of the lower jaw contains the roots of the _____ teeth.

9. The _____ is that part of the anatomic crown that is visible and not covered by gingiva.

10. The height of the clinical crown is determined by the location of the marginal gingiva, which can change over time, especially with _____ as the marginal gingiva recedes toward the root.

anatomic crown	alveolar process	cementum
pulp cavity	clinical crown	mandibular
enamel layer	dentin	gingival recession
cementoenamel junction		

References Chapter 15, Overview of dentitions. In Fehrenbach MJ Popowics T: *Illustrated dental embryology, histology, and anatomy,* ed 5, St. Louis, 2020, Saunders; Chapter 2, Surface anatomy, Fehrenbach, MJ, Herring SW: *Illustrated anatomy of the head and neck,* ed 6, St. Louis, 2021, Saunders.

NOTES

FIGURE 3.6 Enamel with enamel rods (longitudinal section with microanatomic views)

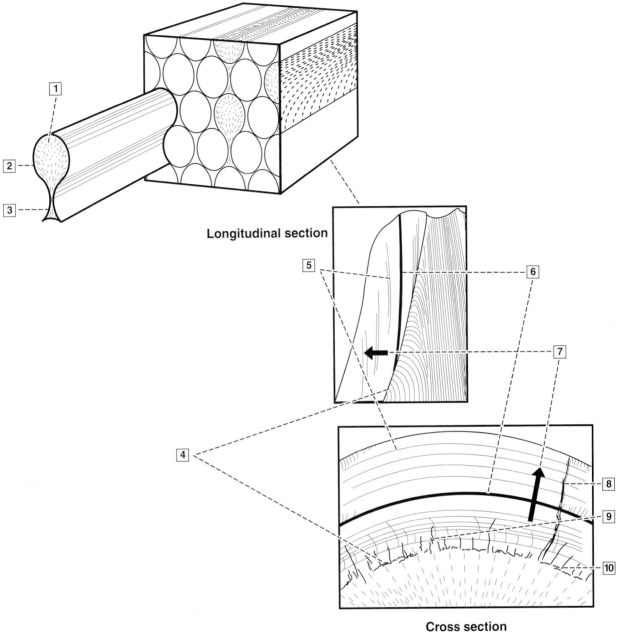

Longitudinal section

Cross section

1	Enamel rod	6	Neonatal line in enamel
2	Head	7	Direction of enamel rod
3	Tail	8	Enamel lamella
4	Dentinoenamel junction (DEJ)	9	Enamel spindle
5	Lines of Retzius	10	Enamel tuft

REVIEW QUESTIONS: Enamel with enamel rods

Fill in the blanks by choosing the appropriate terms from the list below.

1. Mature enamel is a highly mineralized or inorganic material, consisting of mainly _____.

2. Enamel appears more _____ (or lighter) than either dentin or pulp because it is denser than the latter structures, both of which appear more radiolucent (or darker).

3. Surrounding the outer part of each enamel rod is the _____ creating an interprismatic region that has been secreted by ameloblasts; even though similar in structure to the enamel rod, this type of enamel appears different from the rod core on cross sections because of its different crystalline orientation.

4. The _____ are the incremental lines (or striae) in a microscopic section of mature enamel with different orientation depending on the sectioning of the tissue.

5. Associated with the lines of Retzius are the raised imbrication lines and grooves of the _____, which are noted clinically on the nonmasticatory surfaces of some teeth in the oral cavity, and that can be lost through tooth wear except on the protected cervical regions of some teeth.

6. The _____ is a pronounced incremental line of Retzius, which marks the stress or trauma experienced by the ameloblasts during birth, illustrating the sensitivity of the ameloblasts as they form an enamel matrix.

7. The dentinoenamel junction is a junction between mature enamel and dentin that appears scalloped on a cross section of a tooth, with the convex side toward the _____ and the concave side toward the enamel.

8. The _____ are a microscopic feature of mature enamel and represent short dentinal tubules near the dentinoenamel junction that result from odontoblasts that crossed the basement membrane before it mineralized into the dentinoenamel junction.

9. The _____ are a microscopic feature that are noted as small dark brushes with their bases near the dentinoenamel junction in the inner one third of enamel, representing areas of less mineralization from an anomaly of crystallization.

10. The _____ are a microscopic feature that represent partially mineralized vertical sheets of enamel matrix that extend from the dentinoenamel junction near the tooth's cervix to the outer occlusal surface.

radiopaque	perikymata	enamel spindles
interrod enamel	neonatal line	dentin
enamel tufts	enamel lamellae	calcium hydroxyapatite
lines of Retzius		

Reference Chapter 12, Enamel. In Fehrenbach MJ, Popowics T: *Illustrated dental embryology, histology, and anatomy,* ed 5, St. Louis, 2020, Saunders.

FIGURE 3.7   Enamel and dentin development at the dentinoenamel junction (microanatomic views)

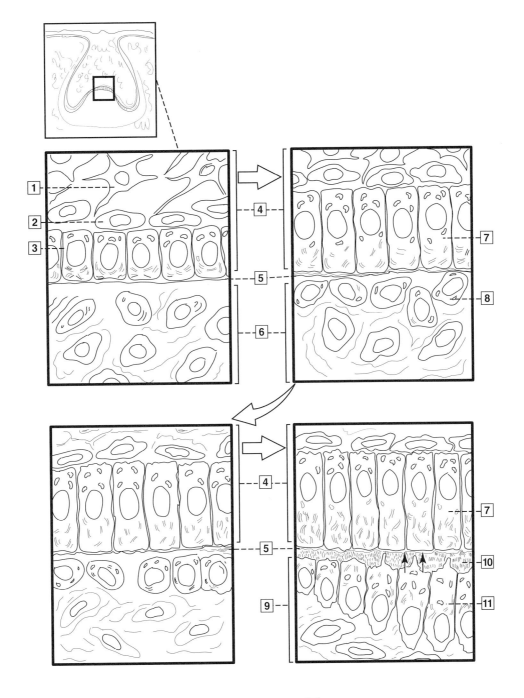

1	Stellate reticulum	**7**	Preameloblast
2	Stratum intermedium	**8**	Outer cell of the dental papilla
3	Inner enamel epithelium (IEE)	**9**	Pulp
4	Enamel organ	**10**	Predentin
5	Basement membrane	**11**	Odontoblast
6	Dental papilla		

REVIEW QUESTIONS: Enamel and dentin development at dentinoenamel junction

Fill in the blanks by choosing the appropriate terms from the list below.

1. The outer cuboidal cells of the enamel organ are the outer enamel epithelium, which will serve as a protective barrier for the rest of the enamel organ during enamel production within the _____ stage.

2. Between the outer enamel epithelium and inner enamel epithelium are the two innermost layers or *dental core*, the _____ and stratum intermedium.

3. One of the innermost layers of the enamel organ is the _____, which is made up of a compressed layer of flat to cuboidal cells.

4. After the formation of the _____ in the bell-shaped enamel organ, these innermost cells grow even more columnar as they elongate and differentiate into preameloblasts, lining up alongside the basement membrane and then undergoing repolarization of the nuclei in each cell.

5. In the future development, the _____ will induce dental papilla cells to differentiate into dentin-forming cells (odontoblasts) and then will themselves differentiate into cells that secrete enamel (ameloblasts).

6. The dental papilla within the concavity of the enamel organ undergoes extensive _____ so that it now consists of two types of tissue in layers, the outer cells of the dental papilla and central cells of the dental papilla.

7. The outer cells of the dental papilla are induced by the preameloblasts to differentiate into _____, undergoing cellular repolarization of their nuclei and starting to line up adjacent to the basement membrane on the opposite side.

8. After differentiation and repolarization, the odontoblasts begin _____, which is the appositional growth of dentin matrix or predentin on their side of the basement membrane.

9. After the differentiation of odontoblasts from the outer cells of the dental papilla and their formation of predentin, the _____ between the preameloblasts and the odontoblasts disintegrates; this is the future dentinoenamel junction.

10. The _____ become, with further tooth development, the primordium of the pulp.

stellate reticulum	dentinogenesis	odontoblasts
preameloblasts	central cells of the dental papilla	stratum intermedium
histodifferentiation	inner enamel epithelium	basement membrane
bell		

References   Chapter 6, Tooth development and eruption. In Fehrenbach MJ, Popowics T: *Illustrated dental embryology, histology, and anatomy,* ed 5, St. Louis, 2020, Saunders; Chapter 13, Dentin and pulp. In Fehrenbach MJ, Popowics T: *Illustrated dental embryology, histology, and anatomy,* ed 5, St. Louis, 2020, Saunders.

ANSWER KEY   1. bell, **2.** stellate reticulum, **3.** stratum intermedium, **4.** inner enamel epithelium, **5.** preameloblasts, **6.** histodifferentiation, **7.** odontoblasts, **8.** dentinogenesis, **9.** basement membrane, **10.** central cells of the dental papilla

FIGURE 3.8 Enamel and dentin apposition at the dentinoenamel junction (microanatomic views)

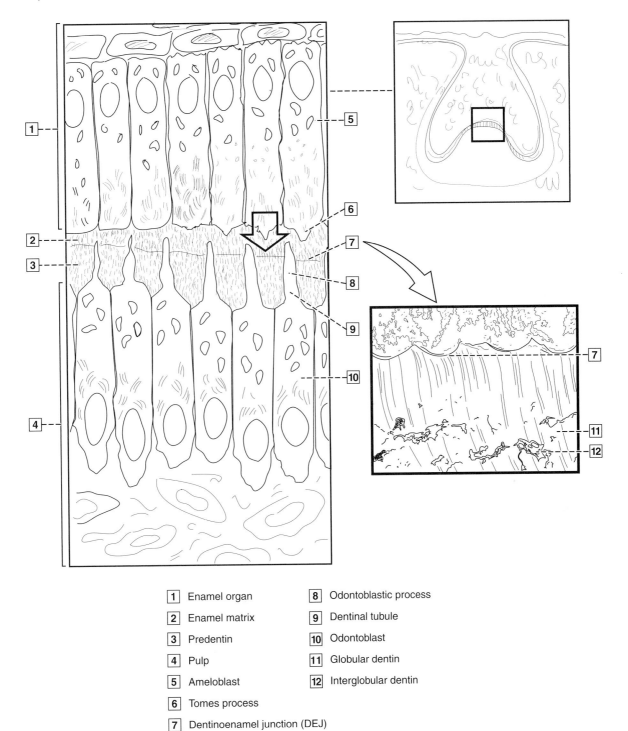

1 Enamel organ		**8** Odontoblastic process
2 Enamel matrix		**9** Dentinal tubule
3 Predentin		**10** Odontoblast
4 Pulp		**11** Globular dentin
5 Ameloblast		**12** Interglobular dentin
6 Tomes process		
7 Dentinoenamel junction (DEJ)		

REVIEW QUESTIONS: Enamel and dentin apposition at dentinoenamel junction

Fill in the blanks by choosing the appropriate terms from the list below.

1. The final stages of odontogenesis include the _____ stage during which the enamel, dentin, and cementum are secreted in successive layers upon those already present.

2. The _____ is reached when the matrices of the hard dental tissue types subsequently fully mineralize to their correct levels.

3. The disintegration of the basement membrane allows the preameloblasts to contact the newly formed predentin, which induces the preameloblasts to differentiate into _____; the calcium hydroxyapatite crystals form in the predentin as highly mineralized globular dentin (darker) with less mineralized interglobular dentin (lighter) between.

4. After differentiation, the ameloblasts begin _____ or the appositional growth of enamel matrix, laying it down on their side of the now disintegrating basement membrane.

5. The enamel matrix is secreted from _____, an angled distal part of each ameloblast that faces the fully disintegrating basement membrane created, as there is group movement of the ameloblasts away from the basement membrane.

6. Continued appositional growth of both types of dental matrix becomes regular and rhythmic, as the cellular bodies of both the odontoblasts and ameloblasts retreat away from the _____, forming their perspective tissue types.

7. The odontoblasts, unlike the ameloblasts, will leave attached cellular extensions in the length of the pre-dentin, the _____ as they move away from the newly formed dentinoenamel junction; the dentinoenamel junction begins to demonstrate its scalloped interface, having its concave side toward the enamel and its convex side toward the dentin.

8. Each odontoblastic process is contained in a mineralized cylinder, the _____.

9. The cell bodies of odontoblasts will remain within the _____ attached by the odontoblastic processes after the appositional growth stage.

10. The _____ of the ameloblasts will be involved in the final phases of the mineralization process but will be lost after eruption of the tooth into the oral cavity.

Tomes process   dentinoenamel junction   pulp
appositional growth   ameloblasts   cell bodies
amelogenesis   maturation stage   dentinal tubule
odontoblastic processes

Reference Chapter 6, Tooth development and eruption. In Fehrenbach MJ, Popowics T: *Illustrated dental embryology, histology, and anatomy,* ed 5, St. Louis, 2020, Saunders.

ANSWER KEY 1. appositional growth, 2. maturation stage, 3. ameloblasts, 4. amelogenesis, 5. Tomes process, 6. dentinoenamel junction, 7. odontoblastic processes, 8. dentinal tubule, 9. pulp, 10. cell bodies

FIGURE 3.9   Dentin (mesiodistal section with microanatomic views)

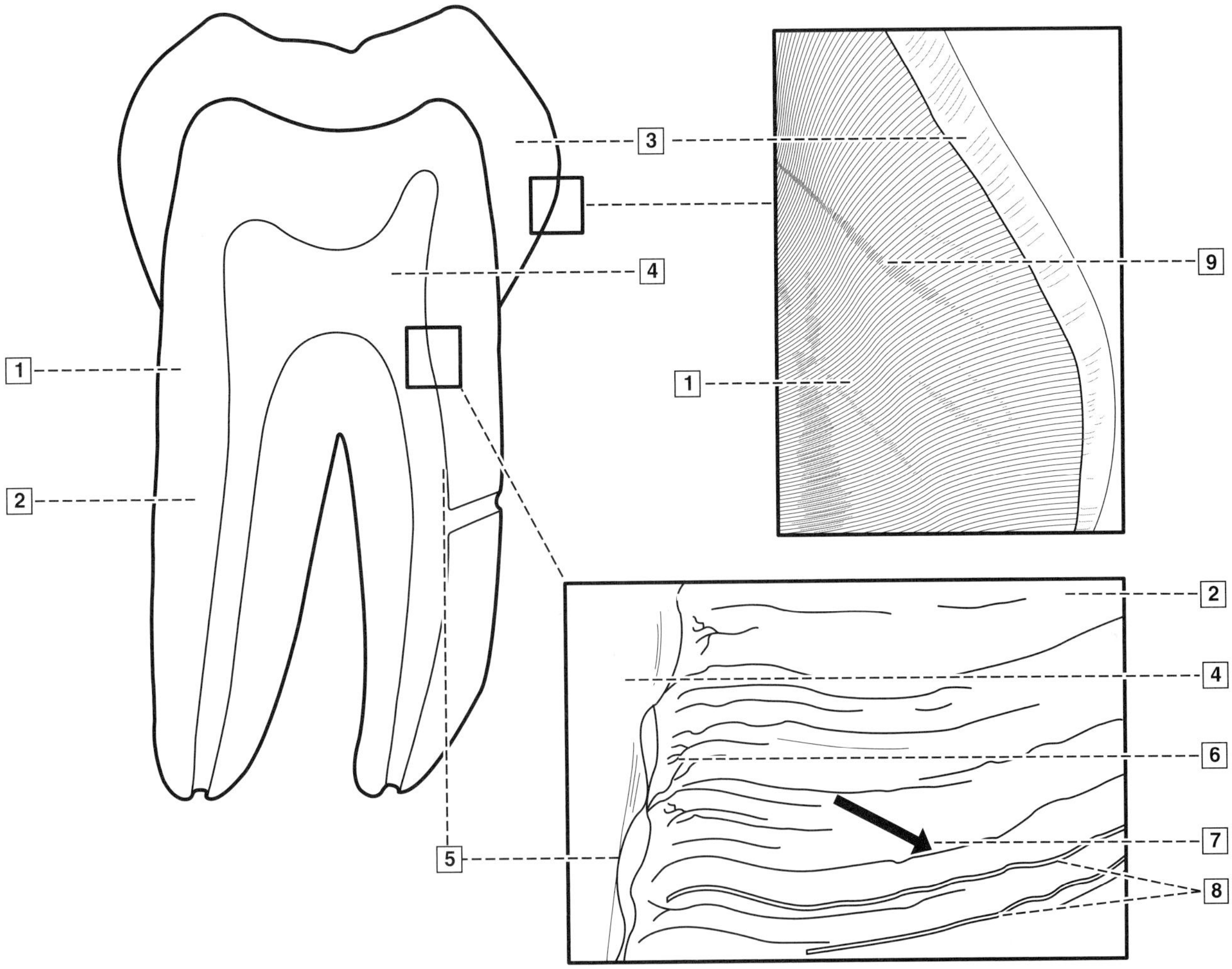

1	Mantle dentin	**6**	Odontoblastic processes
2	Circumpulpal dentin	**7**	Direction of imbrication lines of von Ebner
3	Enamel	**8**	Dentinal tubules
4	Pulp	**9**	Neonatal line in dentin
5	Outer pulpal wall		

REVIEW QUESTIONS: Dentin (mesiodistal section with microanatomic views)

Fill in the blanks by choosing the appropriate terms from the list below.

1. The dentinal tubules are long tubes in the dentin that extend from the dentinoenamel junction in the crown area or dentinocemental junction in the root area to the outer wall of the pulp and are filled with

   _____.

2. The _____ is a long cellular extension located within the dentinal tubule that is still attached to the cell body of the odontoblast within the pulp.

3. Dentin that creates the wall of the dentinal tubule is the _____, which is highly mineralized after dentin maturation.

4. The dentin that is found between the tubules is the _____, which is highly mineralized but less so than peritubular dentin.

5. The _____ is the first predentin that forms and matures within the tooth near the dentinoenamel junction and underneath the enamel.

6. Deep to the mantle dentin is the layer of dentin around the outer wall of pulp, the _____, which makes up the bulk of the dentin in a tooth.

7. The _____ is formed in a tooth before the completion of the apical foramen or foramina of the root, which is the opening(s) in the root's pulp canal and is characterized by its regular pattern of dentinal tubules.

8. The secondary dentin is formed after the completion of the _____ or foramina and continues to form throughout the life of the tooth; it is formed more slowly than primary dentin and thus makes up less of the dentin in the tooth.

9. The _____ are a microscopic feature that appear as incremental lines or bands in a microscopic section of dentin; they are also similar to the incremental lines of Retzius noted in enamel.

10. The Tomes granular layer is a microscopic feature most often found in the peripheral part of dentin beneath the root's cementum, adjacent to the _____.

dentinocemental junction	circumpulpal dentin	apical foramen
mantle dentin	odontoblastic process	peritubular dentin
dentinal fluid	imbrication lines of von Ebner	primary dentin
intertubular dentin		

Reference   Chapter 13, Dentin and pulp. In Fehrenbach MJ, Popowics T: *Illustrated dental embryology, histology, and anatomy,* ed 5, St. Louis, 2020, Saunders.

FIGURE 3.10 Pulp within primary and permanent teeth (mesiodistal sections)

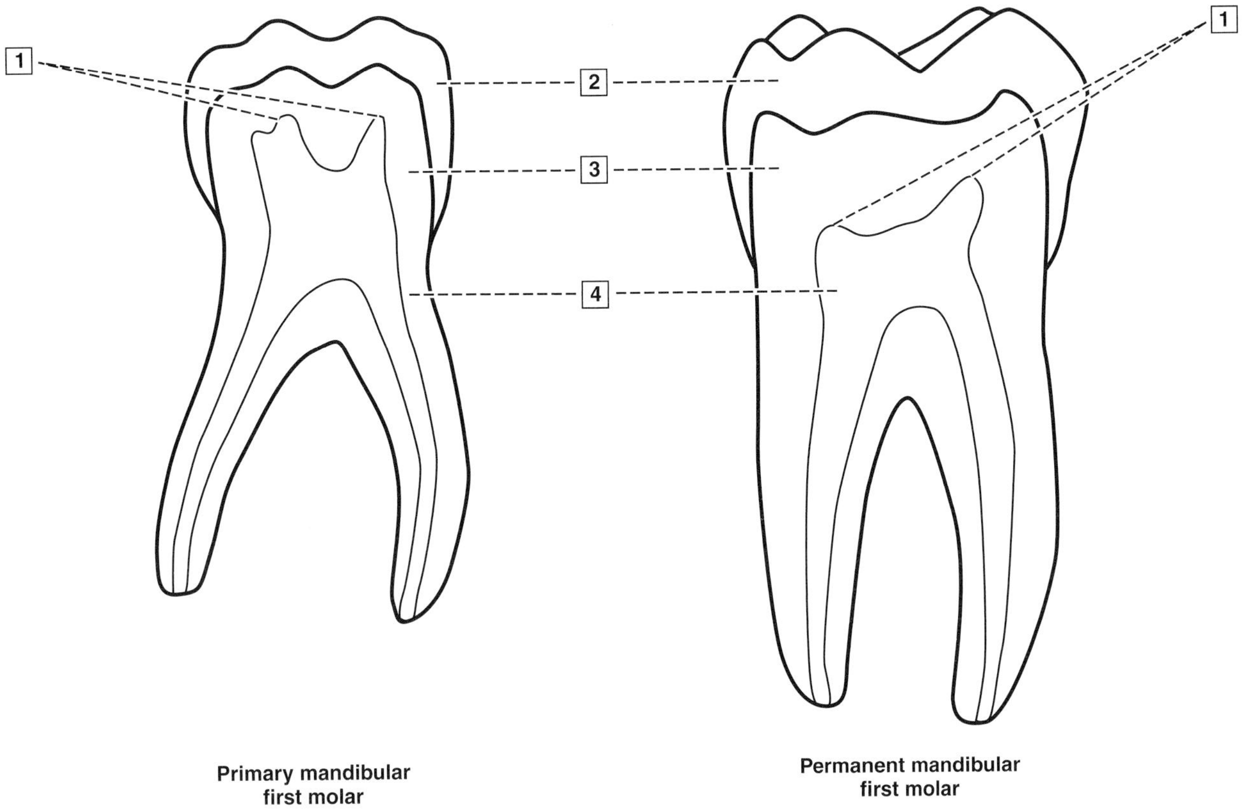
1
2
3
4
1
Primary mandibular first molar
Permanent mandibular first molar

1 Pulp horns
2 Enamel
3 Dentin
4 Pulp cavity

REVIEW QUESTIONS: Pulp within primary and permanent teeth

Fill in the blanks by choosing the appropriate terms from the list below.

1. The _____ is the innermost soft tissue of the tooth and appears radiolucent (or darker) because it is less dense than the radiopaque (or lighter) hard tissue of the tooth.

2. The pulp of a tooth is a connective tissue with all the components of such a tissue such as _____, fibers, and intercellular substance as well as tissue fluid, other cells, lymphatics, vascular system, and nerves.

3. The pulp forms from the _____ during tooth development.

4. The _____ on primary teeth shows that pulp chambers and pulp horns are relatively large in proportion to those of the permanent teeth, especially the mesial pulp horns of the molars.

5. The large mass of pulp is contained within the _____ of the tooth.

6. Smaller extensions of _____ into the cusps of posterior teeth form the pulp horns.

7. The _____ are especially prominent in the permanent dentition under the buccal cusp of premolars and in the primary dentition under the mesiobuccal cusp of molars; in contrast, pulp horns are not found on anterior teeth and all pulp horns recede with age.

8. Overall, the _____ of the primary dentition is thinner than that of the permanent counterparts; however, its thickness between the pulp chambers and the enamel is increased, especially in the primary mandibular second molar.

9. The _____ is relatively thin in comparison to permanent counterparts, but it has consistent thickness overlying the dentin of the crown.

10. The _____ teeth have a whiter tone of enamel on their crowns than the permanent teeth because of the increased opacity of the enamel that covers the underlying yellow dentin.

coronal pulp	pulp cavity	pulp chamber
enamel	central cells of the dental papilla	pulp
primary	pulp horns	fibroblasts
dentin		

References Chapter 13, Dentin and pulp. In Fehrenbach MJ, Popowics T: *Illustrated dental embryology, histology, and anatomy,* ed 5, St. Louis, 2020, Saunders; Chapter 18, Primary dentition. In Fehrenbach MJ, Popowics T: *Illustrated dental embryology, histology, and anatomy,* ed 5, St. Louis, 2020, Saunders.

NOTES

FIGURE 3.11 **Pulp with zones (mesiodistal section with microanatomic view)**

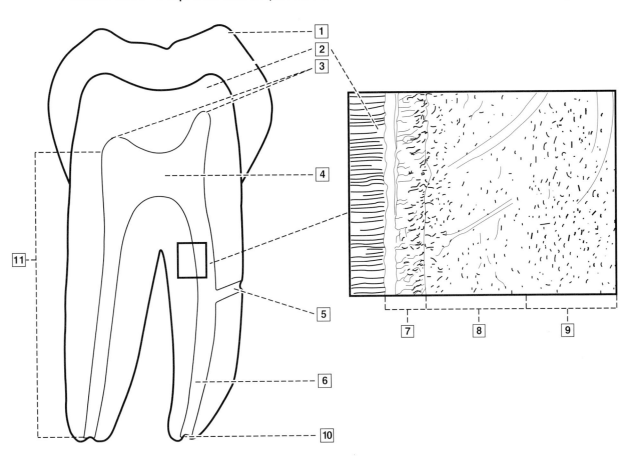

1 Enamel	**6** Radicular pulp within pulp canal
2 Dentin	**7** Odontoblastic layer
3 Pulp horns	**8** Cell-free zone
4 Coronal pulp	**9** Cell-rich zone
5 Accessory canal	**10** Apical foramen
	11 Pulp chamber

REVIEW QUESTIONS: Pulp with zones

Fill in the blanks by choosing the appropriate terms from the list below.

1. In addition to fibroblasts and odontoblasts, the pulp contains undifferentiated mesenchyme type of cells, _____.

2. The fibers present in the pulp are mostly _____ fibers and some reticular fibers since the pulp contains no elastic fibers.

3. The _____ is the part of the pulp located in the crown of the tooth.

4. The _____ (or root pulp) is that part of the pulp located in the root of the tooth within the pulp canal, which is also considered a "root canal" by patients.

5. The _____ is the opening from the pulp into the surrounding periodontal ligament near each apex of the tooth.

6. The _____ or *lateral canals* may be associated with the pulp and are extra openings from the pulp to the periodontal ligament because they are usually located on the lateral surface of the roots of the teeth but this is not always the case since they can be found anywhere along the root surface.

7. The first zone of pulp closest to the dentin is the odontoblastic layer that lines the outer pulpal wall and consists of a layer of the _____ of odontoblasts, whose odontoblastic processes are located in the dentinal tubules of the adjacent dentin.

8. The next zone, nearest to the odontoblastic layer and inward from the dentin, is considered the _____; in reality, this zone consists of fewer cells in contrast to the odontoblastic layer, but it is not entirely cell free.

9. The next zone after the cell-free zone is the _____, inward from dentin; this zone has an increased density of cells compared with the cell-free zone but still does not contain as many cells as the odontoblastic layer.

10. The zone of pulp that is in the center of the pulp chamber is the _____.

collagen	apical foramen	coronal pulp
radicular pulp	pulpal core	cell-free zone
cell-rich zone	accessory canals	cell bodies
dental pulp stem cells		

Reference Chapter 13, Dentin and pulp. In Fehrenbach MJ, Popowics T: *Illustrated dental embryology, histology, and anatomy*, ed 5, St. Louis, 2020, Saunders.

ANSWER KEY 1. dental pulp stem cells, 2. collagen, 3. coronal pulp, 4. radicular pulp, 5. apical foramen, 6. accessory canals, 7. cell bodies, 8. cell-free zone, 9. cell-rich zone, 10. pulpal core

FIGURE 3.12 Periodontium and dentin (mesiodistal section with microanatomic view)

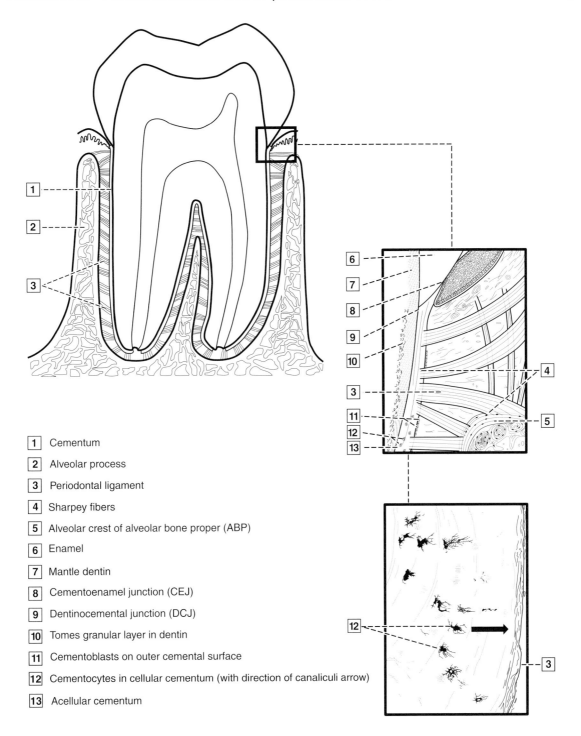

1. Cementum
2. Alveolar process
3. Periodontal ligament
4. Sharpey fibers
5. Alveolar crest of alveolar bone proper (ABP)
6. Enamel
7. Mantle dentin
8. Cementoenamel junction (CEJ)
9. Dentinocemental junction (DCJ)
10. Tomes granular layer in dentin
11. Cementoblasts on outer cemental surface
12. Cementocytes in cellular cementum (with direction of canaliculi arrow)
13. Acellular cementum

REVIEW QUESTIONS: Periodontium and dentin

Fill in the blanks by choosing the appropriate terms from the list below.

1. The periodontium includes the cementum, alveolar process, and _____.

2. The cementum is the part of the periodontium that attaches the teeth to the _____ by anchoring the periodontal ligament.

3. In a healthy situation, the cementum is not clinically visible because it usually covers the entire root, overlying _____ in dentin, a region that is not usually exposed in a healthy oral cavity.

4. Cementum is a hard tissue that is thickest at the tooth's apex or apices and in the interradicular areas of multirooted teeth and thinnest at the _____.

5. The _____ are collagen fibers from the periodontal ligament that are each partially inserted into the outer part of the cementum at 90° or perpendicular (as well as those in alveolar process).

6. After the appositional growth of cementum in layers, the _____ that do not become entrapped in cementum line up along the cemental surface for the entire length of the outer covering of the periodontal ligament so that they can form subsequent layers of cementum if the tooth is injured.

7. The _____ cementum consists of the first layers of cementum deposited at the dentinocemental junction and thus is also referred to as *primary cementum* and contains no embedded cementocytes.

8. The _____ cementum is sometimes referred to as *secondary cementum* because it is deposited later than primary type and thus many embedded cementocytes are found within it.

9. The _____ of the cementocytes within the lacunae are oriented toward the periodontal ligament and contain cementocytic processes that exist to diffuse nutrients from the vascularized periodontal ligament; however, cementocytes far away in the deeper layers may no longer be vital.

10. The width of cellular cementum can change during the life of the tooth, especially at the apex or apices of the tooth; this type of cementum is also common in _____ areas.

alveolar process	cellular	cementoenamel junction
Sharpey fibers	Tomes granular layer	interradicular
cementoblasts	periodontal ligament	cellular
canaliculi		

Reference Chapter 14, Periodontium. In Fehrenbach MJ, Popowics T: *Illustrated dental embryology, histology, and anatomy,* ed 5, St. Louis, 2020, Saunders.

FIGURE 3.13 Dentin and cementum with root development (microanatomic views)

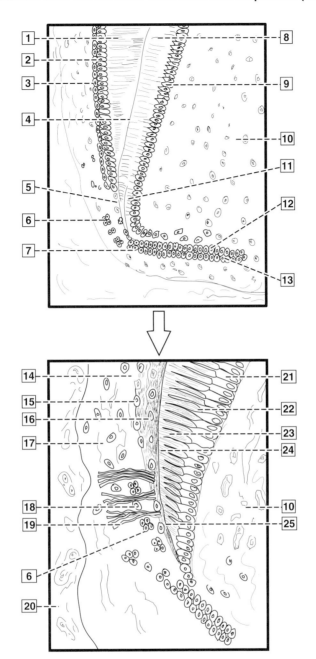

1 Enamel	**7** Disintegration of Hertwig epithelial root sheath
2 Ameloblasts	
3 Stratum intermedium	**8** Coronal dentin
4 Dentinoenamel junction (DEJ)	**9** Odontoblasts
5 Future cementoenamel junction (CEJ)	**10** Pulp
	11 Root dentin
6 Epithelial rests of Malassez	**12** Inner enamel epithelium (IEE)

13 Outer enamel epithelium (OEE)	**19** Formation of periodontal ligament
14 Cementum	**20** Developing alveolar process
15 Cementoblast	**21** Odontoblast
16 Cementocyte	**22** Predentin
17 Dental sac	**23** Root dentin
18 Dental sac cell becoming a cementoblast	**24** Dentinocemental junction (DCJ)
	25 Cementoid

REVIEW QUESTIONS: Dentin and cementum with root development

Fill in the blanks by choosing the appropriate terms from the list below.

1. The process of root development takes place long after the _____ is completely formed and the tooth is starting to erupt into the oral cavity.

2. The structure responsible for root development is the cervical loop, which is the most cervical part of the _____, a bilayer rim that consists of only inner enamel epithelium and outer enamel epithelium.

3. To form the root region, the cervical loop begins to grow deeper into the surrounding _____ of the dental sac, elongating and moving away from the newly completed crown area to enclose more of the dental papilla, forming the Hertwig epithelial root sheath.

4. The function of the _____ is to shape the root(s) by inducing dentin formation in the root so that it is continuous with coronal dentin.

5. After this disintegration of the Hertwig epithelial root sheath, its cells may become the _____; these groups after formation are then located in the mature periodontal ligament.

6. The _____ will produce the periodontium, the supporting tissue types of the tooth, including the cementum, as well as alveolar process and periodontal ligament during tooth development.

7. This disintegration of the Hertwig epithelial root sheath allows the undifferentiated cells of the dental sac to contact the newly formed surface of root dentin, which induces these cells to become immature _____.

8. The cementoblasts move to cover the root dentin area and undergo cementogenesis, laying down cementum matrix or _____.

9. Unlike ameloblasts and odontoblasts, which leave no cellular bodies in their secreted products, many cementoblasts become entrapped by the cementum they produce and become mature _____ in the later stages of appositional growth.

10. As a result of the appositional growth of cementum over the dentin, the _____ is formed in the area where the disintegrating basement membrane between the two tissue types was located.

cementoblasts	dentinocemental junction	ectomesenchyme
dental sac	crown	Hertwig epithelial root sheath
cementoid	enamel organ	cementocytes
epithelial rests of Malassez		

Reference   Chapter 6, Tooth development and eruption. In Fehrenbach MJ, Popowics T: *Illustrated dental embryology, histology, and anatomy,* ed 5, St. Louis, 2020, Saunders.

FIGURE 3.14 Reduced enamel epithelium formation (microanatomic views over new enamel surface)

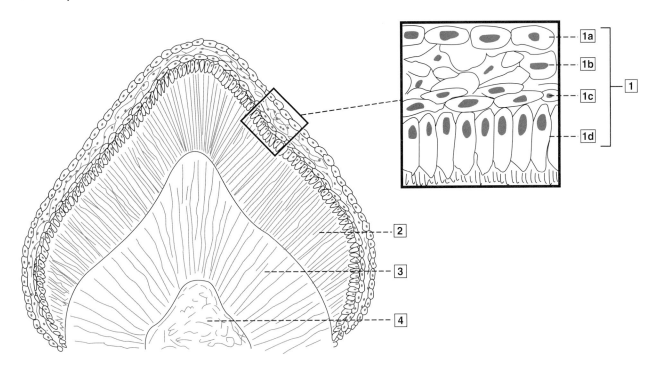

1	Compressed to form reduced enamel epithelium (REE)	**1d**	Ameloblasts
1a	Outer enamel epithelium (OEE)	**2**	Enamel
1b	Stellate reticulum	**3**	Dentin
1c	Stratum intermedium	**4**	Pulp

REVIEW QUESTIONS: Reduced enamel epithelium formation

Fill in the blanks by choosing the appropriate terms from the list below.

1. The _____ eruption of a primary tooth has many stages as the tooth moves into place in the alveolar process of each arch; this is not the same as passive eruption, which occurs with aging, when the gingival tissue recedes, uncovering the clinical root and increasing instead the size of the clinical crown, but no actual tooth movement takes place.

2. After enamel appositional growth ceases in the crown area of each primary or permanent tooth, the _____ place an acellular dental cuticle on the newly formed outer enamel surface.

3. During tooth development, the enamel organ consists of stellate reticulum, stratum intermedium, and _____, along with the ameloblasts from the inner enamel epithelium.

4. The layers of the enamel organ become compressed after enamel appositional growth ceases, forming the _____, which appears as a few layers of flattened cells overlying the enamel surface.

5. The external cells of the reduced enamel epithelium are mostly from the stratum intermedium cells but may also include cellular remnants of the stellate reticulum and outer enamel; thus these undifferentiated epithelial cells will divide and multiply and eventually give rise to the _____ of the tooth.

6. When this formation of the reduced enamel epithelium occurs for a primary tooth, it can then begin to _____ into the oral cavity.

7. To allow for the eruption process, the reduced enamel epithelium first must fuse with the _____ lining the oral cavity; second, enzymes from the epithelium then disintegrate the central part of the fused tissue, leaving a protective epithelial-lined eruption tunnel for the tooth to erupt through the surrounding oral epithelium into the oral cavity.

8. A residue, _____, may form on newly erupted teeth of both dentitions that may leave the teeth extrinsically stained green-gray; this residue consists of the fused tissue of the reduced enamel epithelium and oral epithelium, as well as the dental cuticle placed by the ameloblasts on the newly formed outer enamel surface.

9. Nasmyth membrane easily picks up coloring from food debris but can be removed by _____.

10. With the _____ forming before the root, prevention of traumatic injury to the permanent teeth before they are fully anchored into the jaws is very important.

erupt | reduced enamel epithelium | ameloblasts
Nasmyth membrane | initial junctional epithelium | active
selective polishing | oral epithelium | outer enamel epithelium
crown

Reference Chapter 6, Tooth development and eruption. In Fehrenbach MJ, Popowics T: *Illustrated dental embryology, histology, and anatomy*, ed 5, St. Louis, 2020, Saunders.

FIGURE 3.15   Tooth eruption (microanatomic views)

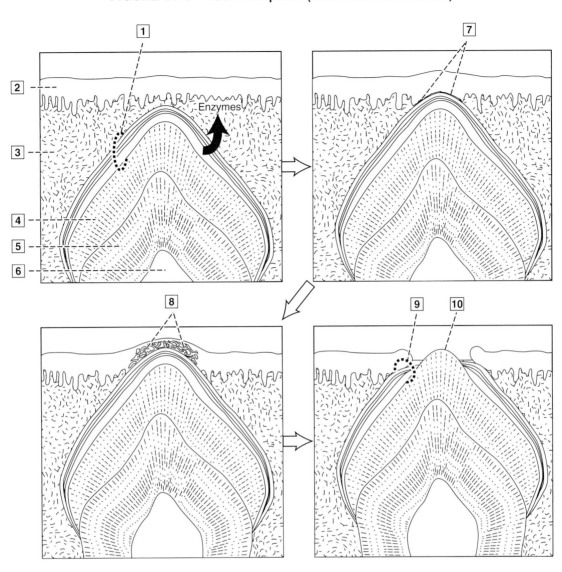

Enzymes

1	Reduced enamel epithelium (REE)	6	Pulp
2	Oral epithelium	7	Fusion of tissue
3	Connective tissue	8	Area of tissue disintegration
4	Enamel	9	Initial junctional epithelium (JE)
5	Dentin	10	Tip of erupting tooth

REVIEW QUESTIONS: Tooth eruption

Fill in the blanks by choosing the appropriate terms from the list below.

1. To allow for the eruption process, the reduced enamel epithelium first must undergo _____ with the oral epithelium lining the oral cavity.

2. Second, the enzymes from the reduced enamel epithelium disintegrate the central part of the fused tissue, leaving a protective epithelial-lined _____ for the tooth to erupt through the surrounding oral epithelium into the oral cavity.

3. The tissue _____ during the eruption process causes the usually present inflammatory response known as "teething," which may be accompanied by tenderness and edema of the local tissue.

4. Instituting thorough homecare can reduce the amount of _____ and thus most of the discomfort associated with these oral changes in infants as their first teeth erupt as well as in young adults when their third molars erupt.

5. Panoramic radiographs of the _____ are important in order to monitor tooth development.

6. A permanent tooth often starts to erupt before the _____ tooth is fully shed, possibly creating problems in spacing but interceptive orthodontic therapy can prevent some of these situations.

7. As a primary tooth actively erupts, the coronal part of the fused epithelial tissue peels off the crown, leaving the cervical part still attached to the neck of the tooth, which can then serve as the initial _____ of the tooth, creating a seal between the tissue and the tooth surface.

8. The initial junctional epithelium of the tooth is replaced by a definitive junctional epithelium as the _____ becomes completely formed.

9. The process of eruption for a succedaneous permanent tooth is the same as for the primary tooth after the widening of the _____.

10. The process of the _____ permanent tooth's eruption is similar to that of a succedaneous one, but no primary tooth is shed to allow for the process as with the succedaneous permanent teeth.

eruption tunnel	inflammation	disintegration
root	gubernacular canal	primary
nonsuccedaneous	fusion	junctional epithelium
mixed dentition		

Reference   Chapter 6, Tooth development and eruption. In Fehrenbach MJ, Popowics T: *Illustrated dental embryology, histology, and anatomy,* ed 5, St. Louis, 2020, Saunders.

FIGURE 3.16   **Permanent dentition development (section of fetal mandible)**

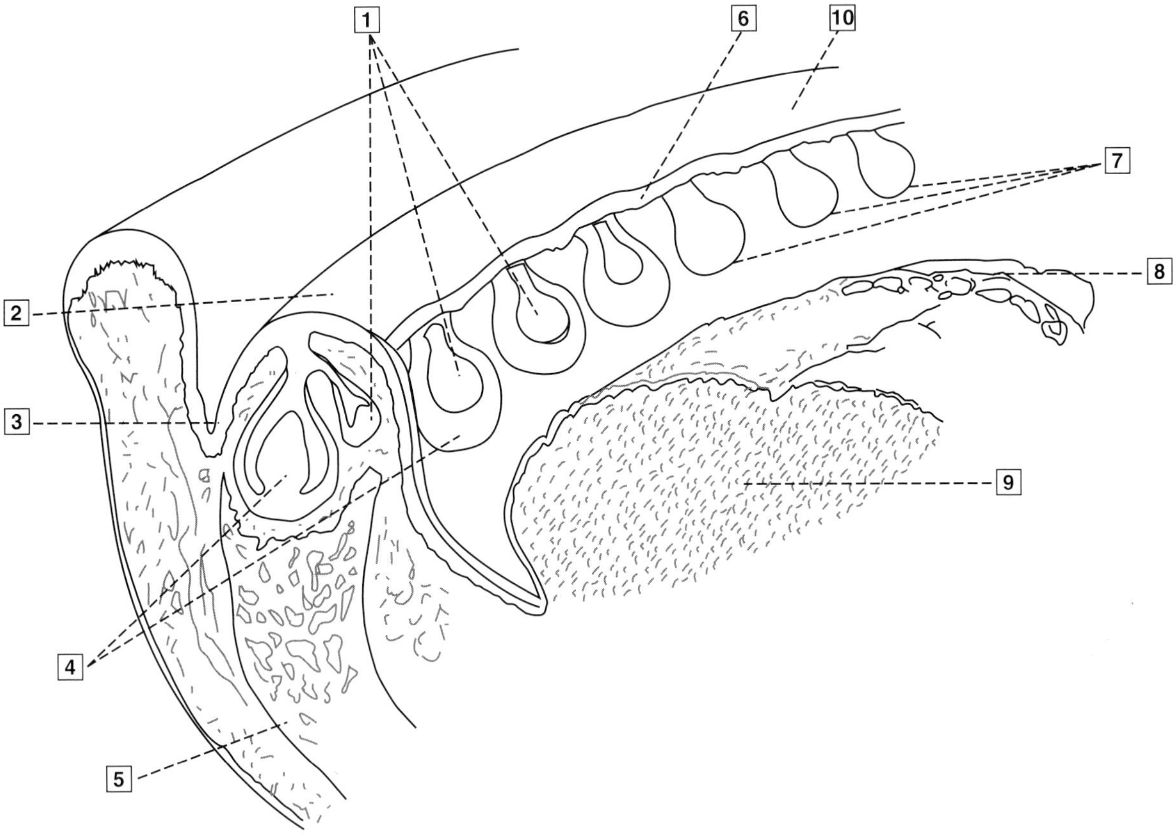

1	Successional dental lamina of permanent teeth primordia	
2	Developing mandibular dental arch	
3	Vestibule	
4	Developing primary teeth	
5	Developing mandible	
6	Oral epithelium (cut to show tooth buds)	
7	Tooth germs of nonsuccedaneous permanent molars	
8	Base of tongue	
9	Body of tongue	
10	Posterior extension of dental lamina	

REVIEW QUESTIONS: Permanent dentition development

Fill in the blanks by choosing the appropriate terms from the list below.

1. To allow for the eruption process, the _____ first must fuse with the oral epithelium lining the oral cavity.

2. When the primary tooth is shed, the succedaneous permanent tooth develops _____ to it.

3. The process involving shedding of the primary tooth consists of differentiation of multinucleated _____ from fused macrophages of the surrounding area, which absorb the alveolar process between the two teeth from their *ruffled borders*.

4. The _____ are formed from undifferentiated mesenchyme; these cells cause mostly primary root resorption with removal of dentin and cementum.

5. Special fibroblasts, now considered _____, destroy any remaining collagen fibers holding the primary tooth within the surrounding periodontal ligament during the shedding process of the primary dentition.

6. The _____ develops only after root formation has been initiated; when established, it must be remodeled to accommodate continued eruptive tooth movement.

7. The process of shedding the primary tooth is intermittent ("tight/loose"), because at the same time that osteoclasts differentiate to resorb bone and odontoblasts differentiate to resorb dental tissue, the always ready _____ and cementoblasts work to replace the resorbed parts of the root as well as the fibroblasts to repair the periodontal ligament.

8. The succedaneous permanent tooth usually erupts into the oral cavity in a position lingual to the roots of the shedding _____ tooth, just as it develops that way.

9. The only exception to the lingual eruption placement is the permanent _____, which move to a more facially placed position as they erupt into the oral cavity.

10. Both succedaneous and nonsuccedaneous permanent teeth erupt in _____ order.

reduced enamel epithelium	osteoclasts	primary
fibroclasts	periodontal ligament	maxillary incisors
lingual	eruption	chronologic
odontoclasts		

Reference Chapter 6, Tooth development and eruption. In Fehrenbach MJ, Popowics T: *Illustrated dental embryology, histology, and anatomy,* ed 5, St. Louis, 2020, Saunders.

FIGURE 3.17   **Multirooted tooth development (apical and cross section views)**

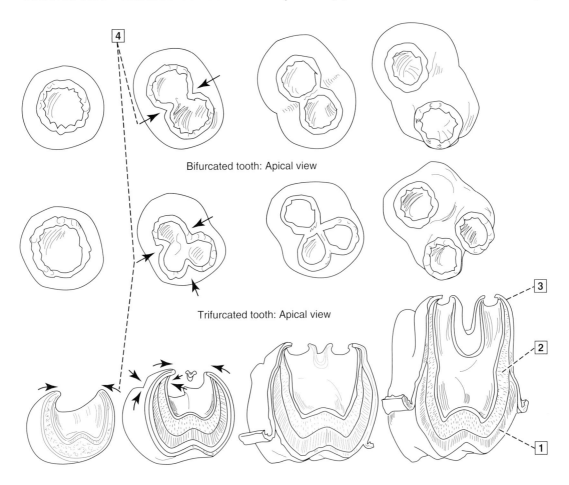

Bifurcated tooth: Apical view

Trifurcated tooth: Apical view

Trifurcated tooth: Cross section

1	Enamel
2	Dentin
3	Pulp
4	Horizontal extensions of cervical loop (arrows)

REVIEW QUESTIONS: Multirooted tooth development

Fill in the blanks by choosing the appropriate terms from the list below.

1. Like anterior teeth, multirooted premolars and molars originate as a _____ on the base of the crown, with this part of the posterior teeth considered the *root trunk*.

2. The cervical cross section of the _____ initially follows the form of the crown; however, the root of a posterior tooth divides from the root trunk into the correct number of root branches for its tooth type.

3. Differential growth of _____ causes the root trunk of the multirooted teeth to divide into two or three roots.

4. During the formation of the enamel organ on a multirooted tooth, elongation of its _____ occurs, which allows the development of long tongue-like horizontal epithelial extensions or flaps within it.

5. Two or three epithelial extensions or flaps can be present on multirooted teeth from the elongation of the cervical loop, depending on the similar number of _____ on the mature tooth.

6. The usually single cervical opening of the coronal _____ is divided into two or three openings by these horizontal extensions from the cervical loop to produce the correct number of roots.

7. On the pulpal surfaces of these openings that correspond to each root, dentin formation starts after the induction of the odontoblasts and _____ of Hertwig epithelial root sheath and the associated basement membrane.

8. The _____ are induced to form cementum on the newly formed dentin only at the periphery of each opening on the pulpal surface corresponding to each root needed.

9. The molars of the _____ of the permanent dentition usually have three roots.

10. The molars of the _____ of the permanent dentition usually have two roots.

disintegration	cervical loop	enamel organ
maxillary arch	single root	cementoblasts
roots	root trunk	mandibular arch
Hertwig epithelial root sheath		

Reference Chapter 6, Tooth development and eruption. In Fehrenbach MJ, Popowics T: *Illustrated dental embryology, histology, and anatomy,* ed 5, St. Louis, 2020, Saunders.

NOTES

FIGURE 3.18 Alveolar process (microanatomic view)

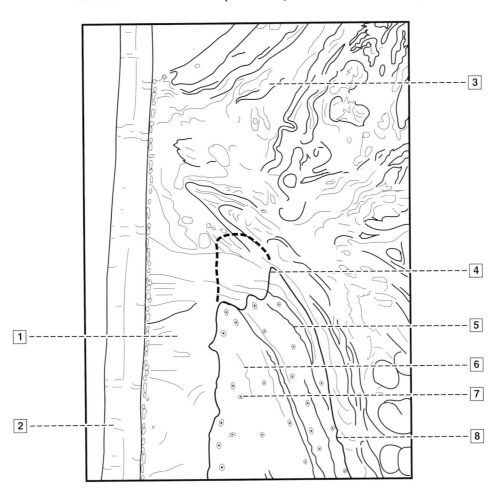

1	Periodontal ligament	**5**	Arrest line
2	Cementum	**6**	Reversal line
3	Gingiva	**7**	Osteocyte in lacuna
4	Alveolar crest with slight resorption (dashed line)	**8**	Howship lacuna

REVIEW QUESTIONS: Alveolar process

Fill in the blanks by choosing the appropriate terms from the list below.

1. The _____ is that part of either the maxillae or mandible that supports and protects the teeth.

2. The alveolar process is that part of the periodontium in which the cementum of the tooth is attached to it through the _____.

3. The _____ is the lining of the tooth socket or alveolus; although it is composed of compact bone, it may also be referred to as the *cribriform plate* because it contains numerous holes where Volkmann canals with its nerves and blood vessels pass from it into the periodontal ligament.

4. The _____ is the most cervical rim of the alveolar bone proper; the alveolar crests of neighboring teeth are also uniform in height along the jaw.

5. The _____ consists of both cortical bone and trabecular bone; the cortical bone consists of a plate of compact bone on both the facial and lingual surfaces of the alveolar process and can also be described as the *cortical plate*.

6. The cell body of the osteocyte is surrounded by bone, except for the space immediately around it, the _____.

7. Within fully mineralized bone are osteocytes, which are entrapped mature osteoblasts; the cytoplasmic processes of the osteocytes radiate outward in all directions in the bone and are located in tubular canals of matrix or _____.

8. The appositional growth, with layered formation of bone along its periphery, is accomplished by the _____, which later become entrapped as osteocytes.

9. The _____ or *resting lines* appear as smooth lines between the layers of bone because of osteoblasts having rested, formed bone, and then rested again after appositional growth, showing the incremental or layered nature of appositional growth.

10. The _____ appear as scalloped lines between the layers of bone showing where bone resorption by osteoclasts has first taken place, followed quickly by appositional growth of new bone.

osteoblasts	alveolar crest	canaliculi
lacuna	alveolar process	periodontal ligament
reversal lines	alveolar bone proper	arrest lines
supporting alveolar bone		

References   Chapter 8, Basic tissue. In Fehrenbach MJ, Popowics T: *Illustrated dental embryology, histology, and anatomy,* ed 5, St. Louis, 2020, Saunders; Chapter 14, Periodontium. In Fehrenbach MJ, Popowics T: *Illustrated dental embryology, histology, and anatomy,* ed 5, St. Louis, 2020, Saunders.

FIGURE 3.19 Periodontal ligament and alveolar process (mesiodistal section)

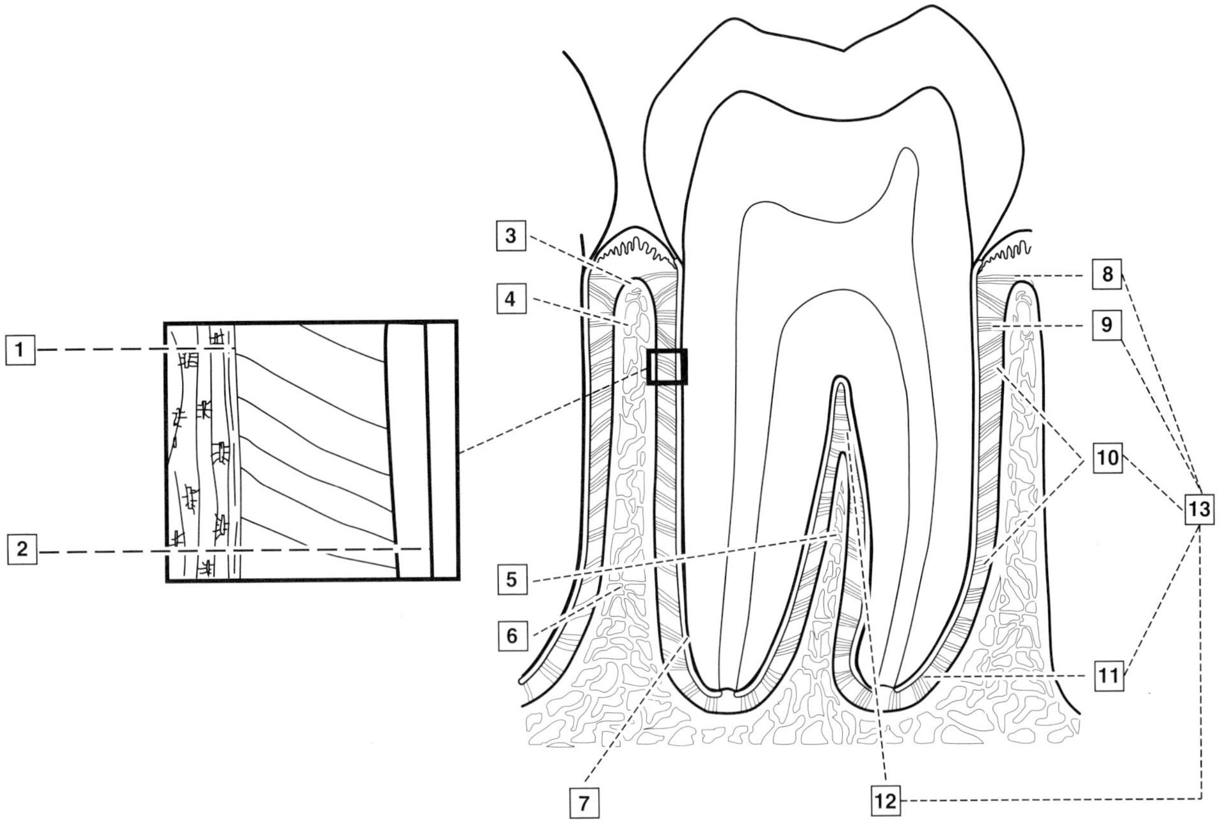

1 Sharpey fibers within alveolar bone proper (ABP)	**8** Alveolar crest group
2 Sharpey fibers within cementum	**9** Horizontal group
3 Alveolar crest	**10** Oblique group
4 Alveolar bone proper (ABP)	**11** Apical group
5 Interradicular septum	**12** Interradicular group
6 Interdental septum	**13** Alveolodental ligament
7 Cementum	

REVIEW QUESTIONS: Periodontal ligament and alveolar process

Fill in the blanks by choosing the appropriate terms from the list below.

1. The _____ consists of cancellous bone (or spongy bone) that is located between the alveolar bone proper and the plates of cortical bone.

2. The alveolar process between two neighboring teeth is the _____; it consists of both the compact bone of the alveolar bone proper and cancellous bone of the trabecular bone.

3. The alveolar process between roots is the _____; it consists of both alveolar bone proper and trabecular bone.

4. The alveolar bone proper consists of plates of compact bone that surround the tooth and assume the shape of the tooth; a part of the alveolar bone proper is seen on radiographs as the _____, which is uniformly radiopaque (or lighter).

5. The ends of the principal fibers that are within either cementum or alveolar bone proper are considered _____.

6. The main principal fiber group is the _____, which consists of five fiber subgroups, the alveolar crest, horizontal, oblique, apical, and interradicular groups on multirooted teeth.

7. The _____ of the alveolodental ligament is attached to the cementum just below the cementoenamel junction and runs in an inferior and outward direction to insert into the alveolar crest of the alveolar bone proper.

8. The horizontal group of the alveolodental ligament function to resist _____ forces, which work to force the tooth to tip mesially, distally, lingually, or facially, and to resist rotational forces; it is located just apical to the alveolar crest subgroup and runs at 90° to the long axis of the tooth from cementum to the alveolar bone proper, just inferior to its alveolar crest.

9. The _____ of the alveolodental ligament is the most numerous of the fiber subgroups and covers the apical two-thirds of the root, with this subgroup running from the cementum in an oblique direction to insert into the alveolar bone proper more coronally; its function is to resist intrusive forces, which try to push the tooth inward as well as rotational forces.

10. The function of the apical group of the alveolodental ligament is to resist _____ forces, which try to pull the tooth in an outward manner, and rotational forces; it radiates from the cementum around the apex of the root to the surrounding alveolar bone proper, forming the base of the alveolus.

lamina dura	tilting	Sharpey fibers
interradicular septum	interdental bone	oblique group
extrusive	alveolar crest group	alveolodental ligament
trabecular bone		

Reference   Chapter 14, Periodontium. In Fehrenbach MJ, Popowics T: *Illustrated dental embryology, histology, and anatomy,* ed 5, St. Louis, 2020, Saunders.

FIGURE 3.20   Interdental ligament (facial tooth surface with mesiodistal section)

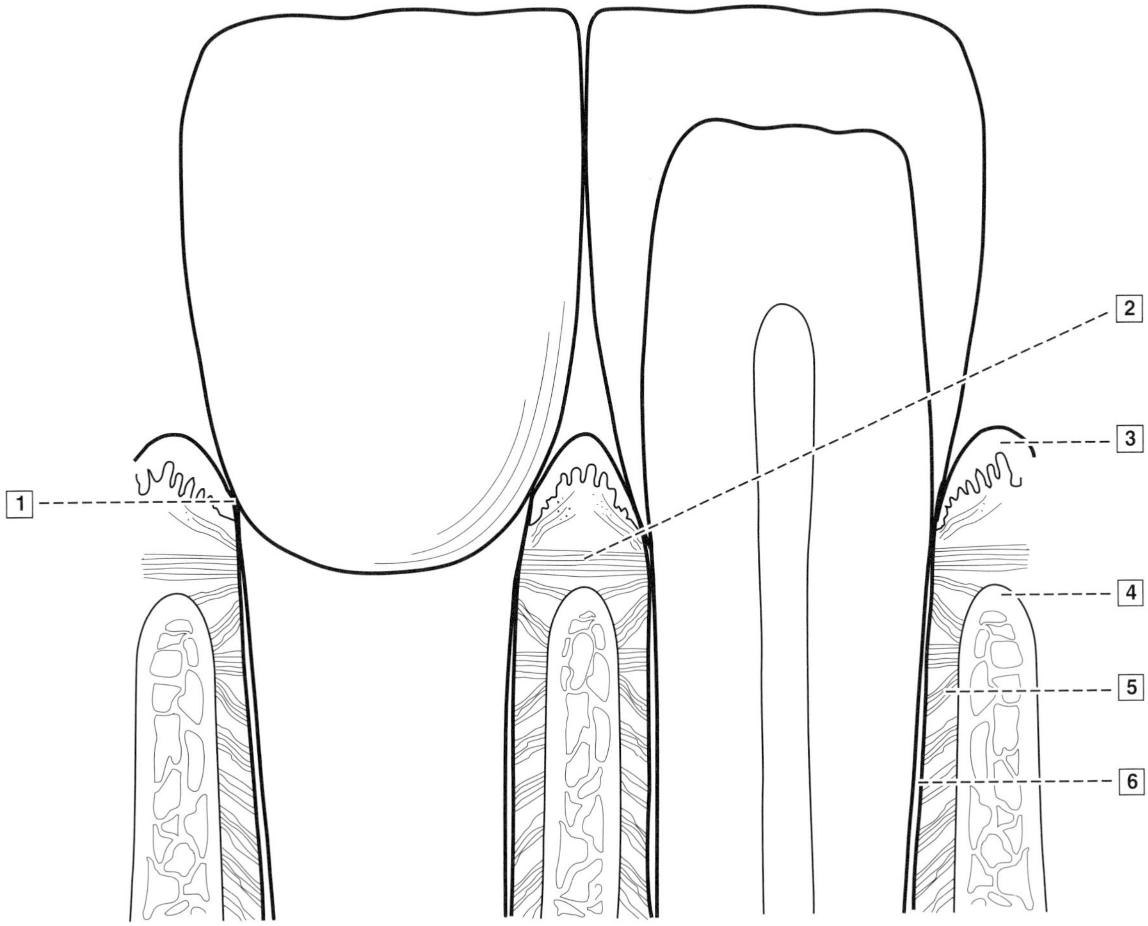

1 Cementoenamel junction (CEJ)

2 Interdental ligament

3 Interdental papilla

4 Alveolar crest

5 Alveolodental ligament

6 Cementum

REVIEW QUESTIONS: Interdental ligament

Fill in the blanks by choosing the appropriate terms from the list below.

1. The periodontal ligament appears on radiographs as the _____, which is a radiolucent (or darker) area located between the denser radiopaque (or lighter) lamina dura of the alveolar bone proper and the similar radiopaque (or lighter) of the cementum.

2. The _____ are not found as individual fibers within the periodontal ligament but are organized into groups or bundles according to their orientation to the mature tooth and related function.

3. The interdental ligament (or transseptal ligament) inserts _____ or interdentally into the cervical cementum of neighboring teeth.

4. The interdental ligament is at a height coronal to the _____ of the alveolar bone proper.

5. The interdental ligament is at a height apical to the base of the _____.

6. The interdental ligament's fibers travel from cementum to cementum without any attachment to the
_____.

7. The interdental ligament helps to hold the teeth in _____.

8. The _____ connects all the teeth of each arch, both maxillary and mandibular.

9. The function of the interdental ligament is to resist _____ or twisting of the tooth in its alveolus.

10. The fibers that are inserted from the interdental ligament into both cementum and alveolar process are considered _____.

principal fibers	junctional epithelium	interproximal contact
periodontal ligament space	Sharpey fibers	interdental ligament
alveolar crest	alveolar process	rotational forces
mesiodentally		

Reference Chapter 14, Periodontium. In Fehrenbach MJ, Popowics T: *Illustrated dental embryology, histology, and anatomy,* ed 5, St. Louis, 2020, Saunders.

NOTES

FIGURE 3.21 Gingival fiber group (interproximal view and labiolingual section)

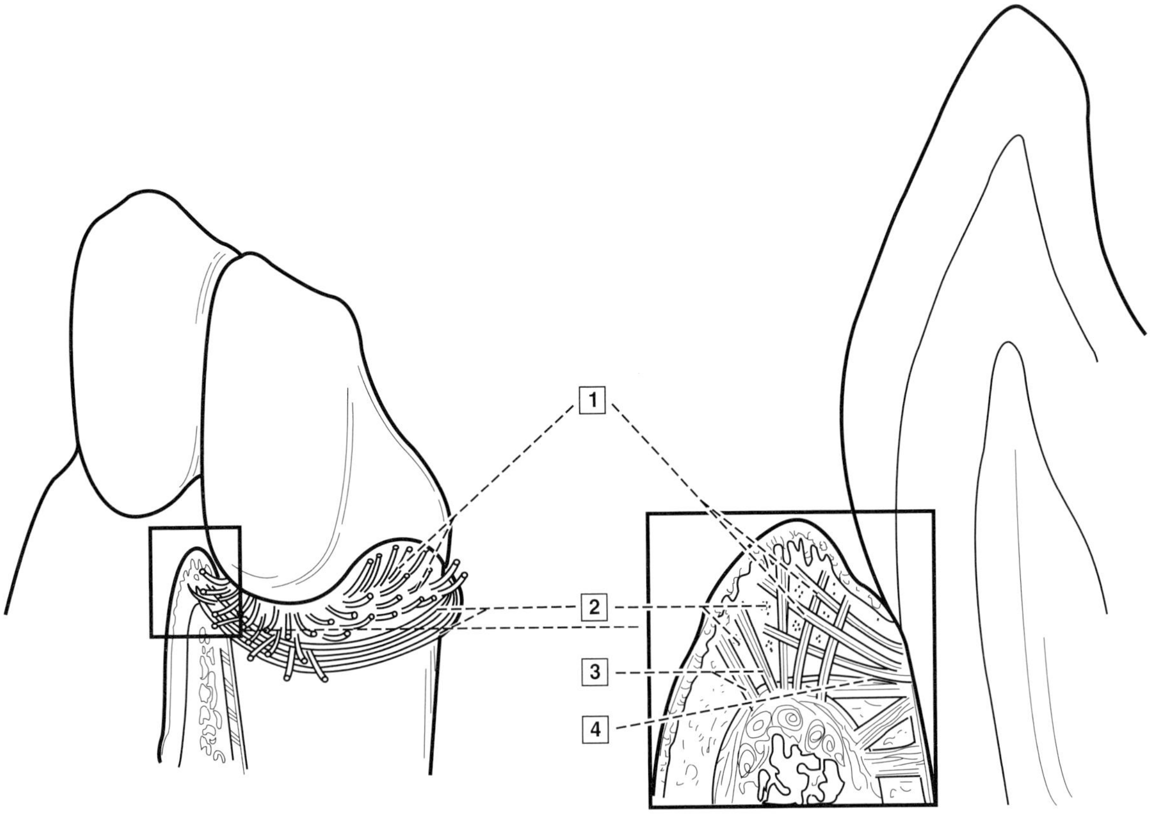

1 Dentogingival ligament
2 Circular ligament
3 Alveologingival ligament
4 Dentoperiosteal ligament

REVIEW QUESTIONS: Gingival fiber group

Fill in the blanks by choosing the appropriate terms from the list below.

1. The _____ is considered by some histologists to be part of the principal fibers of the periodontal ligament.

2. The gingival fiber group is a separate but adjacent group to the _____ and interdental ligament.

3. The gingival fiber group is found within the _____ of the marginal gingiva.

4. The gingival fiber group does not support the tooth in relation to the jaw, resisting any forces of mastication or speech; instead, it supports only the _____ in an effort to maintain its relationship to the tooth.

5. The _____ of the gingival fiber group encircles the tooth as shown on a cross section of a tooth, interlacing with the other gingival fiber subgroups.

6. The dentogingival ligament is the most extensive of the gingival fiber group as it inserts in the cementum on the root apical to the _____ and extends into the lamina propria of the marginal and attached gingiva; thus it has only one mineralized attachment to the cementum.

7. The dentogingival ligament works with the circular ligament to maintain _____, mostly of the marginal gingiva.

8. The _____ radiates from the alveolar crest of the alveolar bone proper and extends coronally into the overlying lamina propria of the marginal gingiva.

9. The alveologingival ligament helps to attach the gingiva to the _____ because of its one mineralized attachment to bone.

10. The _____ runs from the cementum near the cementoenamel junction and then across the alveolar crest to anchor the tooth to the bone and protect the deeper periodontal ligament.

circular ligament	epithelial attachment	alveolar process
dentoperiosteal ligament	gingival fiber group	alveolodental ligament
marginal gingiva	lamina propria	gingival integrity
alveologingival ligament		

Reference   Chapter 14, Periodontium. In Fehrenbach MJ, Popowics T: *Illustrated dental embryology, histology, and anatomy,* ed 5, St. Louis, 2020, Saunders.

NOTES

FIGURE 3.22 Primary dentition chart (occlusal view with facial and lingual views)

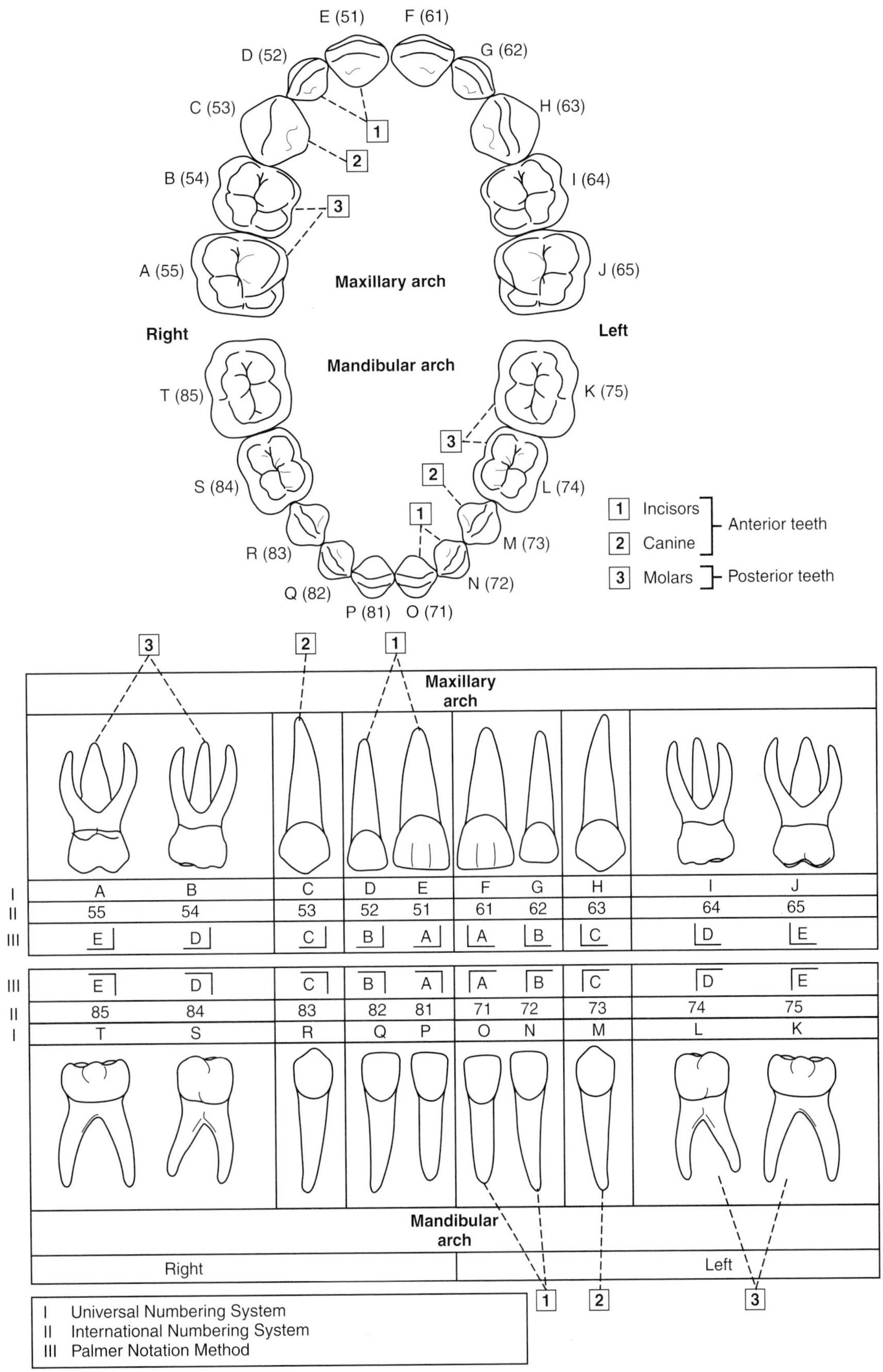
E (51)
F (61)
D (52)
G (62)
C (53)
H (63)
B (54)
I (64)
A (55)
J (65)
1
2
3
Maxillary arch
Right
Left
Mandibular arch
T (85)
K (75)
S (84)
L (74)
R (83)
M (73)
Q (82)
N (72)
P (81)
O (71)
1 Incisors
2 Canine
Anterior teeth
3 Molars
Posterior teeth
Maxillary arch
I: A B C D E F G H I J
II: 55 54 53 52 51 61 62 63 64 65
III: E D C B A A B C D E
III: E D C B A A B C D E
II: 85 84 83 82 81 71 72 73 74 75
I: T S R Q P O N M L K
Mandibular arch
Right
Left
I Universal Numbering System
II International Numbering System
III Palmer Notation Method

REVIEW QUESTIONS: Primary dentition

Fill in the blanks by choosing the appropriate terms from the list below.

1. The tooth types of both arches within the primary dentition, which is also termed the
_____ dentition, include eight incisors, four canines, and eight molars, for a total
of 20 teeth.

2. It is important to note that only the permanent dentition has premolars; in contrast, the primary dentition
does not have _____.

3. The _____ function as instruments for biting and cutting food during mastication
because of their triangular proximal form.

4. The _____ because of their tapered shape and their prominent cusp function to pierce
or tear food during mastication.

5. As the teeth with the largest and strongest crowns, the _____ function in grinding food
during mastication, assisted by the premolars.

6. It is the wide masticatory surface, the occlusal surface of the molars with their prominent
_____, that also help with mastication.

7. Both the primary teeth and the permanent teeth can be designated by either letters or numbers using the
_____.

8. With the Universal Numbering System, the primary teeth are designated from each other in a consecutive
arrangement by using capital letters, *A* through *T*, starting with the maxillary right second molar, moving
_____ and ending with the mandibular right second molar.

9. Another tooth designation system that is commonly used during orthodontic therapy is the
_____, which is also known as the *Military Numbering System*.

10. Within the Palmer Notation Method, the teeth are designated from each other with a right-angle symbol
indicating the _____ and arch, with the tooth number inside.

molars	Universal Numbering System	canines
Palmer Notation Method	cusps	quadrants
deciduous	clockwise	premolars
incisors		

Reference Chapter 15, Overview of dentitions. In Fehrenbach MJ, Popowics T: *Illustrated dental embryology, histology, and anatomy,* ed 5, St. Louis, 2020, Saunders.

FIGURE 3.23   Permanent dentition chart (occlusal view with facial and lingual views)

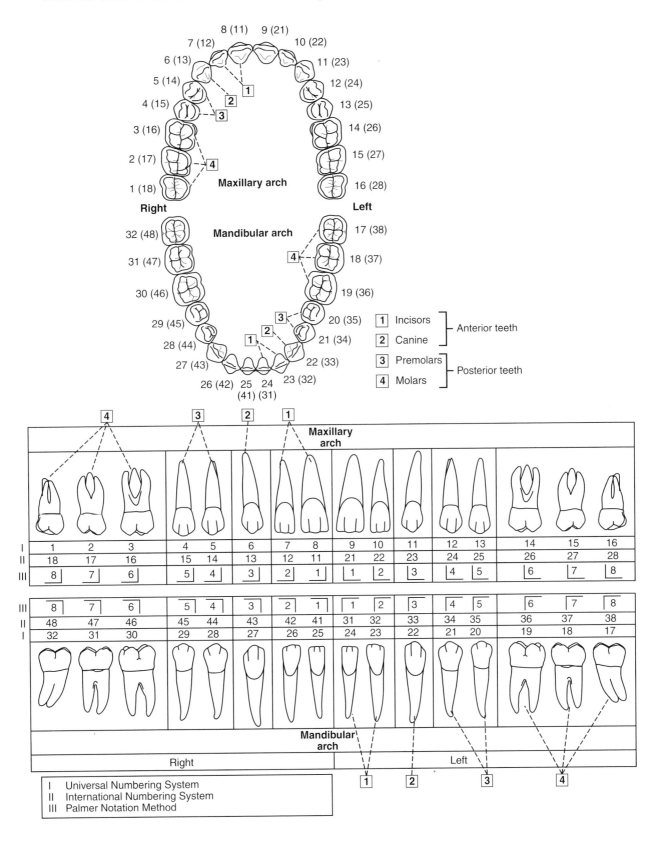

REVIEW QUESTIONS: Permanent dentition

Fill in the blanks by choosing the appropriate terms from the list below.

1. The tooth types of both dental arches within the permanent dentition, which is also called the _____ dentition, include 8 incisors, 4 canines, 8 premolars, and 12 molars, for a total of 32 teeth.

2. Note that only the permanent dentition has _____; in contrast, the primary dentition does not have this tooth type.

3. The premolars, which are found only during the permanent dentition period, function to assist the _____ in grinding food during mastication because of the crown's wide masticatory surface, the occlusal surface.

4. The premolars assist the _____ in piercing and tearing food because of prominent cusps of their crowns during mastication.

5. As the teeth with the largest and strongest crowns, the molars function in grinding food during _____, as assisted by the premolars.

6. The molars of the permanent dentition are _____ because they are without any primary predecessors.

7. Only the anterior teeth and premolars of the permanent dentition are _____ because they have primary predecessors.

8. The permanent teeth are designated from each other by the _____, in a consecutive arrangement as observed from the front and using the digits 1 through 32, starting with the maxillary right third molar, moving clockwise and ending with the mandibular right third molar.

9. The _____ as instituted by the International Standards Organization and World Health Organization has the teeth designated from each other by using a two-digit code with the first digit of the code indicating the quadrant and the second indicating the toot's position in this quadrant.

10. Using the International Numbering System, the second digit, which indicates the tooth, the digits *1* through *8* are used for the permanent teeth, with this designation using the _____ and numbering in a distal direction.

Universal Numbering System	International Numbering System	midline
molars	secondary	mastication
nonsuccedaneous	succedaneous	canines
premolars		

Reference Chapter 15, Overview of dentitions. In Fehrenbach MJ, Popowics T: *Illustrated dental embryology, histology, and anatomy,* ed 5, St. Louis, 2020, Saunders.

FIGURE 3.24   Orientational tooth surface terms

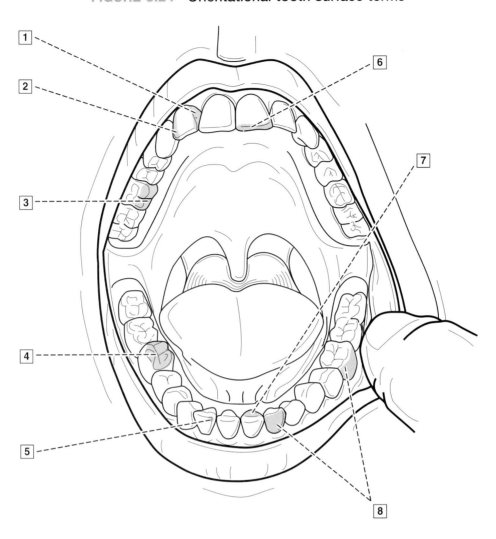

1 Mesial surface		**5** Proximal surface with contact area
2 Distal surface		**6** Incisal surface
3 Palatal surface		**7** Lingual surface
4 Occlusal surface		**8** Facial surfaces: labial surface and buccal surface

REVIEW QUESTIONS: Orientational tooth surface terms

Fill in the blanks by choosing the appropriate terms from the list below.

1. The tooth surface closest to the surface of the face is _____.

2. The facial tooth surfaces closest to the lips are _____.

3. The facial tooth surfaces closest to the inner cheek are _____.

4. The tooth surfaces closest to the _____ are lingual.

5. Those lingual surfaces closest to the palate on the maxillary arch are sometimes also considered
   _____.

6. The _____ surface is the chewing surface on the most superior surface of the crown;
   it is the incisal surface for anterior teeth.

7. The masticatory surface is the chewing surface on the most superior surface of the crown; it is the
   _____ surface for posterior teeth.

8. The surface closest to the _____ is mesial.

9. The surface farthest away from the midline is _____.

10. Either the mesial or the distal surfaces between adjacent teeth are considered _____.

midline	facial	palatal
distal	labial	occlusal
masticatory	buccal	proximal
tongue		

Reference Chapter 15, Overview of dentitions. In Fehrenbach MJ, Popowics T: *Illustrated dental embryology, histology, and anatomy,* ed 5, St. Louis, 2020, Saunders.

NOTES

FIGURE 3.25 **Embrasures of teeth**

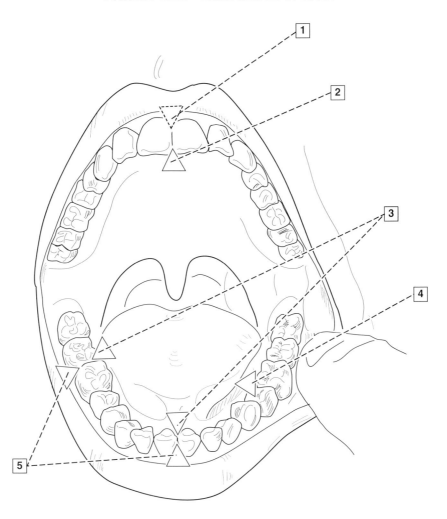

1 Apical embrasure (with loss of tissue)

2 Incisal embrasure

3 Lingual embrasures

4 Occlusal embrasure

5 Facial embrasures

REVIEW QUESTIONS: Embrasures of teeth

Fill in the blanks by choosing the appropriate terms from the list below.

1. When two teeth in the same arch come into contact, their curvatures next to the contact areas form spaces considered _____; these consist of triangular-shaped spaces between two teeth, created by the sloping away of the mesial and distal surfaces and may diverge facially, lingually, occlusally, or apically with loss of tissue.

2. The embrasures are continuous with the _____ between the teeth and there is an increasing angle of the occlusal embrasures anteroposteriorly.

3. The embrasures form _____ between teeth to direct food away from the gingiva.

4. The embrasures also provide a mechanism for teeth to be more _____.

5. The embrasures also protect the _____ from undue frictional trauma but still provide the proper degree of stimulation to the tissue.

6. The area where the crowns of adjacent teeth in the same arch physically touch each adjacent proximal surface is the _____.

7. The _____ or *crest of curvature* is the greatest elevation of the tooth either incisocervically or occlusocervically on a specific surface of the crown when viewing its profile from the labial or buccal and the lingual.

8. It is noted when viewing teeth overall that the proximal _____ curvature is greatest on the anterior teeth and the least on the posterior teeth.

9. The cementoenamel junction curvature is approximately similar on _____ and distal surfaces of the two teeth that face each other.

10. On any given tooth, the height of the cementoenamel junction curvature is greater on the mesial aspect of that tooth than it is on the _____.

gingiva	contact area	interproximal spaces
spillways	self-cleansing	cementoenamel junction
mesial	embrasures	distal
height of contour		

Reference Chapter 15, Overview of dentitions. In Fehrenbach MJ, Popowics T: *Illustrated dental embryology, histology, and anatomy,* ed 5, St. Louis, 2020, Saunders.

FIGURE 3.26   Maxillary right central incisor (lingual, labial, and incisal views)

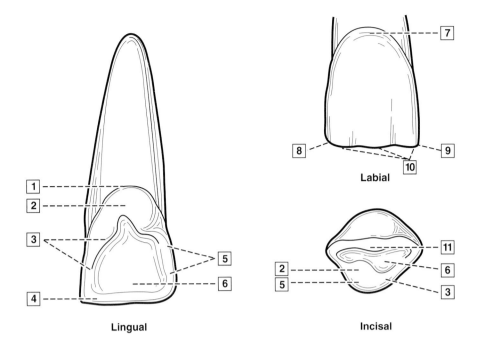

Lingual

Labial

Incisal

1	Cementoenamel junction	7	Imbrication lines
2	Cingulum	8	Distoincisal angle
3	Mesial marginal ridge	9	Mesioincisal angle
4	Linguoincisal ridge	10	Mamelons
5	Distal marginal ridge	11	Incisal ridge
6	Lingual fossa		

REVIEW QUESTIONS: Maxillary central incisor

Fill in the blanks by choosing the appropriate terms from the list below.

1. The permanent maxillary central incisors erupt between 7 and 8 years of age with root completion at age 10, usually after the _____.

2. They are the most prominent teeth in the permanent dentition because of both their large size and their _____ position.

3. They are the largest of all the incisors and the two usually share a mesial _____.

4. The maxillary central incisor has a single conical _____, smooth and slightly straight, usually with a rounded apex; the root shape on the cervical cross section is roughly triangular, with the base at the labial aspect, being slightly wider on the labial surface and narrower at the lingual.

5. From the labial view, the _____ is nearly straight with two labial developmental depressions that may extend the length of the crown from the cervical to the incisal.

6. The overall mesial outline from the labial view is slightly rounded with a sharp mesioincisal _____ in comparison with the distoincisal one.

7. On the lingual surface, the single _____ is wide and well developed in size as well as being located slightly off center toward the distal.

8. From the lingual view, the mesial _____ is longer than the distal one.

9. The single _____ is wide yet shallow and is located immediately incisal to the cingulum.

10. There may be a vertically placed palatogingival or _____, which originates in the lingual pit and extends cervically and slightly distally onto the cingulum.

angle	anterior arch	marginal ridge
linguogingival groove	contact area	lingua fossa
root	cingulum	incisal ridge
maxillary central incisors		

Reference   Chapter 16, Permanent anterior teeth. In Fehrenbach MJ, Popowics T: *Illustrated dental embryology, histology, and anatomy,* ed 5, St. Louis, 2020, Saunders.

NOTES

FIGURE 3.27 Maxillary right lateral incisor (lingual and incisal views)

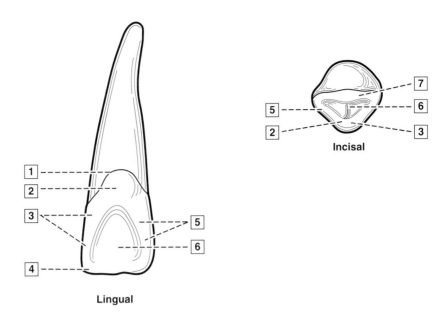

Incisal

Lingual

1	Cementoenamel junction
2	Cingulum
3	Mesial marginal ridge
4	Linguoincisal ridge
5	Distal marginal ridge
6	Lingual fossa
7	Incisal ridge

REVIEW QUESTIONS: Maxillary lateral incisor

Fill in the blanks by choosing the appropriate terms from the list below.

1. The permanent maxillary lateral incisors erupt between 8 and 9 years of age with root completion at age 11, usually after the _____.

2. The _____ of a maxillary lateral incisor has the greatest degree of variation in the form of any permanent tooth except for the third molars.

3. It has a prominent, yet centered and narrower _____ than does a maxillary central incisor on the lingual surface.

4. It has a deeper _____ on the lingual surface than does the maxillary central incisor.

5. The longer mesial _____ on the lingual surface is nearly straight, and the shorter distal one is quite straight.

6. The _____ is noticeably well developed in size as noted from the lingual view.

7. A(n) _____ is more common on a lateral than on a maxillary central incisor and is located on the incisal surface of the cingulum, along the lingual groove.

8. The vertical _____ is more common on the tooth than on a maxillary central incisor as seen from the lingual view and originates in the lingual pit and extends cervically and slightly distally onto the cingulum; it may also extend onto the root surface, where the root shape on the cervical cross section is oval (or ovoid or egg shaped).

9. Similar to a maxillary central incisor, the _____ on a lateral is more curved on the mesial surface than the distal surface of this tooth as noted from the proximal.

10. The _____ is usually labial to the long axis of the tooth as noted in its proximal view features.

linguoincisal ridge   lingual pit   crown

cementoenamel junction   marginal ridge   linguogingival groove

cingulum   incisal ridge   lingual fossa

maxillary central incisors

Reference   Chapter 16, Permanent anterior teeth. In Fehrenbach MJ, Popowics T: *Illustrated dental embryology, histology, and anatomy,* ed 5, St. Louis, 2020, Saunders.

NOTES

FIGURE 3.28 Mandibular right central incisor (lingual and incisal views)

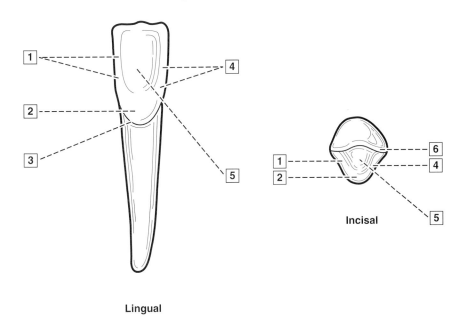

Lingual

Incisal

1	Mesial marginal ridge
2	Cingulum
3	Cementoenamel junction
4	Distal marginal ridge
5	Lingual fossa
6	Incisal ridge

REVIEW QUESTIONS: Mandibular central incisor

Fill in the blanks by choosing the appropriate terms from the list below.

1. The permanent mandibular central incisors erupt between 6 and 7 years of age with root completion at age 9, usually before the _____; the root shape is elliptical (or elongated oval) on cervical cross section.

2. Due to its smallness, the tooth has only one antagonist in the _____.

3. The crown outline of a mandibular central incisor is quite _____ from the labial view, having a fan shape.

4. The _____ of a mandibular central incisor is narrower on the lingual surface than on the labial surface, which is the reverse of the labial view.

5. Overall, the lingual surface is less pronounced and has a small, centered _____.

6. On the lingual surface, the single _____ is barely noticeable.

7. Because the cingulum is centered, the faint mesial and distal _____ have the same length.

8. The _____ curvature is higher incisally on the mesial surface than on the distal surface.

9. The _____ is usually at 90° or perpendicular to the labiolingual axis of the crown of the tooth and overall is just lingual to the long axis of the root.

10. They are the smallest and simplest teeth of the permanent dentition; thus, they are smaller than the lateral incisors of the _____.

lingual fossa	marginal ridges	crown
mandibular arch	maxillary central incisors	maxillary arch
symmetrical	cingulum	incisal ridge
cementoenamel junction		

Reference Chapter 16, Permanent anterior teeth. In Fehrenbach MJ, Popowics T: *Illustrated dental embryology, histology, and anatomy,* ed 5, St. Louis, 2020, Saunders.

NOTES

FIGURE 3.29 Mandibular right lateral incisor (lingual and incisal views)

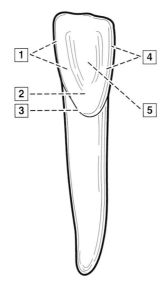

Lingual

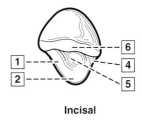

Incisal

1	Mesial marginal ridge
2	Cingulum
3	Cementoenamel junction
4	Distal marginal ridge
5	Lingual fossa
6	Incisal ridge

REVIEW QUESTIONS: Mandibular lateral incisor

Fill in the blanks by choosing the appropriate terms from the list below.

1. The permanent mandibular lateral incisors erupt between 7 and 8 years of age with root completion at age 10, usually after the _____; the root shape is elliptical (or elongated oval) on cervical cross section.

2. From both the labial and lingual views, the _____ appears tilted or twisted distally in regard to the long axis of the tooth.

3. The mesioincisal _____ of the incisal ridge is sharper than the distoincisal ridge from the labial view.

4. The small single _____ lies just distal to the long axis of the root on its lingual surface.

5. On the lingual surface, both the mesial and distal _____ are more developed than on a mandibular central incisor, although the mesial one is longer than the distal one.

6. A single _____ is present on the lingual surface of the tooth.

7. A(n) _____ is rarely present on a mandibular lateral incisor, although it happens more often than on a mandibular central incisor.

8. The height of the _____ curvature is greater on the mesial surface than on the distal surface.

9. The crown of a mandibular lateral incisor is not as _____, as that of the central incisor of the same arch.

10. The tooth has a single root and like the mandibular central incisor has pronounced _____, especially on the distal surface.

symmetrical	lingual fossa	crown
cementoenamel junction	root concavities	lingual pit
angle	marginal ridges	mandibular central incisors
cingulum		

Reference Chapter 16, Permanent anterior teeth. In Fehrenbach MJ, Popowics T: *Illustrated dental embryology, histology, and anatomy,* ed 5, St. Louis, 2020, Saunders.

NOTES

FIGURE 3.30   Maxillary right canine (lingual and incisal views)

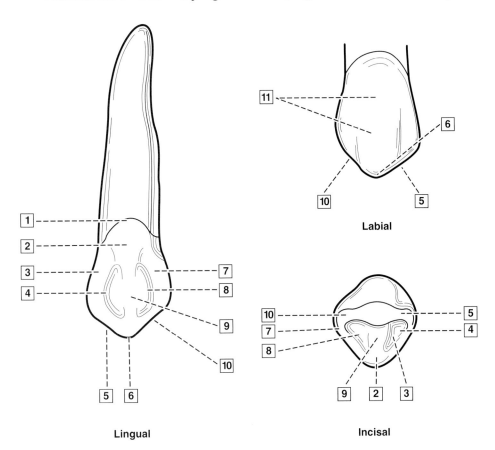

Labial

Lingual

Incisal

1	Cementoenamel junction	7	Distal marginal ridge
2	Cingulum	8	Distolingual fossa
3	Mesial marginal ridge	9	Lingual ridge
4	Mesiolingual fossa	10	Distal cusp slope
5	Mesial cusp slope	11	Labial ridge
6	Cusp tip		

REVIEW QUESTIONS: Maxillary canine

Fill in the blanks by choosing the appropriate terms from the list below.

1. The permanent maxillary canines erupt between 11 and 12 years of age with root completion between ages 13 and 15, usually after the _____, the maxillary incisors, and possibly the maxillary premolars.

2. The long _____ is single and has a blunt apex; it is the longest one in the maxillary arch; the root shape is oval (or ovoid or egg-shaped) on cervical cross section.

3. The _____ on the lingual surface is more developed and larger than that of a central incisor of the same arch, making the tooth stronger during mastication.

4. A maxillary canine does somewhat resemble a mandibular canine; however, the cusp is more developed and larger, and the _____ is sharper as on all maxillary teeth.

5. All lingual surface features of the maxillary canine are more prominent than those of the mandibular canine, including the _____ and marginal ridge.

6. The lingual surface has prominent mesial and distal _____, with one on each side of the cingulum.

7. The tooth has a shallow but visible _____ and distolingual fossa on the lingual surface.

8. The cingulum and the incisal half of the lingual surface are sometimes separated by a shallow lingual groove, and this groove may contain a _____ near its center or it may be present without the lingual groove.

9. The _____ curves higher incisally on the mesial surface than on the distal surface.

10. The _____ seem to form a nearly straight line and the mesial marginal ridge is longer than the distal marginal ridge.

lingual ridge	root	cingulum
mesiolingual fossa	cusp slopes	mandibular canines
lingual pit	cusp tip	marginal ridges
cementoenamel junction		

Reference Chapter 16, Permanent anterior teeth. In Fehrenbach MJ, Popowics T: *Illustrated dental embryology, histology, and anatomy,* ed 5, St. Louis, 2020, Saunders.

NOTES

FIGURE 3.31 **Mandibular right canine (lingual and incisal views)**

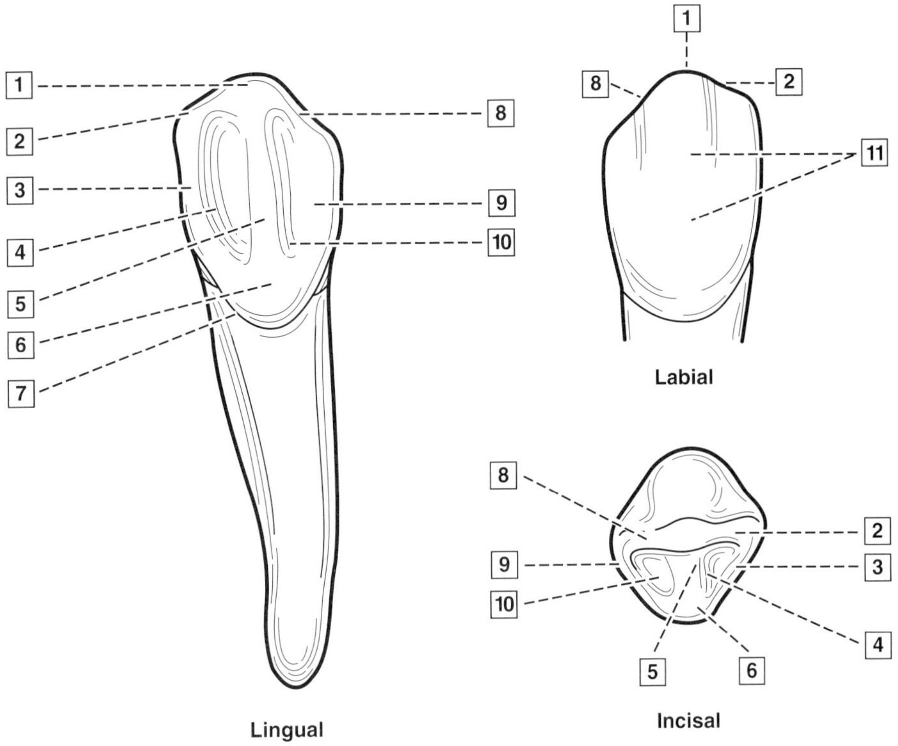

Labial

Lingual

Incisal

1 Cusp tip		**7** Cementoenamel junction	
2 Mesial cusp slope		**8** Distal cusp slope	
3 Mesial marginal ridge		**9** Distal marginal ridge	
4 Mesiolingual fossa		**10** Distolingual fossa	
5 Lingual ridge		**11** Labial ridge	
6 Cingulum			

REVIEW QUESTIONS: Mandibular canine

Fill in the blanks by choosing the appropriate terms from the list below.

1. The permanent mandibular canines erupt between 9 and 10 years of age with root completion between ages 12 and 14, usually before the maxillary canines and after most of the _____ have erupted.

2. The lingual surface of the crown of a mandibular canine is less pronounced than that of a maxillary canine and has a less developed _____ as well as the two marginal ridges.

3. The single _____ of a mandibular canine may be as long as that of a maxillary canine, but it is usually somewhat shorter, although it is still the longest of the mandibular arch; the root shape is oval (or ovoid or egg-shaped) on the cervical cross section.

4. The _____ outline is shorter and rounder than the mesial outline, similar to that of a maxillary canine.

5. The mesial _____ of a mandibular canine is shorter than the one on the distal cusp when first erupted as noted from the labial view.

6. The lingual surface is less pronounced, except for the faintly demarcated features of a _____, mesial marginal ridge, distal marginal ridge, and two lingual fossae, the distolingual fossa and mesiolingual fossa.

7. Rarely are there _____ or lingual grooves on the lingual surface.

8. The _____ is more lingually inclined without incisal wear, unlike the labially placed one on a cusp of the maxillary canine.

9. The _____ curvature on the mesial surface is more toward the incisal when compared to the same surface of a maxillary canine.

10. From the incisive view, the mesial _____ is longer than the distal marginal one.

lingual pits	cementoenamel junction	distal
cusp tip	lingual ridge	cingulum
root	cusp slope	incisors
marginal ridge		

Reference Chapter 16, Permanent anterior teeth. In Fehrenbach MJ, Popowics T: *Illustrated dental embryology, histology, and anatomy,* ed 5, St. Louis, 2020, Saunders.

NOTES

FIGURE 3.32   Maxillary right first premolar (mesial, buccal, and occlusal views)

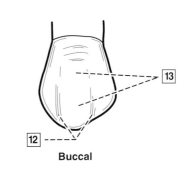

Buccal

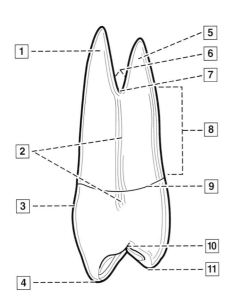

Mesial

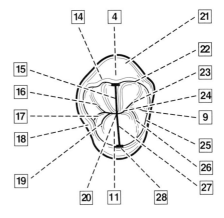

Occlusal

1 Buccal root	11 Lingual cusp	20 Central groove
2 Mesial developmental depression	12 Buccal development depressions	21 Buccal cusp ridge of the buccal cusp
3 Buccal cervical ridge	13 Buccal ridge	22 Mesial cusp ridge of the buccal cusp
4 Buccal cusp	14 Distal cusp ridge of buccal cusp	23 Mesiobuccal triangular groove
5 Lingual root	15 Lingual cusp ridge of buccal cusp (buccal triangular ridge)	24 Mesial triangular fossa (with mesial pit)
6 Furcation crotch area	16 Distobuccal triangular groove	25 Mesial marginal ridge
7 Furcation	17 Distal triangular fossa (with distal pit)	26 Mesiolingual triangular groove
8 Root trunk	18 Distal marginal ridge	27 Lingual triangular ridge
9 Cementoenamel junction	19 Distolingual triangular groove	28 Transverse ridge
10 Mesial marginal groove		

REVIEW QUESTIONS: Maxillary first premolar

Fill in the blanks by choosing the appropriate terms from the list below.

1. The permanent maxillary first premolars erupt between 10 and 11 years of age with root completion between ages 12 and 13, distal to the _____ or their arch space, and thus are the succedaneous replacements for the primary maxillary first molars.

2. Most maxillary first premolars are _____ having two root branches in the apical third, with both a buccal root and a lingual root or *palatal root*; the root shape on the cervical cross section is elliptical (or elongated oval), which is an elongated oval, but may be slightly altered by proximal root concavities.

3. A distinct mesial _____ is present on the root trunk of the maxillary first premolar, extending from the contact area to the bifurcation.

4. The pulp cavity for a two-rooted tooth usually shows two pulp horns (one for each cusp) and two _____ (one for each root).

5. From the buccal view, the _____ of a maxillary first premolar is the widest mesiodistally of all the premolars.

6. This tooth is the only tooth in the permanent dentition that has a buccal cusp with the mesial _____ longer than the distal one.

7. The shorter _____ is sharp but not as sharp as the buccal cusp and is offset toward the mesial.

8. The _____ curvature is more occlusally located on the mesial surface than on the distal surface.

9. Extending mesiodistally, across the occlusal table of the maxillary first premolar, there is a long _____, evenly dividing the tooth buccolingually.

10. The _____ triangular fossa, which surrounds the mesiobuccal triangular groove, is deeper than the shallower distal triangular fossa, which surrounds the distobuccal triangular groove, with the deepest parts of these fossae being the occlusal developmental pits, mesial and distal.

bifurcated	cusp slope	pulp canals
mesial	crown	root concavity
central groove	cementoenamel junction	primary maxillary canines
lingual cusp		

Reference Chapter 17, Permanent posterior teeth. In Fehrenbach MJ, Popowics T: *Illustrated dental embryology, histology, and anatomy,* ed 5, St. Louis, 2020, Saunders.

FIGURE 3.33 **Maxillary right second premolar (mesial and occlusal views)**

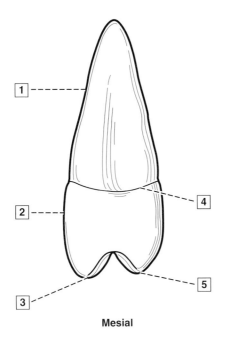

Mesial

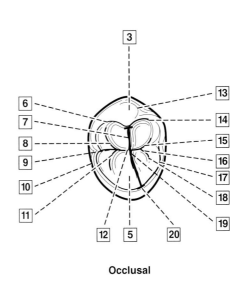

Occlusal

1	Root	**8**	Distobuccal triangular groove	**15**	Mesiobuccal triangular groove
2	Buccal cervical ridge	**9**	Distal triangular fossa (with distal pit)	**16**	Mesial triangular fossa (with mesial pit)
3	Buccal cusp	**10**	Distal marginal ridge	**17**	Mesial marginal ridge
4	Cementoenamel junction	**11**	Distolingual triangular groove	**18**	Mesiolingual triangular groove
5	Lingual cusp	**12**	Central groove	**19**	Lingual triangular ridge
6	Distal cusp ridge of buccal cusp	**13**	Buccal cusp ridge of the buccal cusp	**20**	Transverse ridge
7	Lingual cusp ridge of buccal cusp (buccal triangular ridge)	**14**	Mesial cusp ridge of the buccal cusp		

REVIEW QUESTIONS: Maxillary second premolar

Fill in the blanks by choosing the appropriate terms from the list below.

1. The permanent maxillary second premolars erupt between 10 and 12 years of age with root completion between ages 12 and 14, distal to the permanent maxillary first premolars, and thus are the succedaneous replacements for the _____.

2. A maxillary second premolar resembles a first premolar, except that its _____ is less angular and more rounded.

3. Unlike a maxillary first premolar, a maxillary second premolar usually has only a single _____; its root shape on the cervical cross section is elliptical (or elongated oval), which is an elongated oval, but may be slightly altered by proximal root concavities.

4. The pulp cavity of this tooth has two _____ and one single pulp canal.

5. The _____ of a maxillary second premolar is neither as long nor as sharp as that of a maxillary first premolar.

6. All lingual surface features of a maxillary second premolar are similar to those of a maxillary first premolar; one exception is that the _____ is larger, almost the same height as the buccal cusp on a maxillary second premolar, and slightly displaced to the mesial.

7. The mesial surface of a maxillary second premolar is similar to that of a maxillary first premolar, except that the cusps are closer to having the same size and no mesial _____ is present on the crown and root surfaces.

8. Both the contact areas and _____ marginal ridge are more cervically located than those on a maxillary first premolar.

9. The _____ is shorter on a maxillary second premolar than on a maxillary first premolar and ends in a mesial pit and distal pit, which are closer together and thus more to the middle of the occlusal table.

10. A maxillary second premolar has numerous _____ radiating from the central groove, giving the tooth a more wrinkled appearance compared with a maxillary first premolar.

developmental depression	supplemental grooves	mesial
central groove	root	crown
pulp horns	lingual cusp	primary maxillary second molars
buccal cusp		

Reference Chapter 17, Permanent posterior teeth. In Fehrenbach MJ, Popowics T: *Illustrated dental embryology, histology, and anatomy,* ed 5, St. Louis, 2020, Saunders.

FIGURE 3.34 Mandibular right first premolar (mesial and occlusal views)

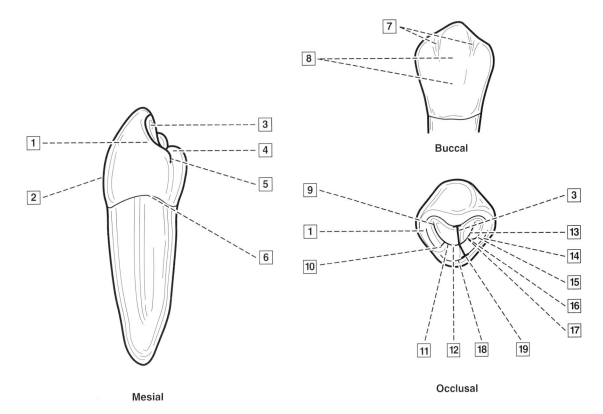

Buccal

Mesial

Occlusal

1	Mesial marginal ridge	11	Mesial fossa (with mesial pit)
2	Buccal cervical ridge	12	Central groove
3	Buccal triangular ridge	13	Distobuccal triangular groove
4	Lingual cusp	14	Distal marginal ridge
5	Mesiolingual groove	15	Distal marginal groove
6	Cementoenamel junction	16	Distolingual triangular groove
7	Buccal development depressions	17	Distal fossa (with distal pit)
8	Buccal ridge	18	Lingual triangular ridge
9	Mesiobuccal triangular groove	19	Transverse ridge
10	Mesiolingual groove		

REVIEW QUESTIONS: Mandibular first premolar

Fill in the blanks by choosing the appropriate terms from the list below.

1. The permanent mandibular first premolars erupt between 10 and 12 years of age with root completion between ages 12 and 13, distal to the permanent mandibular canines, and thus are the _____ replacements for the primary mandibular first molars.

2. A mandibular first premolar resembles a mandibular _____ in many more ways than it does a mandibular second premolar but both can have the same root shape on the cervical cross section: either oval (or ovoid or egg-shaped) or elliptical (or elongated oval) but these shapes may be slightly altered by the presence of proximal root concavities.

3. A mandibular first premolar has a(n) _____ that is long and sharp and is the only functional cusp during occlusion, which is similar to a mandibular canine.

4. The _____ of a mandibular first premolar is usually small and nonfunctioning and is similar in appearance to the cingulum found on some maxillary canines.

5. The outline of the _____ of a mandibular first premolar from the buccal view is nearly symmetrical.

6. The mesial _____ of the buccal cusp is shorter than the distal cusp.

7. Because the lingual cusp is small, most of the _____ can be seen from the lingual view.

8. From the proximal view, the mesial _____ is nearly parallel to the angulation of the transverse ridge at a more cervical level.

9. The _____ curvature is more occlusal on the mesial surface.

10. The crown outline of the mandibular first premolar is diamond-shaped from the occlusal with a notch in the mesial outline at the _____.

mesiolingual groove	canine	lingual cusp
crown	cusp slope	occlusal surface
marginal ridge	succedaneous	cementoenamel junction
buccal cusp		

Reference Chapter 17, Permanent posterior teeth. In Fehrenbach MJ, Popowics T: *Illustrated dental embryology, histology, and anatomy,* ed 5, St. Louis, 2020, Saunders.

NOTES

ANSWER KEY 1. succedaneous, 2. canine, 3. buccal cusp, 4. lingual cusp, 5. crown, 6. cusp slope, 7. occlusal surface, 8. marginal ridge, 9. cementoenamel junction, 10. mesiolingual groove

FIGURE 3.35   Mandibular right second premolar (mesial and occlusal views of cusp types)

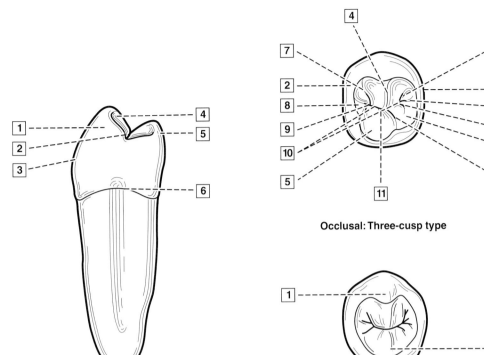

Mesial

Occlusal: Three-cusp type

Occlusal: Two-cusp type

1	Buccal cusp	10	Central groove
2	Mesial marginal ridge	11	Central pit
3	Buccal cervical ridge	12	Distobuccal triangular groove
4	Buccal triangular ridge	13	Distal marginal ridge
5	Mesiolingual cusp	14	Distolingual cusp
6	Cementoenamel junction (CEJ)	15	Distal marginal groove
7	Mesiobuccal triangular groove	16	Distal fossa (with distal pit)
8	Mesial marginal groove	17	Lingual groove
9	Mesial fossa (with mesial pit)	18	Lingual cusp

REVIEW QUESTIONS: Mandibular second premolar

Fill in the blanks by choosing the appropriate terms from the list below.

1. The permanent mandibular second premolars erupt between 11 and 12 years of age with root completion between ages 13 and 14, distal to the _____, and thus are the succedaneous replacements for the primary mandibular second molars.

2. Unlike mandibular first premolars, the more common three-cusp type has three cusps, one large _____ composed of the three buccal lobes and two smaller lingual cusps composed of the two lingual lobes.

3. Similar to mandibular first premolars, the less common two-cusp type has a larger buccal cusp and a single smaller _____; the general shape of the crown outline of a mandibular second premolar is nearly square, especially in the three-cusp type, than a mandibular first premolar.

4. The _____ of the three-cusp type shows three pointed pulp horns; the root shape on the cervical cross section can be either oval (or ovoid or egg-shaped) or elliptical (or elongated oval) but these shapes may be slightly altered by the presence of proximal root concavities.

5. The lingual cusp or cusps, depending on the type, are longer, causing less of the _____ to be seen from the lingual view.

6. From the proximal view, the mesial _____ is perpendicular or 90° to the long axis of the tooth and there is no mesiolingual groove present.

7. On the three-cusp type, the cusps are separated by two developmental grooves, a V-shaped _____, and a linear lingual groove.

8. The central groove on the two-cusp type is most often crescent-shaped, forming a U-shaped groove pattern on the _____; less often, the central groove may be straight, forming an H-shaped groove pattern on the same tooth surface.

9. On the three-cusp type, a deep _____ is located at the junction of the central groove and the lingual groove, toward the lingual.

10. The central groove of the two-cusp type has its terminal ends centered in the mesial fossa and distal fossa, which are circular depressions having _____ radiating from them and none of the two-cusp types have a lingual groove or central pit.

marginal ridge
supplemental grooves
central groove
occlusal surface

pulp cavity
buccal cusp
lingual cusp

mandibular first premolars
central pit
occlusal table

Reference Chapter 17, Permanent posterior teeth. In Fehrenbach MJ, Popowics T: *Illustrated dental embryology, histology, and anatomy,* ed 5, St. Louis, 2020, Saunders.

FIGURE 3.36 Maxillary right first molar (lingual, mesial, and occlusal views)

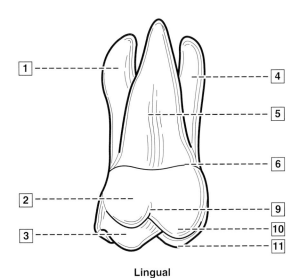

Lingual

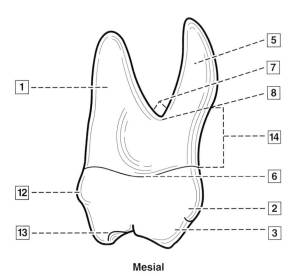

Mesial

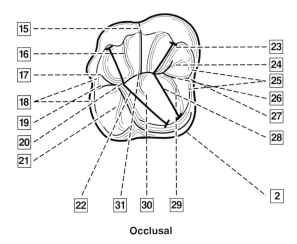

Occlusal

1 Mesiobuccal root

2 Cusp of Carabelli

3 Mesiolingual cusp

4 Distobuccal root

5 Lingual root

6 Cementoenamel junction

7 Furcation crotch area

8 Furcation

9 Distolingual groove

10 Distolingual cusp

11 Distobuccal cusp

12 Cervical ridge

13 Mesiobuccal cusp

14 Root trunk

15 Buccal groove

16 Mesial ridge of distobuccal cusp

17 Distobuccal triangular developmental groove

18 Distal marginal ridge

19 Distal triangular fossa

20 Distal fossa (with distal pit)

21 Distolingual cusp ridge

22 Oblique ridge

23 Mesiobuccal cusp ridge

24 Mesiobuccal triangular groove

25 Mesial marginal ridge

26 Mesial fossa (with mesial pit)

27 Mesial marginal ridge groove

28 Transverse ridge

29 Mesiolingual triangular groove

30 Mesiolingual cusp ridge

31 Central groove with central pit

REVIEW QUESTIONS: Maxillary first molar

Fill in the blanks by choosing the appropriate terms from the list below.

1. The permanent maxillary first molars erupt between 6 and 7 years of age with root completion between ages 9 and 10, _____ to the primary maxillary second molars and thus nonsuccedaneous because there are no primary predecessors.

2. These teeth are the first permanent teeth to erupt into the _____.

3. The maxillary first molar is the largest tooth in the maxillary arch, and has the largest _____ in the permanent dentition.

4. The three _____ of maxillary first molars are larger, more divergent than those of the second molars, and are more complex in form than those of the maxillary premolars.

5. The _____ or lingual root is the largest and longest, inclines lingually, and extends beyond the crown outline with a banana-like curvature toward the buccal.

6. The pulp cavity of a maxillary first molar usually has one _____ for each major cusp.

7. From the buccal view, the occlusal outline of a maxillary first molar is divided symmetrically by the _____.

8. A developmental groove extends between the two buccal cusps, runs apically about halfway to the cementoenamel junction, and is parallel to the long axis of the tooth, where it can fade out or end in a _____.

9. The _____ is initially with a primary maxillary second molar until that tooth is shed; later the tooth's contact is with the permanent second premolar after that tooth erupts.

10. From the lingual view, since it is the largest cusp on the occlusal surface, the _____ outline is much longer and larger, but the cusp is not as sharp as the distolingual cusp; commonly arising from the lingual surface of this cusp is a fifth nonfunctioning cusp, the cusp of Carabelli.

buccal groove	buccal pit	crown
mesiolingual cusp	palatal	distal
mesial contact	roots	maxillary arch
pulp horn		

Reference Chapter 17, Permanent posterior teeth. In Fehrenbach MJ, Popowics T: *Illustrated dental embryology, histology, and anatomy,* ed 5, St. Louis, 2020, Saunders.

NOTES

FIGURE 3.37 Maxillary second molar: rhomboidal crown outline (lingual, mesial, and occlusal views)

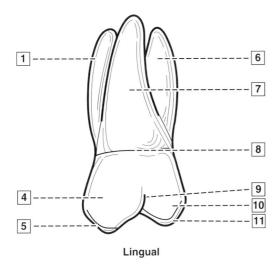

Lingual

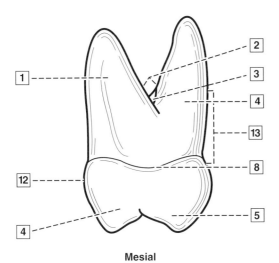

Mesial

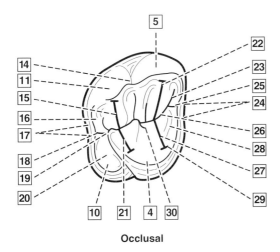

Occlusal

1	Mesiobuccal root
2	Furcation crotch area
3	Furcation
4	Mesiolingual cusp
5	Mesiobuccal cusp
6	Distobuccal root
7	Lingual root
8	Cementoenamel junction
9	Distolingual groove
10	Distolingual cusp
11	Distobuccal cusp
12	Cervical ridge
13	Root trunk
14	Buccal groove
15	Distobuccal cusp ridge
16	Distobuccal triangular groove
17	Distal marginal ridge
18	Distal marginal ridge groove
19	Distal fossa (with distal pit)
20	Distolingual cusp ridge
21	Oblique ridge
22	Mesiobuccal cusp ridge
23	Mesiobuccal triangular groove
24	Mesial marginal ridge
25	Mesial marginal ridge groove
26	Mesial fossa (with mesial pit)
27	Mesiolingual cusp ridge
28	Mesiolingual triangular groove
29	Transverse ridge
30	Central groove with central pit

REVIEW QUESTIONS: Maxillary second molar

Fill in the blanks by choosing the appropriate terms from the list below.

1. The permanent maxillary second molars erupt between 12 and 13 years of age with root completion between ages 14 and 16, _____ to the permanent maxillary first molars and thus nonsuccedaneous, having no primary predecessors.

2. The _____ usually has four cusps similar to the four major cusps of the maxillary first molar, but it can also have three cusps.

3. The three _____ on maxillary second molars are smaller than the maxillary first molars, less divergent, and placed at a more parallel position than on the maxillary first molars.

4. The pulp cavity of a maxillary second molar consists of a(n) _____ and three main pulp canals, one for each of the three roots.

5. The more common rhomboidal type has four sides with opposite sides parallel; this type is similar to that of the maxillary _____ but with an even more accentuated outline.

6. The heart-shaped type is less common and is similar to the typical maxillary _____.

7. However, the defining _____ is less prominent on the maxillary second molar than on the maxillary first molar, as seen on the occlusal table of the tooth.

8. An increased number of _____ are usually present on the occlusal table of the maxillary second molar, making it seem wrinkled.

9. With the heart-shaped type, the _____ is quite small with the other three cusps completely overshadowing it.

10. It is important to note that no _____ for the maxillary second molar is present until the maxillary third molar possibly erupts and moves into occlusion.

oblique ridge   supplemental grooves   distal

distal contact area   pulp chamber   crown

first molar   roots   third molar

distolingual cusp

Reference Chapter 17, Permanent posterior teeth. In Fehrenbach MJ, Popowics T: *Illustrated dental embryology, histology, and anatomy,* ed 5, St. Louis, 2020, Saunders.

NOTES

FIGURE 3.38 Mandibular right first molar (lingual, mesial, and occlusal views)

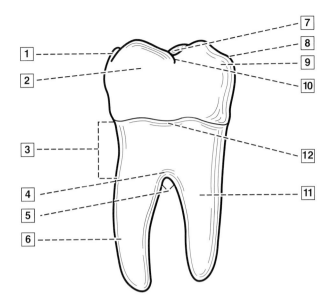

Lingual

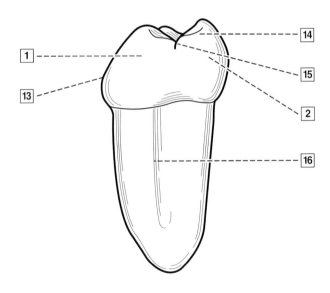

Mesial

Occlusal

1	Mesiobuccal cusp
2	Mesiolingual cusp
3	Root trunk
4	Furcation
5	Furcation crotch area
6	Mesial root
7	Distobuccal cusp
8	Distal cusp
9	Distolingual cusp
10	Lingual groove
11	Distal root
12	Cementoenamel junction
13	Cervical ridge
14	Mesial marginal ridge
15	Mesial marginal ridge groove
16	Mesial fluting
17	Mesiobuccal groove
18	Mesiobuccal cusp ridge
19	Mesial triangular fossa (with mesial pit)
20	Mesiolingual cusp ridge
21	Distobuccal cusp ridge
22	Distobuccal groove
23	Distal cusp ridge
24	Distal marginal ridge
25	Distal marginal ridge groove
26	Distal triangular fossa (with distal pit)
27	Distolingual cusp ridge
28	Central groove with central pit

REVIEW QUESTIONS: Mandibular first molar

Fill in the blanks by choosing the appropriate terms from the list below.

1. The permanent mandibular first molars erupt between 6 and 7 years of age with root completion between ages 9 and 10, distal to the primary mandibular second molars and thus are _____, having no primary predecessors.

2. These teeth are usually the first _____ to erupt in the oral cavity.

3. The _____ of a mandibular first molar usually has five cusps, three buccal and two lingual.

4. The two roots, mesial and distal, of a mandibular first molar, are larger and more _____ than on the mandibular second molar, leaving them widely separated buccally and no longer parallel to each other.

5. There is the presence of _____, an elongated developmental depression noted on many surfaces of the root branches, especially noted on the mesial surface of the mesial root; however, it is not observed on the distal surface of the distal root.

6. The pulp cavity of a mandibular first molar is more likely to have three _____, distal, mesiobuccal, and mesiolingual and five pulp horns.

7. The mesiobuccal groove extends straight cervically to a point about midway occlusocervically, but slightly mesial to the center mesiodistally, and usually ends in the _____.

8. A(n) _____, which has a mesiodistally-oriented roundness in the cervical third of the buccal surface, is apparent; it is usually more prominent in its mesial part.

9. The _____ is the smallest cusp and has a sharp tip.

10. The Y-shaped groove pattern is formed on the _____ around the cusps by the mesio-buccal groove, distobuccal groove, and lingual groove; it also has three fossae, which includes a large central fossa, smaller mesial triangular fossa, and distal triangular fossa, with associated pits.

crown	fluting	permanent teeth
occlusal table	divergent	nonsuccedaneous
distal cusp	buccal cervical ridge	buccal pit
pulp canals		

Reference Chapter 17, Permanent posterior teeth. In Fehrenbach MJ, Popowics T: *Illustrated dental embryology, histology, and anatomy,* ed 5, St. Louis, 2020, Saunders.

FIGURE 3.39 Mandibular right second molar (lingual, mesial, and occlusal views)

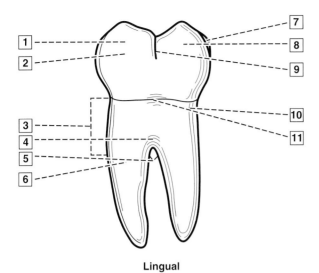

Lingual

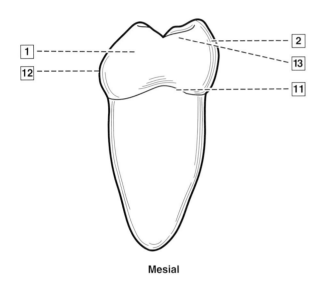

Mesial

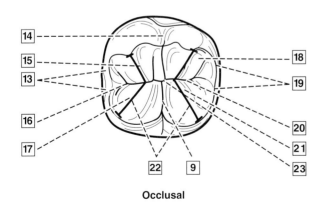

Occlusal

1	Mesiobuccal cusp
2	Mesiolingual cusp
3	Root trunk
4	Furcation
5	Furcation crotch area
6	Mesial root
7	Distobuccal cusp
8	Distolingual cusp

9	Lingual groove
10	Distal root
11	Cementoenamel junction
12	Cervical ridge
13	Mesial marginal ridge
14	Buccal groove

15	Mesiobuccal cusp ridge
16	Mesial triangular fossa (with mesial pit)
17	Mesiolingual cusp ridge
18	Distobuccal cusp ridge
19	Distal marginal ridge
20	Distal triangular fossa (with distal pit)

21	Distolingual cusp ridge
22	Transverse ridges
23	Central groove with central pit

REVIEW QUESTIONS: Mandibular second molar

Fill in the blanks by choosing the appropriate terms from the list below.

1. The permanent mandibular second molars erupt between 11 and 13 years of age with root completion between ages 14 and 15, _____ to the permanent mandibular first molars and thus nonsuccedaneous, having no primary predecessors.

2. The _____ measurements of a mandibular second molar are generally smaller than those of a first molar, and the four cusps of a second molar are nearly equal in size compared with the five cusps of different sizes of a mandibular first molar.

3. The two _____ of a second molar are smaller, shorter, and less divergent in placement than those of a mandibular first molar, being more parallel to each other.

4. Although the pulp cavity of a mandibular second molar can have two of these (one for each root), it is more likely to have three _____, similar to a mandibular first molar, including distal, mesiobuccal, and mesiolingual ones (the latter two being together in the mesial root).

5. From the buccal view, the _____ divides the same-sized mesiobuccal cusp and distobuccal cusp of a mandibular second molar.

6. The occlusal surface of a mandibular second molar is considerably different from that of a mandibular first molar because there is no _____ and all cusps present are of equal size.

7. A cross-shaped groove pattern is formed where the well-defined central groove is crossed by the buccal groove and lingual groove, dividing the _____ into four parts that are nearly equal.

8. On the occlusal table there are three _____ present, central, mesial, and distal.

9. The cusp slopes on a mandibular second molar are less smooth than those on a mandibular first molar because second molars have an increased number of _____.

10. Unlike a mandibular first molar, this tooth has two _____; the triangular ridges of the mesiobuccal and mesiolingual cusps meet to form these structures, as do the distobuccal and distolingual cusps.

crown	distal cusp	occlusal pits
supplemental grooves	distal	transverse ridges
occlusal table	roots	pulp canals
buccal groove		

Reference Chapter 17, Permanent posterior teeth. In Fehrenbach MJ, Popowics T: *Illustrated dental embryology, histology, and anatomy,* ed 5, St. Louis, 2020, Saunders.

ANSWER KEY 1. distal, 2. crown, 3. roots, 4. pulp canals, 5. buccal groove, 6. distal cusp, 7. occlusal table, 8. occlusal pits, 9. supplemental grooves, 10. transverse ridges

FIGURE 4.1 Skull bones (anterior view)

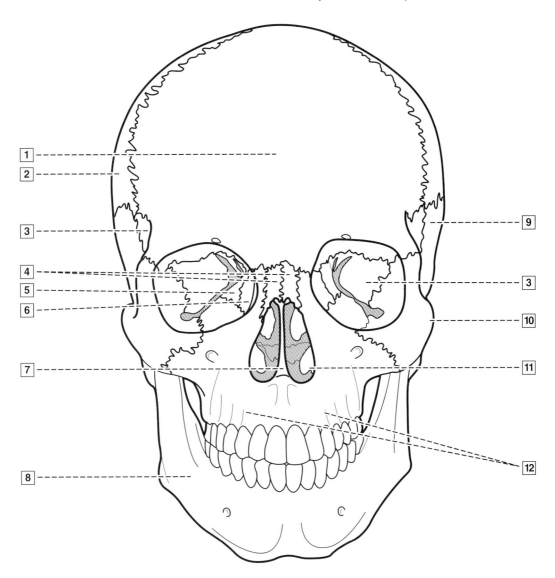

1	Frontal bone	7	Vomer
2	Parietal bone	8	Mandible
3	Sphenoid bones	9	Temporal bone
4	Nasal bone	10	Zygomatic bone
5	Ethmoid bone	11	Inferior nasal concha
6	Lacrimal bone	12	Maxillae

REVIEW QUESTIONS: Skull bones

Fill in the blanks by choosing the appropriate terms from the list below.

1. The _____ is a single cranial bone of the skull with four sides that forms the posterior part of the skull and the base of the cranium that articulates with the first cervical vertebra atlas.

2. The _____ is a single fused cranial bone of the skull that forms the anterior part of the skull superior to the eyes and includes the majority of the forehead as well the roof of each orbit.

3. Each _____ is one of a pair of cranial bones of the skull that articulate with each other at the sagittal suture and that together form the greater part of the right and left lateral walls and roof of the skull.

4. Each _____ is one of a pair of cranial bones of the skull that together form the lateral walls of the skull and part of the base of the skull with each bone composed of three parts that include the squamous, tympanic, and petrous.

5. The _____ is a single midline cranial bone of the skull in the shape of a bat or butterfly located; it assists the formation of the base of the cranium and the lateral borders of the skull as well as the floors and walls of each of the orbits.

6. The _____ is a single midline cranial bone of the skull that includes two unpaired plates, the perpendicular plate and cribriform plate, which cross over each other.

7. Each _____ is a small oblong paired facial bone of the skull that lies side by side, fused to each other to form the bridge of the nose in the midline superior to the piriform aperture, the anterior opening of the nasal cavity.

8. Each _____ or *zygoma* is one of a pair of facial bones of the skull in the shape of a diamond, which together form the majority of the cheekbones or *malar* surface and also help form the lateral walls and floor of the orbit; it is composed of three processes, the frontal, temporal, and maxillary.

9. The _____ is one of a pair of facial bones of the skull that fuse developmentally and together form the upper jaw; each has a body and four processes that include the frontal, zygomatic, palatine, and alveolar processes.

10. The _____ is a single fused facial bone of the skull that forms the lower jaw and is the only freely movable bone of the skull, having an articulation with the paired temporal bones at each temporomandibular joint.

frontal bone	ethmoid bone	zygomatic bone
parietal bone	mandible	maxilla
sphenoid bone	temporal bone	occipital bone
nasal bone		

Reference   Chapter 3, Skeletal system. In Fehrenbach MJ, Herring SW: *Illustrated anatomy of the head and neck,* ed 6, St. Louis, 2021, Saunders.

ANSWER KEY 1. occipital bone, 2. frontal bone, 3. parietal bone, 4. temporal bone, 5. sphenoid bone, 6. ethmoid bone, 7. nasal bone, 8. zygomatic bone, 9. maxilla, 10. mandible

FIGURE 4.2   Skull bones with landmarks (lateral view)

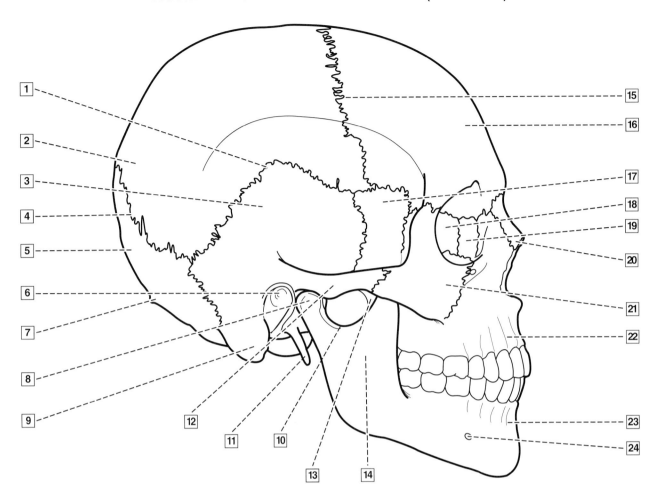

1 Squamosal suture	**9** Mastoid process of temporal bone	**17** Sphenoid bone
2 Parietal bone	**10** Mandibular fossa of mandible	**18** Ethmoid bone
3 Temporal bone	**11** Styloid process of temporal bone	**19** Lacrimal bone
4 Lambdoidal suture	**12** Zygomatic process of temporal bone	**20** Nasal bone
5 Occipital bone	**13** Pterygoid process of sphenoid bone	**21** Zygomatic bone
6 External acoustic meatus of temporal bone	**14** Mandibular ramus	**22** Maxilla
7 External occipital protuberance of occipital bone	**15** Coronal suture	**23** Mandible
8 Condyloid process of mandible	**16** Frontal bone	**24** Mental foramen of mandible

REVIEW QUESTIONS: Skull bones

Fill in the blanks by choosing the appropriate terms from the list below.

1. The paired _____ extends across the skull, between the frontal bone and each parietal bone; it is also the location of the diamond-shaped anterior fontanelle or "soft spot" in a newborn that generally remains open until closure at about 2 years of age.

2. The single _____ extends from the anterior to posterior of the skull at the midline between the parietal bones, is in line with the sagittal plane of the skull, and also generally perpendicular to the coronal suture of the skull.

3. The single _____ is located between the occipital bone and each parietal bone, which is typically more serrated looking than the others and resembles an upside-down V-shape in anatomic position.

4. The paired _____ is arched and located between the temporal bone and the parietal bone on each side.

5. The tympanic part of the temporal bone forms most of the _____, a short canal leading to the tympanic cavity that is located posterior to the articular fossa when intact.

6. On the inferior aspect of the petrous part of the temporal bone and posterior to the external acoustic meatus is the _____, a large roughened projection that is composed of air spaces or mastoid air cells that communicate with the middle ear and that serves as a site for the attachment of the large cervical muscles including the sternocleidomastoid muscle.

7. Inferior and medial to the external acoustic meatus and on the petrous part of the temporal bone is a long pointed projection, the _____, which is a structure that serves as a site for attachment of tongue and pharyngeal muscles.

8. Inferior to the greater wing of the sphenoid bone is the _____, a site of attachment for certain muscles of mastication; it consists of the flattened lateral pterygoid plate and the thinner medial pterygoid plate; the pterygoid fossa lies between the two plates.

9. Each paired _____ is an irregular thin plate of bone located posterior to the frontal processes of the maxillae that forms a small part of the anterior medial wall of the orbit and is considered the smallest and most fragile of all of the facial bones.

10. The _____ is a large and more posterior projection that consists of two parts, the mandibular condyle and the constricted part that supports it, the neck of the mandible.

mastoid process   sagittal suture   condyloid process
lambdoidal suture   external acoustic meatus   coronal suture
lacrimal bone   squamosal suture   pterygoid process
styloid process

Reference   Chapter 3, Skeletal system. In Fehrenbach MJ, Herring SW: *Illustrated anatomy of the head and neck,* ed 6, St. Louis, 2021, Saunders.

FIGURE 4.3 Skull bones with landmarks (inferior view of upper skull)

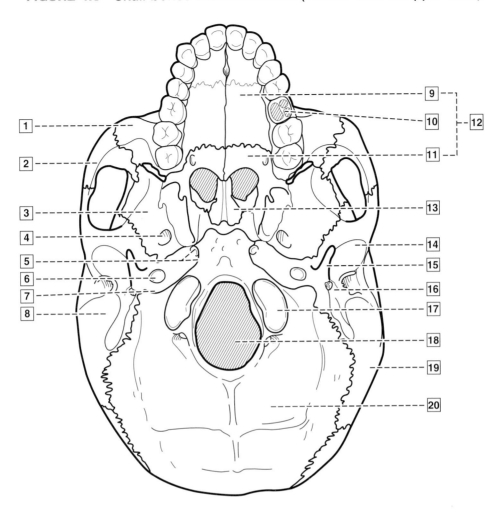

1	Zygomatic process of the maxilla	**8**	Mastoid process of temporal bone	**15**	Styloid process of temporal bone
2	Zygomatic bone	**9**	Palatine process of the maxilla	**16**	Stylomastoid foramen of temporal bone
3	Sphenoid bone	**10**	Alveolar process of the maxilla	**17**	Occipital condyle of occipital bone
4	Foramen ovale of sphenoid bone	**11**	Horizontal plate of the palatine bone	**18**	Foramen magnum of occipital bone
5	Foramen lacerum	**12**	Hard palate	**19**	Temporal bone
6	Carotid canal of temporal bone	**13**	Vomer	**20**	Occipital bone
7	Jugular foramen	**14**	Mandibular fossa of mandible		

REVIEW QUESTIONS: Skull bones

Fill in the blanks by choosing the appropriate terms from the list below.

1. The floor of the nasal cavity is formed from the two separate bones of the hard palate; the hard palate is formed by the two palatine processes of the maxilla anteriorly and the two horizontal plates of the _____(s) posteriorly, with an articulation at the median palatine suture.

2. The larger anterior opening on the sphenoid bone is the _____, which is for the mandibular nerve of the fifth cranial or trigeminal nerve to pass to and from the brain.

3. The large irregularly shaped _____ when intact is filled with cartilage; it is located between the sphenoid bone, apex of petrous part of the temporal bone, and basilar part of the occipital bone.

4. A round opening, the _____, is located in the petrous part of the temporal bone posterolateral to the foramen lace rum and carries the internal carotid artery and carotid plexus of nerves, which is a network of intersecting sympathetic that run parallel to the carotid artery into the head.

5. Immediately posterior to the styloid process is the _____, an opening through which the seventh cranial or facial nerve exits from the skull to the face.

6. The _____ is located just medial to the styloid process and through which passes the internal jugular vein and three cranial nerves, including the ninth cranial nerve or glossopharyngeal nerve, the tenth cranial nerve or vagus nerve, and the eleventh cranial nerve or accessory nerve.

7. The largest opening on the inferior view of the skull is the _____ of the occipital bone, through which the spinal cord, vertebral arteries, and eleventh cranial nerve or accessory nerve pass.

8. On the lateral part of the occipital bone and anterior to each side of the foramen magnum is the _____, which is a curved and smooth projection that has an articulation with the atlas, the first cervical vertebra of the vertebral column.

9. On the inferior surface of the zygomatic process of the temporal bone is the _____, which is located posterior to the articular eminence; together they comprise the parts of the bony surface that articulate with the mandible on each side at the temporomandibular joint.

10. The _____ is a thin and flat single midline facial bone of the skull, which is almost trapezoidal in shape and forms the posterior and inferior part of the nasal septum.

occipital condyle	carotid canal	foramen lacerum
foramen ovale	jugular foramen	articular fossa
stylomastoid foramen	palatine bone	foramen magnum
vomer		

Reference Chapter 3, Skeletal system. In Fehrenbach MJ, Herring SW: *Illustrated anatomy of the head and neck*, ed 6, St. Louis, 2021, Saunders.

FIGURE 4.4   Skull bones with landmarks (internal view)

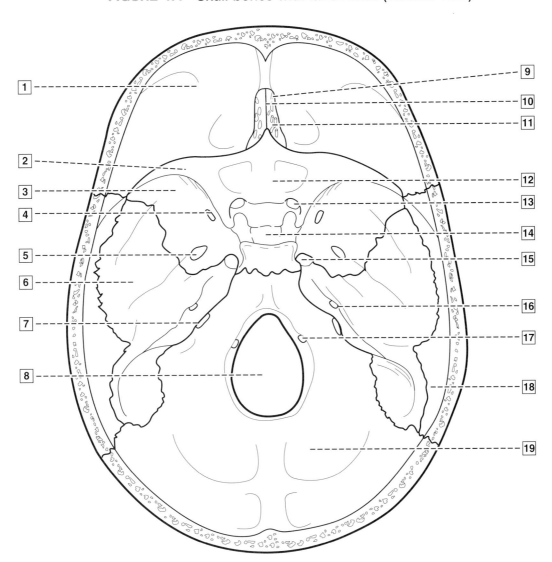

1 Frontal bone	**8** Foramen magnum of occipital bone	**14** Sella turcica of sphenoid bone
2 Lesser wing of sphenoid bone	**9** Ethmoid bone	**15** Foramen lacerum
3 Greater wing of sphenoid bone	**10** Crista galli of ethmoid bone	**16** Internal acoustic meatus of temporal bone
4 Foramen rotundum of sphenoid bone	**11** Cribriform plate of ethmoid bone	**17** Hypoglossal canal of occipital bone
5 Foramen ovale of sphenoid bone	**12** Sphenoid bone	**18** Parietal bone
6 Temporal bone	**13** Optic foramen of sphenoid bone	**19** Occipital bone
7 Jugular foramen		

REVIEW QUESTIONS: Skull bones

Fill in the blanks by choosing the appropriate terms from the list below.

1. The perforated _____ has numerous foramina for the first cranial nerve or olfactory nerve.

2. The _____ carries the maxillary nerve of the fifth cranial nerve or trigeminal nerve.

3. As with an external skull surface view, the _____ of the occipital bone is also present on the superior view of the internal skull, along with other nearby foramina, and carries the spinal cord, vertebral arteries, and the eleventh cranial nerve or accessory nerve.

4. The _____ is the passageway for the seventh cranial nerve or facial nerve and the eighth cranial or vestibulocochlear nerve.

5. The anterolateral process of the midline cranial bone of the skull, the _____, helps form the orbital apex.

6. The large posterolateral process of the midline cranial bone of the skull is the _____.

7. The _____ is a bony canal that is located in the occipital bone of the skull and transmits the twelfth cranial nerve or the hypoglossal nerve.

8. The round opening in the orbital apex is the _____, which lies between the two roots of the lesser wing of the sphenoid bone, which has the second cranial or optic nerve as well as the ophthalmic artery passes through it to reach the eyeball.

9. The _____ is a saddle-shaped depression on the superior surface of the body of the sphenoid bone, with its deepest part, the hypophyseal fossa, containing the pituitary gland.

10. The _____ is a wedge-shaped vertical midline continuation of the perpendicular plate of the ethmoid bone superiorly into the cranial cavity; it serves as an attachment for layers covering the brain.

internal acoustic meatus	crista galli	sella turcica
hypoglossal canal	cribriform plate	lesser wing of the sphenoid bone
greater wing of the sphenoid bone	optic canal	foramen rotundum
foramen magnum		

References   Chapter 3, Skeletal system. In Fehrenbach MJ, Herring SW: *Illustrated anatomy of the head and neck,* ed 6, St. Louis, 2021, Saunders; Chapter 8, Head and neck. In Drake R, Vogl AW, Mitchell AWM: *Gray's anatomy for students,* ed 4, Philadelphia, 2020, Churchill Livingstone.

NOTES

FIGURE 4.5 Skull bones with landmarks (midsagittal section)

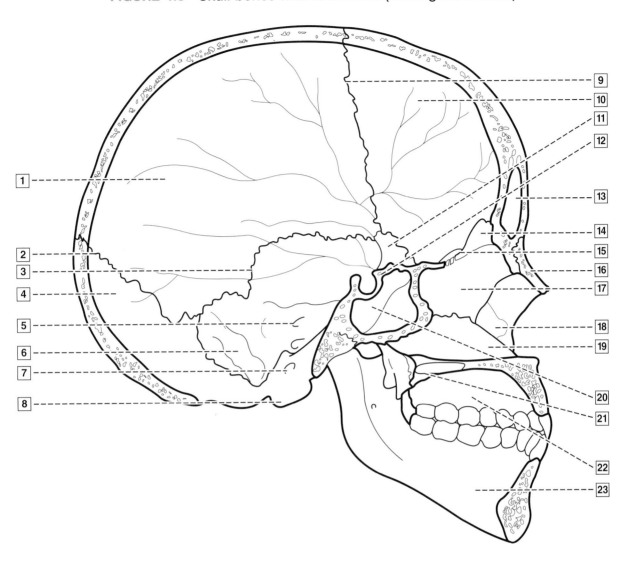

1 Parietal bone	**9** Coronal suture	**17** Perpendicular plate of ethmoid bone
2 Lambdoidal suture	**10** Frontal bone	**18** Inferior nasal concha
3 Squamosal suture	**11** Sphenoid bone	**19** Vomer
4 Occipital bone	**12** Sella turcica of sphenoid bone	**20** Sphenoidal sinus of sphenoid bone
5 Internal acoustic meatus of temporal bone	**13** Frontal sinus of frontal bone	**21** Palatine bone
6 Temporal bone	**14** Crista galli of ethmoid bone	**22** Maxilla
7 Hypoglossal canal of occipital bone	**15** Cribriform plate of ethmoid bone	**23** Mandible
8 Occipital condyle of occipital bone	**16** Nasal bone	

REVIEW QUESTIONS: Skull bones

Fill in the blanks by choosing the appropriate terms from the list below.

1. The pyramid-shaped body of each _____ has four surfaces that include the orbital, nasal, infratemporal, and facial surfaces; each body contains a maxillary sinus, which is an air-filled space or paranasal sinus.

2. The _____ occludes with each maxilla by way of their respective mandibular and maxillary arches of the dentition.

3. The _____ are paired facial bones that project from the maxillae to form a part of the lateral walls of the nasal cavity.

4. Each _____ is relatively square, like a curved plate, and has four borders; each bone is located posterior to the frontal bone, forming the greater part of the right and left lateral walls and the roof of the skull.

5. Lateral and anterior to the foramen magnum are the paired condyles, curved and smooth projections of the _____.

6. The _____ articulates with the zygomatic and parietal bones as well as the occipital and sphenoid bones, and also the mandible.

7. The _____ fit between the frontal processes of the maxillae and thus articulate with the maxillae laterally as well as the frontal bone superiorly at the single frontonasal suture.

8. The paired _____ are located within the frontal bone just superior to the nasal cavity and are asymmetric, with the left and right always separated by a septum.

9. The paired _____ are located deep within the body of the sphenoid bone and are frequently asymmetric due to the lateral displacement of the intervening septum.

10. The horizontal plates of the _____ inferiorly form the posterior part of the hard palate and superiorly the floor of the nasal cavity; anteriorly they join with the maxillae.

maxilla	mandible	palatine bones
parietal bone	sphenoidal sinuses	temporal bone
occipital bone	inferior nasal conchae	nasal bones
frontal sinuses		

Reference Chapter 3, Skeletal system. In Fehrenbach MJ, Herring SW: *Illustrated anatomy of the head and neck,* ed 6, St. Louis, 2021, Saunders.

FIGURE 4.6 Orbital region with features (anterior view of left orbit)

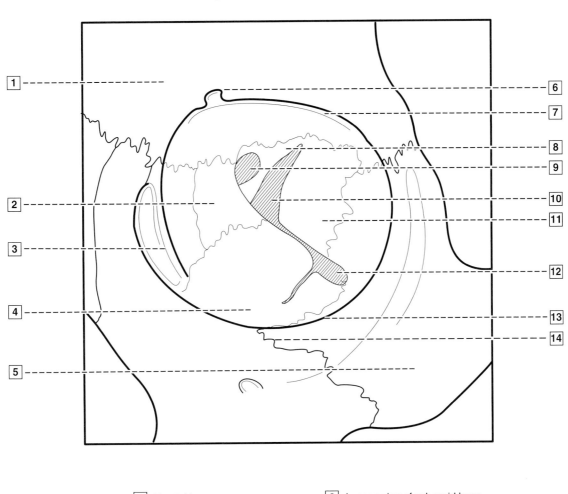

1 Frontal bone	**8**	Lesser wing of sphenoid bone
2 Ethmoid bone	**9**	Optic canal of sphenoid bone
3 Lacrimal bone	**10**	Superior orbital fissure of sphenoid bone
4 Maxilla	**11**	Greater wing of sphenoid bone
5 Zygomatic bone	**12**	Inferior orbital fissure
6 Supraorbital notch of frontal bone	**13**	Infraorbital rim
7 Supraorbital rim	**14**	Zygomaticomaxillary suture

REVIEW QUESTIONS: Orbital region

Fill in the blanks by choosing the appropriate terms from the list below.

1. The _____ contains and protects the eyeball and is a prominent feature of the anterior part of the skull.

2. The round opening in the orbital apex is the _____.

3. The optic canal lies between the two roots of the _____.

4. Lateral to the optic canal is the curved and slitlike _____, which is located between the greater and lesser wings of the sphenoid bone.

5. The inferior orbital fissure can also be noted between the _____ and the maxilla.

6. The _____ connects the orbit with both the infratemporal and pterygopalatine fossae; both the infraorbital and zygomatic nerves, which are branches of the maxillary nerve, and infraorbital artery enter the orbit through this structure.

7. The _____ forms the anterior part of the lateral wall of the orbit.

8. The orbital surfaces of the _____ create the roof or superior wall of the orbit.

9. The _____ forms the greatest part of the medial wall of the orbit.

10. The _____ is located at the anterior medial corner of the orbit.

optic canal	orbit	lacrimal bone
superior orbital fissure	frontal bone	zygomatic bone
greater wing of the sphenoid bone	ethmoid bone	lesser wing of the sphenoid bone
inferior orbital fissure		

Reference   Chapter 3, Skeletal system. In Fehrenbach MJ, Herring SW: *Illustrated anatomy of the head and neck,* ed 6, St. Louis, 2021, Saunders.

NOTES

FIGURE 4.7   Nasal region with features (anterior view)

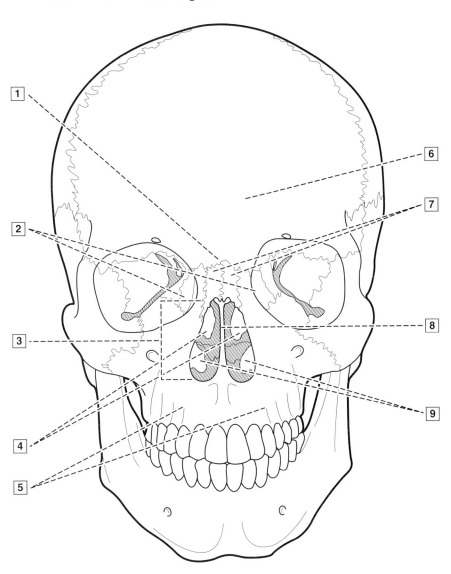

1	Nasion	6	Frontal bone
2	Lacrimal bones	7	Nasal bones
3	Piriform aperture	8	Nasal septum
4	Middle nasal conchae	9	Inferior nasal conchae
5	Maxillae		

REVIEW QUESTIONS: Nasal region

Fill in the blanks by choosing the appropriate terms from the list below.

1. The _____ is the superior part of the respiratory tract and is located between the orbits, having both lateral walls and a floor with anterior and posterior openings.

2. The bridge of the nose is formed from the paired _____.

3. Each lateral wall of the nasal cavity has three projecting structures or turbinates that extend inward, including the superior nasal concha, the _____, and the inferior nasal concha.

4. The vertical partition, the _____, divides the nasal cavity into two parts.

5. Anteriorly, the nasal septum is formed by both the perpendicular plate of the _____ superiorly and the nasal septal cartilage inferiorly.

6. The posterior parts of the nasal septum are formed by the _____.

7. The _____ is a separate facial bone of the skull that forms off the lateral wall of the nasal cavity.

8. The _____, a midpoint cephalometric landmark, is located at the junction of the frontal bone and nasal bones.

9. The anterior opening of the nasal cavity, the _____, is large and triangular.

10. The floor of the nasal cavity is formed from the two separate bones of the hard palate, the palatine processes of the _____ anteriorly and the horizontal plates of the palatine bones posteriorly.

nasal cavity	nasal septum	nasion
ethmoid bone	vomer	piriform aperture
nasal bones	inferior nasal concha	maxillae
middle nasal concha		

References Chapter 3, Skeletal system. In Fehrenbach MJ, Herring SW: *Illustrated anatomy of the head and neck,* ed 6, St. Louis, 2021, Saunders; Chapter 1, Face and neck regions. In Fehrenbach MJ, Popowics T: *Illustrated dental embryology, histology, and anatomy,* ed 5, St. Louis, 2020, Saunders.

NOTES

FIGURE 4.8 Nasal cavity with landmarks (sagittal section of lateral wall)

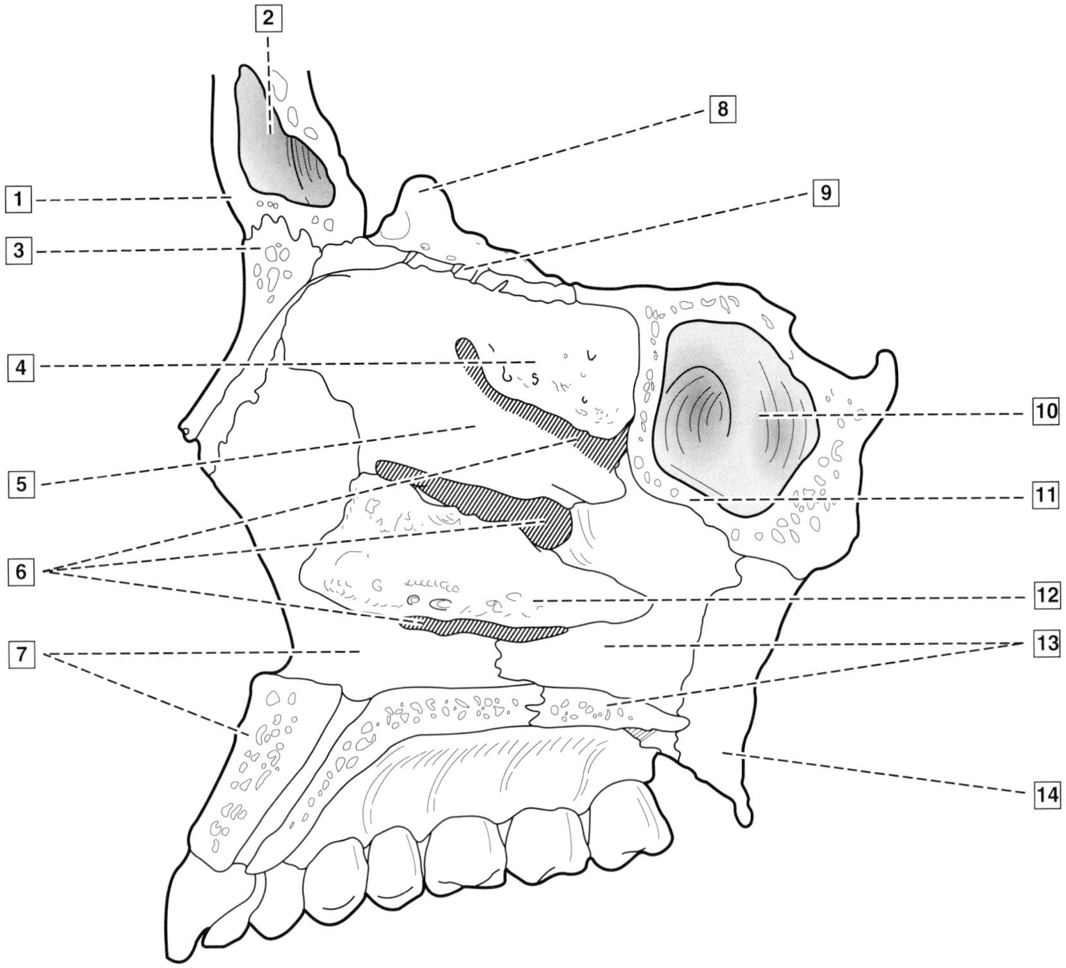

1 Frontal bone	8 Crista galli of ethmoid bone
2 Frontal sinus of frontal bone	9 Cribriform plate of ethmoid bone
3 Nasal bone	10 Sphenoidal sinus of sphenoid bone
4 Superior nasal concha of ethmoid bone	11 Sphenoid bone
5 Middle nasal concha of ethmoid bone	12 Inferior nasal concha
6 Nasal meatuses: superior, middle, inferior	13 Palatine bone
7 Maxilla	14 Medial pterygoid plate of pterygoid process of sphenoid bone

REVIEW QUESTIONS: Nasal cavity

Fill in the blanks by choosing the appropriate terms from the list below.

1. Each _____ communicates with and drains into the nasal cavity by a constricted canal to the middle nasal meatus, the frontonasal duct.

2. Each lateral wall of the nasal cavity has three projecting structures or turbinates that extend inward from the maxilla that include the _____, the middle nasal concha, and the inferior nasal concha.

3. The lateral walls of the nasal cavity are mainly formed by the _____.

4. Protected by each nasal concha is an air channel, the _____, with each having openings through which the paranasal sinuses or nasolacrimal duct communicates with the nasal cavity.

5. When intact, the anterior openings to the nasal cavities are the _____, bordered laterally by the cartilaginous alae and the large deeper posterior openings are choanae or posterior nasal apertures.

6. A vertical midline continuation of the perpendicular plate superiorly into the cranial cavity is the wedge-shaped _____.

7. The horizontal _____ is within the inner surface of the cranial cavity and seen on the superior aspect of the ethmoid bone and surrounding the crista galli, is perforated by numerous foramina to allow the passage of the olfactory nerves for the sense of smell.

8. The vertical plates of the _____ form a part of the lateral walls of the nasal cavity.

9. The _____ are paired facial bones of the skull that project from the maxillae to form a part of the lateral walls of the nasal cavity.

10. The _____ communicate with and drain into the nasal cavity through an opening superior to each superior nasal concha.

palatine bones	superior nasal concha	inferior nasal conchae
frontal sinus	maxillae	cribriform plate
nares	crista galli	sphenoidal sinuses
nasal meatus		

References   Chapter 3, Skeletal system. In Fehrenbach MJ, Herring SW: *Illustrated anatomy of the head and neck,* ed 6, St. Louis, 2021, Saunders; Chapter 11, Head and neck structures. In Fehrenbach MJ, Popowics T: *Illustrated dental embryology, histology, and anatomy,* ed 5, St. Louis, 2020, Saunders.

NOTES

ANSWER KEY 1. frontal sinus, 2. superior nasal concha, 3. maxillae, 4. nasal meatus, 5. nares, 6. crista galli, 7. cribriform plate, 8. palatine bones, 9. inferior nasal conchae, 10. sphenoidal sinuses

FIGURE 4.9 Occipital bone with landmarks (inferior, lateral, and posterior views)

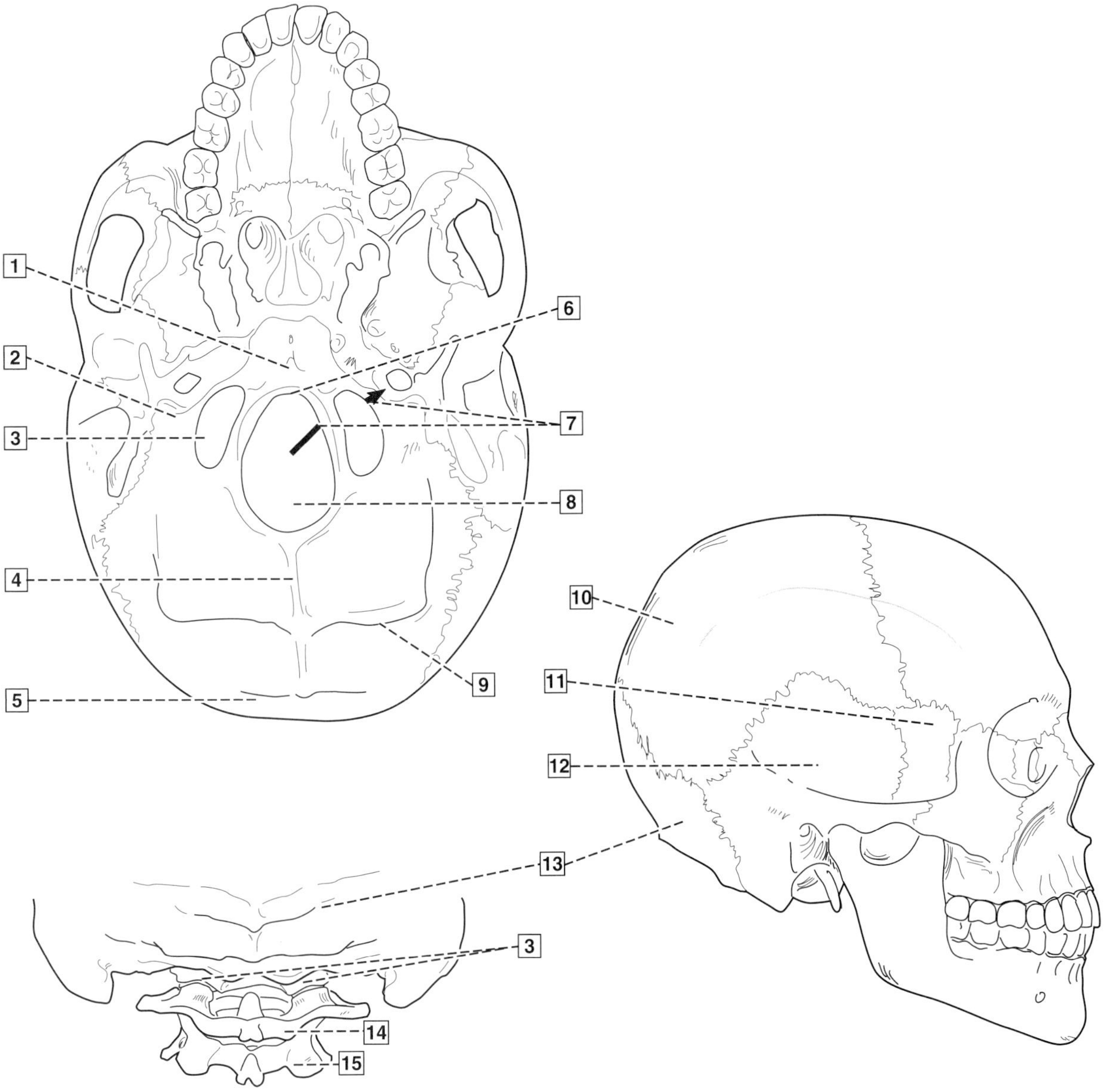

1	Pharyngeal tubercle	6	Basilar part	11	Sphenoid bone
2	Jugular notch of occipital bone	7	Hypoglossal canal	12	Temporal bone
3	Occipital condyle(s)	8	Foramen magnum	13	Occipital bone
4	External occipital protuberance	9	Inferior nuchal line	14	Atlas (first cervical vertebra)
5	Superior nuchal line	10	Parietal bone	15	Axis (second cervical vertebra)

REVIEW QUESTIONS: Occipital bone

Fill in the blanks by choosing the appropriate terms from the list below.

1. The _____ is a single cranial bone of the skull.

2. The occipital bone articulates with the _____, temporal bones, and sphenoid bone of the skull.

3. The occipital bone also articulates with the first cervical vertebra or _____.

4. On the external surface of the occipital bone from an inferior view, it can be noted that the _____ is completely formed by this bone.

5. Lateral and anterior to the foramen magnum are the _____, a pair of curved and smooth projections on the occipital bone.

6. On the stout _____, a four-sided plate anterior to the foramen magnum has a midline projection on the occipital bone, the pharyngeal tubercle.

7. When tilting the skull, the prominent openings anterior and lateral to the foramen magnum are noted on the inferior view of the occipital bone, the paired _____.

8. The _____ of the occipital bone, which forms the medial part of the jugular foramen (the lateral part is from the temporal bone), is noted on the inferior view.

9. The occipital bone is an irregular bone with _____ sides that is somewhat curved.

10. The occipital bone forms the posterior part of the skull and the base of the _____.

jugular notch	foramen magnum	parietal bones
cranium	hypoglossal canals	four
occipital condyles	occipital bone	basilar part
atlas		

Reference   Chapter 3, Skeletal system. In Fehrenbach MJ, Herring SW: *Illustrated anatomy of the head and neck,* ed 6, St. Louis, 2021, Saunders.

NOTES

FIGURE 4.10   Frontal bone with landmarks (lateral view of skull with anterior and inferior views of disarticulated bone)

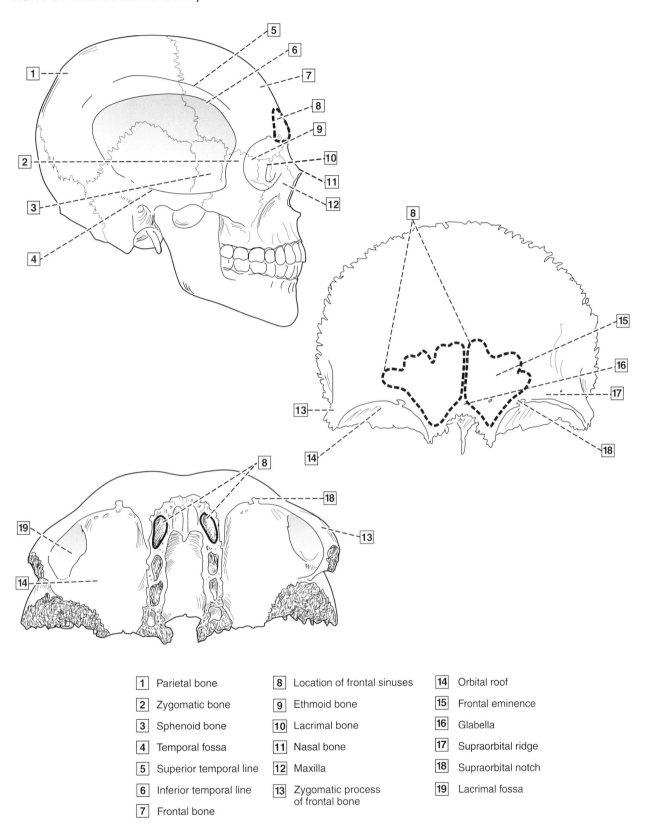

1	Parietal bone	**8**	Location of frontal sinuses	**14**	Orbital roof
2	Zygomatic bone	**9**	Ethmoid bone	**15**	Frontal eminence
3	Sphenoid bone	**10**	Lacrimal bone	**16**	Glabella
4	Temporal fossa	**11**	Nasal bone	**17**	Supraorbital ridge
5	Superior temporal line	**12**	Maxilla	**18**	Supraorbital notch
6	Inferior temporal line	**13**	Zygomatic process of frontal bone	**19**	Lacrimal fossa
7	Frontal bone				

REVIEW QUESTIONS: Frontal bone

Fill in the blanks by choosing the appropriate terms from the list below.

1. The _____ is a single cranial bone of the skull that forms the anterior part of the skull superior to the eyes in the frontal region and includes the majority of the forehead as well as the roof of each orbit.

2. The frontal bone articulates with the _____, sphenoid bone, lacrimal bones, nasal bones, ethmoid bone and zygomatic bones as well as the maxillae.

3. The frontal bone's part of the superior temporal line and _____ is noted when the bone is viewed from the lateral aspect.

4. Internally, the frontal bone contains the paired paranasal sinuses, the _____.

5. The _____ is located on the medial part of the supraorbital ridge of the frontal bone and is where the supraorbital artery and nerve travel from the orbit to the frontal region.

6. Between the supraorbital ridges of the frontal bone is the _____, the smooth elevated area between the eyebrows.

7. Lateral to the orbit is a projection, the orbital surface of the _____ of the frontal bone.

8. From the inferior view of the frontal bone, each _____ is noted and is located just internal to the lateral part of the supraorbital rim.

9. Each lacrimal fossa of the frontal bone contains the _____, which produces lacrimal fluid or *tears.*

10. The curved elevations over the superior part of the orbit are the _____ of the frontal bone, subjacent to the eyebrows.

lacrimal gland	lacrimal fossa	zygomatic process
frontal sinuses	parietal bones	supraorbital ridges
inferior temporal line	supraorbital notch	glabella
frontal bone		

Reference   Chapter 3, Skeletal system. In Fehrenbach MJ, Herring SW: *Illustrated anatomy of the head and neck,* ed 6, St. Louis, 2021, Saunders.

NOTES

ANSWER KEY   1. frontal bone, 2. parietal bones, 3. inferior temporal line, 4. frontal sinuses, 5. supraorbital notch, 6. glabella, 7. zygomatic process, 8. lacrimal fossa, 9. lacrimal gland, 10. supraorbital ridges

FIGURE 4.11 Parietal bones with landmarks (posterior view)

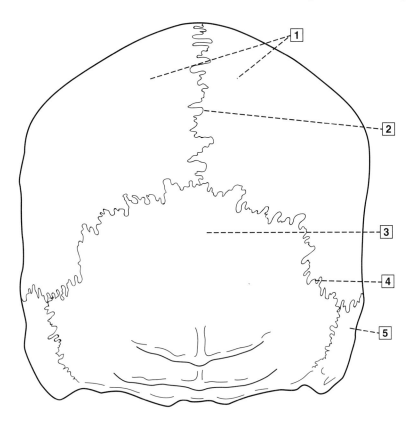

1 Parietal bones

2 Sagittal suture

3 Occipital bone

4 Lambdoidal suture

5 Temporal bone

REVIEW QUESTIONS: Parietal bones

Fill in the blanks by choosing the appropriate terms from the list below.

1. The _____ are paired cranial bones of the skull.

2. The two parietal bones articulate with each other at the single _____, which extends from the anterior to the posterior of the skull at the midline between the bones and is parallel to the sagittal plane of the skull.

3. The parietal bones are located posterior to the _____.

4. The two parietal bones together form the greater part of the right and left lateral walls and the roof of the _____.

5. The parietal bones also articulate with other bones of the skull including the occipital bone, frontal bone, temporal bone, and _____ bone.

6. The paired parietal bones articulate with the occipital bone at the single _____, which is typically more serrated looking than the other sutures, resembling an upside-down V-shape in anatomic position.

7. Each parietal bone has _____ borders and is relatively square and shaped like a curved plate.

8. The external surface of the parietal bone is convex, smooth, and marked near the center by the _____, which indicates the point where ossification commenced.

9. The _____, which is the longest and thickest part of each parietal bone articulates with the bone of the opposite side at the sagittal suture.

10. The point where the sagittal suture intersects the lambdoidal suture is called the _____.

parietal eminence	sagittal suture	skull
sagittal border	lambda	frontal bone
four	parietal bones	lambdoidal suture
sphenoid		

References Chapter 3, Skeletal system. In Fehrenbach MJ, Herring SW: *Illustrated anatomy of the head and neck,* ed 6, St. Louis, 2021, Saunders; Chapter 8, Head and neck. In Drake R, Vogel AW, Mitchell AWM: *Gray's anatomy for students,* ed 4, Philadelphia, 2020, Churchill Livingstone.

NOTES

FIGURE 4.12   Temporal bone(s) with parts and landmarks (lateral view of disarticulated bone and inferior views of disarticulated bone and upper skull)

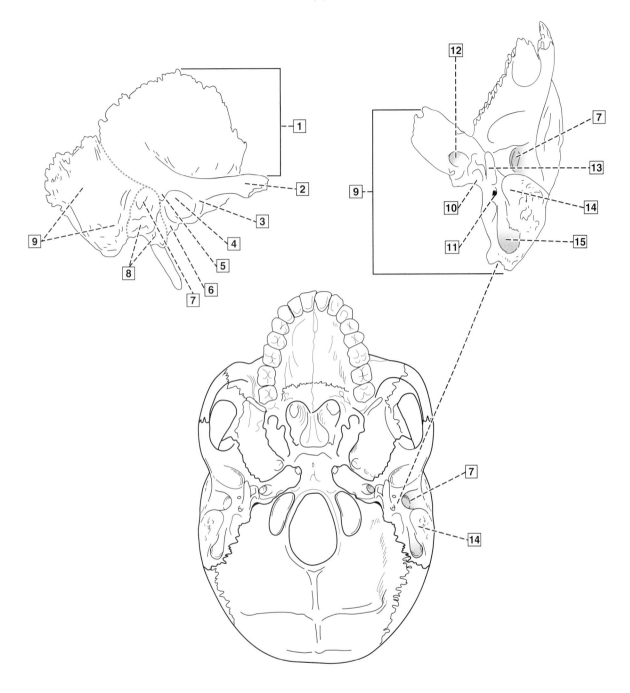

1 Squamous part	**6** Petrotympanic fissure	**11** Stylomastoid foramen
2 Zygomatic process	**7** External acoustic meatus	**12** Carotid canal
3 Articular eminence	**8** Tympanic part	**13** Styloid process
4 Articular fossa	**9** Petrous part	**14** Mastoid process
5 Postglenoid process	**10** Jugular notch	**15** Mastoid notch

REVIEW QUESTIONS: Temporal bone(s)

Fill in the blanks by choosing the appropriate terms from the list below.

1. The _____ are paired cranial bones that form the lateral walls of the skull in the temporal region.

2. The temporal bones are part of the base of the _____ in the auricular region.

3. Each temporal bone is deep to the _____, the superficial side of the head posterior to each eye.

4. Each temporal bone articulates with the zygomatic bone and the parietal bone as well as the occipital bone, sphenoid bone, and the _____.

5. Each temporal bone is composed of _____ parts including the squamous, tympanic, and petrous parts.

6. The small irregularly shaped _____ of the temporal bone is associated with the ear canal and forms most of the external acoustic meatus.

7. The large fan-shaped flat part on each of the temporal bones is the _____ of the temporal bone.

8. The _____ of the temporal bone is inferiorly located and helps form the cranial floor.

9. Anterior to the articular fossa of the temporal bone is the _____ and posterior is the postglenoid process, with the tympanic part separated from the petrous part by the petrotympanic fissure, through which the chorda tympani nerve emerges.

10. On the inferior aspect of the petrous part of the temporal bone and posterior to the external acoustic meatus is a large roughened projection, the _____.

three	temple	skull
mandible	petrous part	squamous part
tympanic part	temporal bones	articular eminence
mastoid process		

Reference Chapter 3, Skeletal system. In Fehrenbach MJ, Herring SW: *Illustrated anatomy of the head and neck,* ed 6, St. Louis, 2021, Saunders.

NOTES

FIGURE 4.13 Sphenoid bone with landmarks (superior view of internal skull surface, lateral view of disarticulated bone, inferior and lateral views of upper skull)

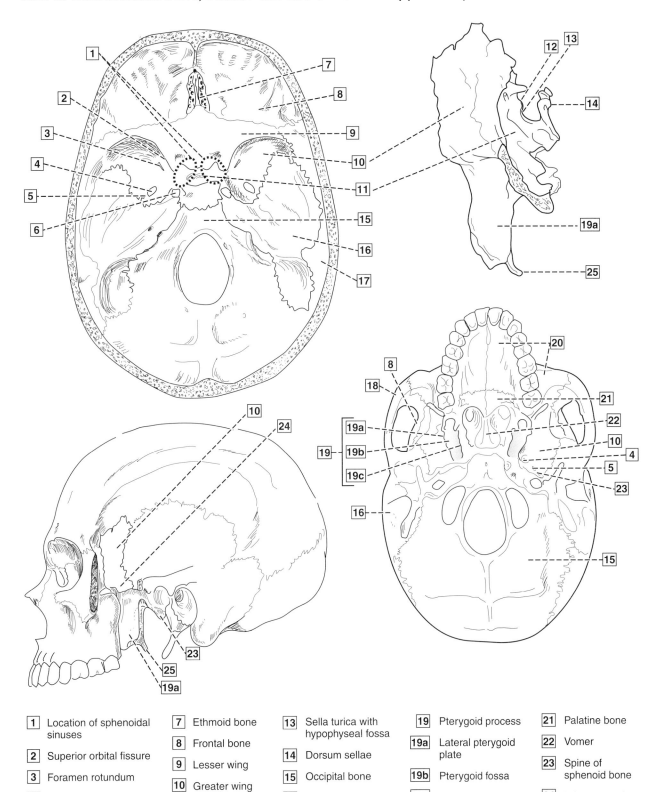

1 Location of sphenoidal sinuses	**7** Ethmoid bone	**13** Sella turica with hypophyseal fossa	**19** Pterygoid process
2 Superior orbital fissure	**8** Frontal bone	**14** Dorsum sellae	**19a** Lateral pterygoid plate
3 Foramen rotundum	**9** Lesser wing	**15** Occipital bone	**19b** Pterygoid fossa
4 Foramen ovale	**10** Greater wing	**16** Temporal bone	**19c** Medial pterygoid plate
5 Foramen spinosum	**11** Body	**17** Parietal bone	**20** Maxilla
6 Foramen lacerum	**12** Tuberculum sellae	**18** Zygomatic bone	

21 Palatine bone	
22 Vomer	
23 Spine of sphenoid bone	
24 Infratemporal crest	
25 Hamulus of medial pterygoid plate	

REVIEW QUESTIONS: Sphenoid bone

Fill in the blanks by choosing the appropriate terms from the list below.

1. The _____ is a midline cranial bone of the skull and thus is internally wedged between several other bones in the anterior part of the cranium, looking like a bat with its wings extended or butterfly taking wing.

2. The sphenoid bone articulates with the frontal, parietal, ethmoid, temporal, zygomatic, maxillae, palatine, vomer, and _____ bones, helping to connect the cranial skeleton to the facial skeleton.

3. The sphenoid bone consists of a(n) _____ and its three paired processes and has a number of features and openings.

4. The body of the sphenoid bone articulates on its anterior surface with the _____ and posteriorly with the basilar part of the occipital bone.

5. The posterolateral process of the sphenoid bone is the _____.

6. A sharp pointed area, the (angular) _____ of the sphenoid bone, is located at the posterior corner of each greater wing of the sphenoid bone.

7. Each greater wing of the sphenoid bone is divided into two smaller surfaces by the _____, the temporal and infratemporal surfaces.

8. The depression of the _____ is located lateral to the lateral pterygoid plate of the sphenoid bone.

9. The _____, a thin curved process, is the inferior termination of the medial pterygoid plate of the sphenoid bone.

10. The vertical pterygomaxillary fissure is located between the lateral pterygoid plate of the _____ of the sphenoid bone and the maxillary tuberosity on the maxilla; it gives passage to part of the maxillary artery and vein.

hamulus	pterygoid process	occipital
infratemporal fossa	ethmoid bone	greater wing
spine	sphenoid bone	infratemporal crest
body		

Reference Chapter 3, Skeletal system. In Fehrenbach MJ, Herring SW: *Illustrated anatomy of the head and neck,* ed 6, St. Louis, 2021, Saunders.

NOTES

FIGURE 4.14 Ethmoid bone with landmarks (anterior view of skull and disarticulated bone, anterolateral view, anterior view of internal skull surface)

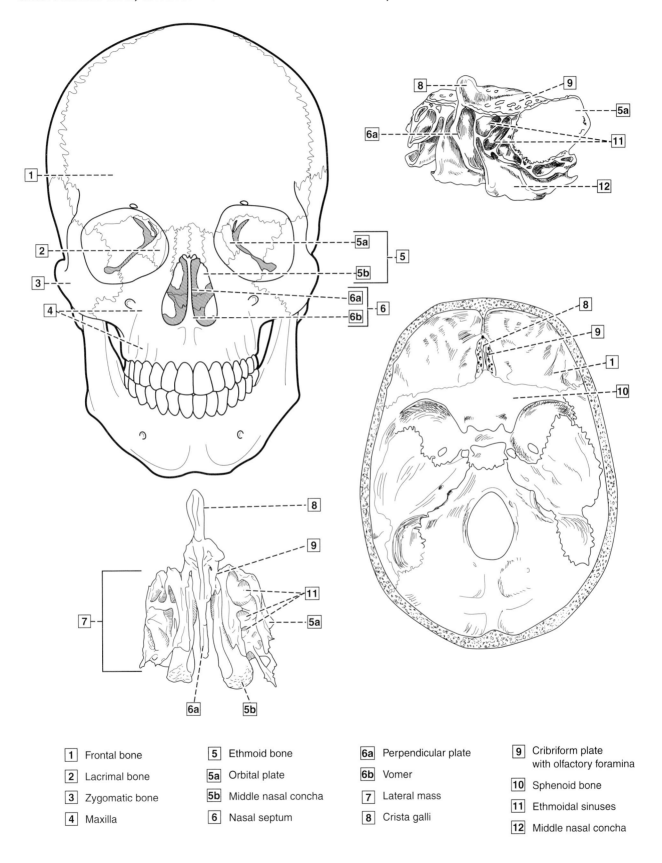

1 Frontal bone	**5** Ethmoid bone	**6a** Perpendicular plate	**9** Cribriform plate with olfactory foramina
2 Lacrimal bone	**5a** Orbital plate	**6b** Vomer	**10** Sphenoid bone
3 Zygomatic bone	**5b** Middle nasal concha	**7** Lateral mass	**11** Ethmoidal sinuses
4 Maxilla	**6** Nasal septum	**8** Crista galli	**12** Middle nasal concha

REVIEW QUESTIONS: Ethmoid bone

Fill in the blanks by choosing the appropriate terms from the list below.

1. The _____ is a single midline cranial bone of the skull.

2. The ethmoid bone is located anterior to the sphenoid bone in the anterior part of the

   _____.

3. The ethmoid bone articulates with the frontal, sphenoid, lacrimal bones and the maxillae, as well as adjoins the _____ at its inferior and posterior borders.

4. The ethmoid bone has two unpaired plates that form it, the midline vertical perpendicular plate and the horizontal _____, which cross over one another.

5. The cribriform plate within the inner surface of the cranial cavity can be seen on the superior surface of the ethmoid bone surrounding the _____; it is perforated by numerous foramina to allow the passage of olfactory nerves for the sense of smell.

6. The lateral part of the ethmoid bone forms the superior nasal and middle nasal _____ on each side that projects inward within the nasal cavity (in that order as part of the lateral nasal wall) as well as forms the paired orbital plate.

7. The _____ of the ethmoid bone forms the medial orbital wall.

8. Between the orbital plate and each set of the two conchae are the _____ or *ethmoid air cells*, which are a variable number of small cavities in the lateral mass of the ethmoid bone that are partly completed by the surrounding articulated bones; the posterior ethmoid air cells open into the superior nasal meatus, and the middle and anterior ethmoid air cells open into the middle nasal meatus.

9. The _____ of the ethmoid bone is viewed within the structure of the nasal cavity and assists the nasal septal cartilage and vomer in forming the nasal septum.

10. A vertical midline continuation of the perpendicular plate superiorly into the _____ is the wedge-shaped crista galli on the ethmoid bone, which serves as an attachment for layers covering the brain.

perpendicular plate	ethmoidal sinuses	ethmoid bone
cranial cavity	cribriform plate	cranium
conchae	vomer	crista galli
orbital plate		

Reference   Chapter 3, Skeletal system. In Fehrenbach MJ, Herring SW: *Illustrated anatomy of the head and neck,* ed 6, St. Louis, 2021, Saunders.

FIGURE 4.15 Vomer with landmarks (medial wall of nasal cavity and lateral view of disarticulated bone)

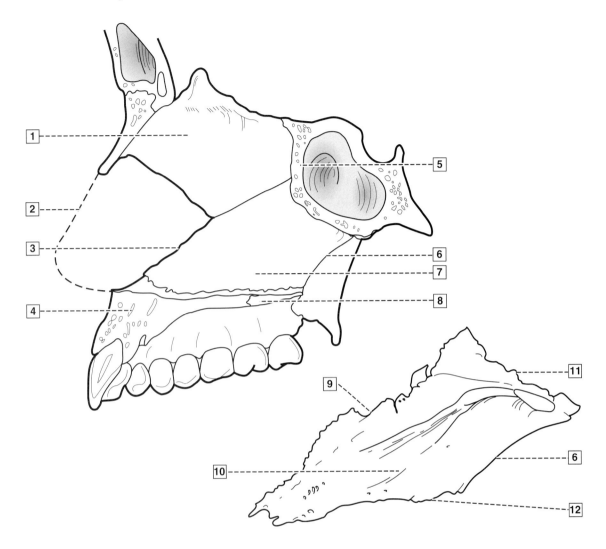

1 Ethmoid bone	**5** Sphenoid bone	**9** Anterior border
2 Location of nasal septal cartilage	**6** Posterior (free) border	**10** Nasopalatine groove
3 Articulation with nasal septal cartilage	**7** Vomer	**11** Superior border
4 Maxilla	**8** Palatine bone	**12** Inferior border

REVIEW QUESTIONS: Vomer

Fill in the blanks by choosing the appropriate terms from the list below.

1. The _____ is a thin and flat single midline facial bone of the skull.

2. The vomer is almost _____ in shape.

3. The vomer forms the posterior part of the _____, with the anterior and superior parts formed by cartilage and the ethmoid bone.

4. The perpendicular plate of the _____ is viewed within the structure of the nasal cavity and assists the nasal septal cartilage and vomer in forming the nasal septum.

5. The floor of the nasal cavity is formed from the bones of the hard palate, the palatine processes of the maxillae anteriorly and the horizontal plates of the _____ posteriorly.

6. The vomer articulates with the perpendicular plate of the ethmoid bone on the superior half of its anterior border, with its inferior half grooved for the inferior margin of the nasal septal cartilage; it also articulates with the _____ on its superior border.

7. The posterior border of the vomer is free of bony articulation and also has no _____ attachments.

8. The vomer is located within the _____ and its articulations are noted on a lateral view of the bone.

9. On each lateral surface is the _____ in which the nasopalatine nerve and branches of the sphenopalatine blood vessels travel.

10. The vomer is not a cranial bone but is considered a(n) _____.

palatine bones	vomer	muscle
facial bone	nasal septum	midsagittal plane
nasopalatine groove	sphenoid bone	trapezoidal
ethmoid bone		

Reference Chapter 3, Skeletal system. In Fehrenbach MJ, Herring SW: *Illustrated anatomy of the head and neck,* ed 6, St. Louis, 2021, Saunders.

NOTES

FIGURE 4.16 Lacrimal bones, nasal bones, and inferior nasal conchae (anterior view)

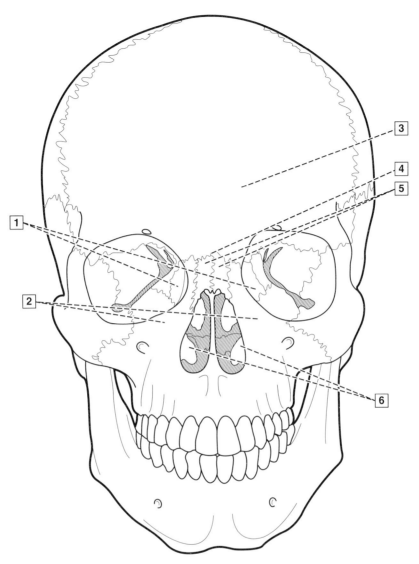

1	Lacrimal bones	**4**	Frontonasal suture
2	Maxillae	**5**	Nasal bones
3	Frontal bone	**6**	Inferior nasal conchae

REVIEW QUESTIONS: Lacrimal bones, nasal bones, and inferior nasal conchae

Fill in the blanks by choosing the appropriate terms from the list below.

1. Each paired _____ is an irregular thin plate of bone that forms a small part of the anterior medial wall of the orbit of the skull.

2. Each lacrimal bone as a facial bone of the skull articulates with both the ethmoid bone and the _____, as well as the maxilla.

3. The nasolacrimal duct is formed at the junction of the lacrimal bone and _____.

4. Lacrimal fluid or *tears* from the lacrimal gland are drained through the nasolacrimal duct into the _____.

5. The _____ are small oblong paired facial bones that lie side by side, fused to each other to form the bridge of the nose in the midline superior to the piriform aperture; the fusion line between the two bones is the *internasal suture.*

6. The nasal bones fit between the frontal processes of the maxillae and thus articulate with the frontal bone superiorly at the _____ and the maxillae laterally.

7. The _____ are paired facial bones of the skull that project from the maxillae to form a part of the lateral walls of the nasal cavity.

8. Unlike the superior and middle nasal conchae that also project from the maxillae, the inferior nasal conchae are two separate _____.

9. The inferior nasal conchae articulate with the ethmoid, lacrimal, and _____ as well as the maxillae.

10. The medial surface of each inferior nasal concha is convex, perforated by numerous apertures, and traversed by _____ for blood vessels.

longitudinal grooves	palatine bones	inferior nasal meatus
maxilla	frontal bone	inferior nasal conchae
facial bones	lacrimal bone	nasal bones
frontonasal suture		

References   Chapter 3, Skeletal system. In Fehrenbach MJ, Herring SW: *Illustrated anatomy of the head and neck,* ed 6, St. Louis, 2021, Saunders; Chapter 8, Head and neck. In Drake R, Vogel AW, Mitchell AWM: *Gray's anatomy for students,* ed 4, Philadelphia, 2020, Churchill Livingstone.

NOTES

FIGURE 4.17 Zygomatic bone(s) with landmarks (lateral and anterior views)

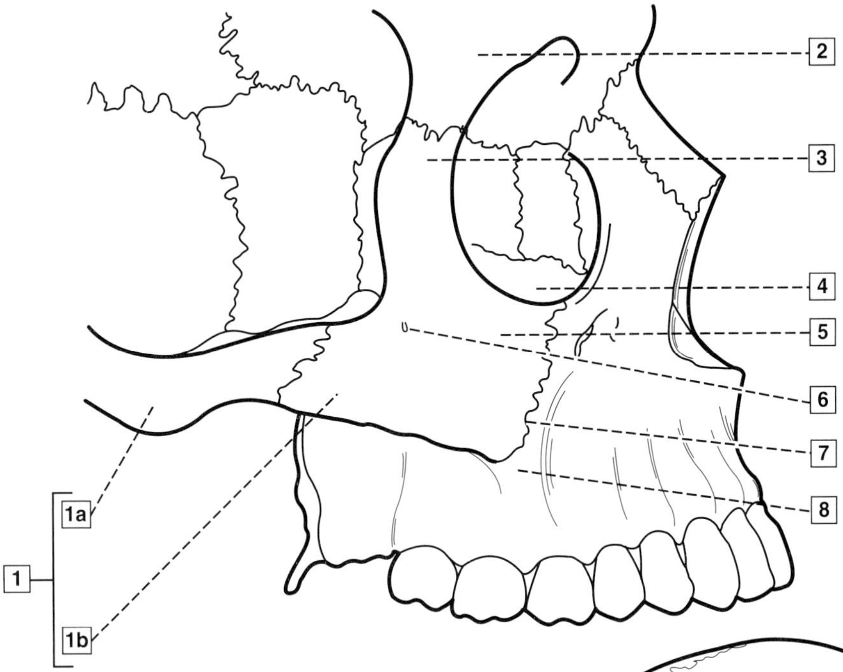

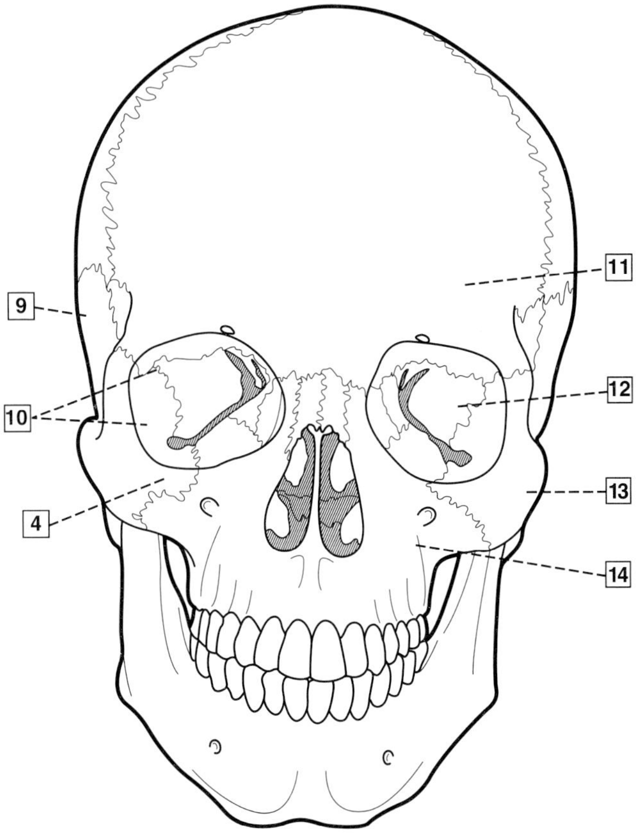

1	Zygomatic arch
1a	Zygomatic process of temporal bone
1b	Temporal process of zygomatic bone
2	Zygomatic process of frontal bone
3	Frontal process of zygomatic bone
4	Infraorbital rim
5	Maxillary process of zygomatic bone
6	Zygomaticomaxillary foramen
7	Zygomaticomaxillary suture
8	Zygomatic process of maxilla
9	Temporal bone
10	Lateral orbital wall
11	Frontal bone
12	Sphenoid bone
13	Zygomatic bone
14	Maxilla

REVIEW QUESTIONS: Zygomatic bone(s)

Fill in the blanks by choosing the appropriate terms from the list below.

1. The _____ or *zygoma* is a paired facial bone of the skull that forms the majority of the cheekbone or *malar surface.*

2. The zygomatic bones articulate with the frontal, temporal, and sphenoid bones as well as the

_____.

3. Each zygomatic bone is diamond-shaped and composed of _____ processes with similarly named associated bony articulations including the frontal, temporal, and maxillary processes.

4. The orbital surface of the _____ of the zygomatic bone forms the anterior lateral orbital wall, usually with a small foramen, the zygomaticofacial foramen, opening onto its lateral surface.

5. The _____ of the zygomatic bone forms the zygomatic arch along with the zygomatic process of the temporal bone, with an equally small zygomaticotemporal foramen present on its posterior surface.

6. The orbital surface of the _____ of the zygomatic bone forms the lateral part of the infra-orbital rim and a small part of the anterior part of the lateral orbital wall.

7. The zygomatic bone helps to form the lateral wall and floor of the _____.

8. Each of the three processes of the zygomatic bone helps to form structures of the

_____.

9. The zygomaticotemporal nerve serves as an afferent nerve for the skin of the temporal region and pierces the temporal process of the zygomatic bone at the _____.

10. The zygomaticofacial nerve serves as an afferent nerve for the skin of the cheek and pierces the frontal process of the zygomatic bone at the _____.

zygomaticotemporal foramen	three	zygomatic bone
orbit	zygomaticofacial foramen	maxillae
skull	maxillary process	frontal process
temporal process		

Reference Chapter 3, Skeletal system. In Fehrenbach MJ, Herring SW: *Illustrated anatomy of the head and neck,* ed 6, St. Louis, 2021, Saunders; Chapter 8, Nervous system. In Fehrenbach MJ, Herring SW: *Illustrated anatomy of the head and neck,* ed 6, St. Louis, 2021, Saunders.

NOTES

ANSWER KEY 1. zygomatic bone, 2. maxillae, 3. three, 4. frontal process, 5. temporal process, 6. maxillary process, 7. orbit, 8. skull, 9. zygomaticotemporal foramen, 10. zygomaticofacial foramen

FIGURE 4.18   Palatine bone(s) and maxillae with landmarks (hard palate view, posteroinferior skull view, and posterolateral view of disarticulated bone)

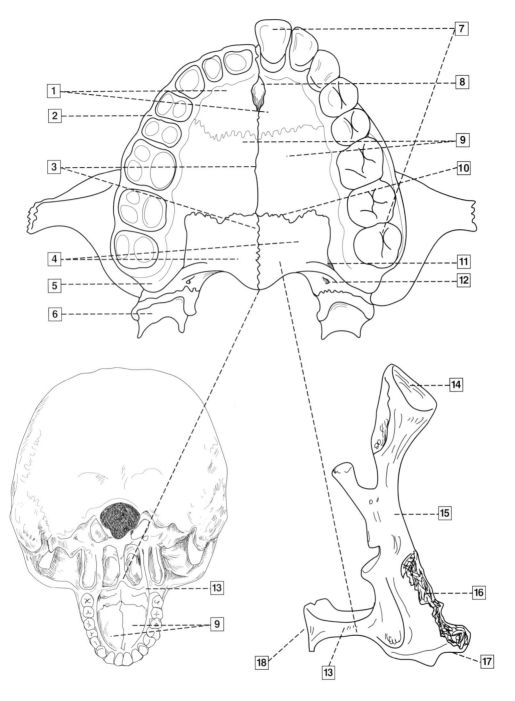

1 Palatine processes of maxilla	**7** Maxillary teeth	**13** Horizontal plate of palatine bone
2 Alveolar process of maxilla	**8** Incisive foramen	**14** Orbital process at apex of orbit
3 Median palatine suture	**9** Maxillae	**15** Vertical plate of palatine bone
4 Horizontal plates of the palatine bones	**10** Transverse suture	**16** Pyramidal process of palatine bone
5 Maxillary tuberosity	**11** Greater palatine foramen	**17** Articulation with palatal process of maxilla at transverse palatine suture
6 Sphenoid bone	**12** Lesser palatine foramen	**18** Articulation with contralateral palatine bone at median palatine suture

REVIEW QUESTIONS: Palatine bone(s) and maxillae

Fill in the blanks by choosing the appropriate terms from the list below.

1. The _____ are paired bones of the skull that form the posterior part of the hard palate and the floor of the nasal cavity; anteriorly they join with the maxillae.

2. Each palatine bone is somewhat L-shaped and thus consists of two plates, the _____ and vertical plate.

3. The horizontal plates of each palatine bone form inferiorly the posterior part of the _____.

4. The _____ of each palatine bone forms a part of the lateral walls of the nasal cavity, and each plate contributes a small part of the bone to the orbital apex.

5. The palatine bones serve as a link between the _____ and the sphenoid bone with which they both articulate.

6. The two horizontal plates of the palatine bones articulate with each other at the posterior part of the _____.

7. The two horizontal plates of each palatine bone articulate anteriorly with the palatine processes of the maxillae at the _____.

8. The larger _____ is located in the posterolateral region of each horizontal plate of the palatine bones, usually superior to apices of the maxillary second or third molars, and transmits the greater palatine nerve and blood vessels, serving as a landmark for the administration of the greater palatine nerve block.

9. A smaller opening near the greater palatine foramen, the _____, transmits the lesser palatine nerve and blood vessels to the soft palate and tonsils.

10. The paired _____ is the opening between the sphenoid bone and orbital processes of each palatine bone; it opens into the nasal cavity and gives passage to branches from the pterygopalatine ganglion, the nasopalatine nerves and posterior superior nasal nerves as well as the sphenopalatine artery from the maxillary artery.

vertical plate	greater palatine foramen	maxillae
sphenopalatine foramen	palatine bones	horizontal plate
median palatine suture	lesser palatine foramen	hard palate
transverse palatine suture		

Reference Chapter 3, Skeletal system. In Fehrenbach MJ, Herring SW: *Illustrated anatomy of the head and neck*, ed 6, St. Louis, 2021, Saunders.

FIGURE 4.19 Maxillae with landmarks (anterior view)

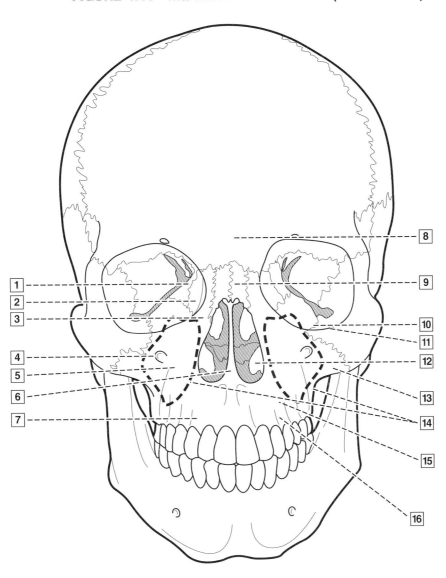

1	Ethmoid bone	6	Vomer	11	Infraorbital rim
2	Lacrimal bone	7	Alveolar process of maxilla	12	Inferior nasal concha
3	Frontal process of maxilla	8	Frontal bone	13	Zygomatic process of maxilla
4	Infraorbital foramen	9	Nasal bone	14	Location of maxillary sinus
5	Body of maxilla	10	Infraorbital sulcus	15	Canine fossa
				16	Canine eminence

REVIEW QUESTIONS: Maxillae

Fill in the blanks by choosing the appropriate terms from the list below.

1. The _____ or upper jaw consists of two maxilla or maxillary bones.

2. The two parts of the maxillae are fused together at the _____.

3. Each maxilla articulates with the _____, lacrimal, nasal, inferior nasal concha, vomer, sphenoid, ethmoid, palatine, and zygomatic bones.

4. Each maxilla has a body and _____ processes, which includes the frontal, zygomatic, palatine, and alveolar processes.

5. The _____ of the maxilla has four surfaces: the orbital, nasal, infratemporal, and facial surfaces.

6. Each of the bodies of the maxillae contains the _____, which are air-filled spaces or paranasal sinuses.

7. The paired maxilla together form the upper _____ as the facial bones of the skull that contain the maxillary teeth.

8. From the anterior view, each _____ of the maxilla articulates with the frontal bone.

9. The infraorbital sulcus becomes the infraorbital canal, and finally terminates on the facial surface of each maxilla as the _____.

10. An elongated depression, the _____, is just posterosuperior to each of the roots of the maxillary canines.

maxillary sinuses	canine fossa	four
body	jaw	intermaxillary suture
frontal process	infraorbital foramen	maxillae
frontal bone		

Reference   Chapter 3, Skeletal system. In Fehrenbach MJ, Herring SW: *Illustrated anatomy of the head and neck,* ed 6, St. Louis, 2021, Saunders.

NOTES

FIGURE 4.20   Maxilla with landmarks (cutaway lateral aspect)

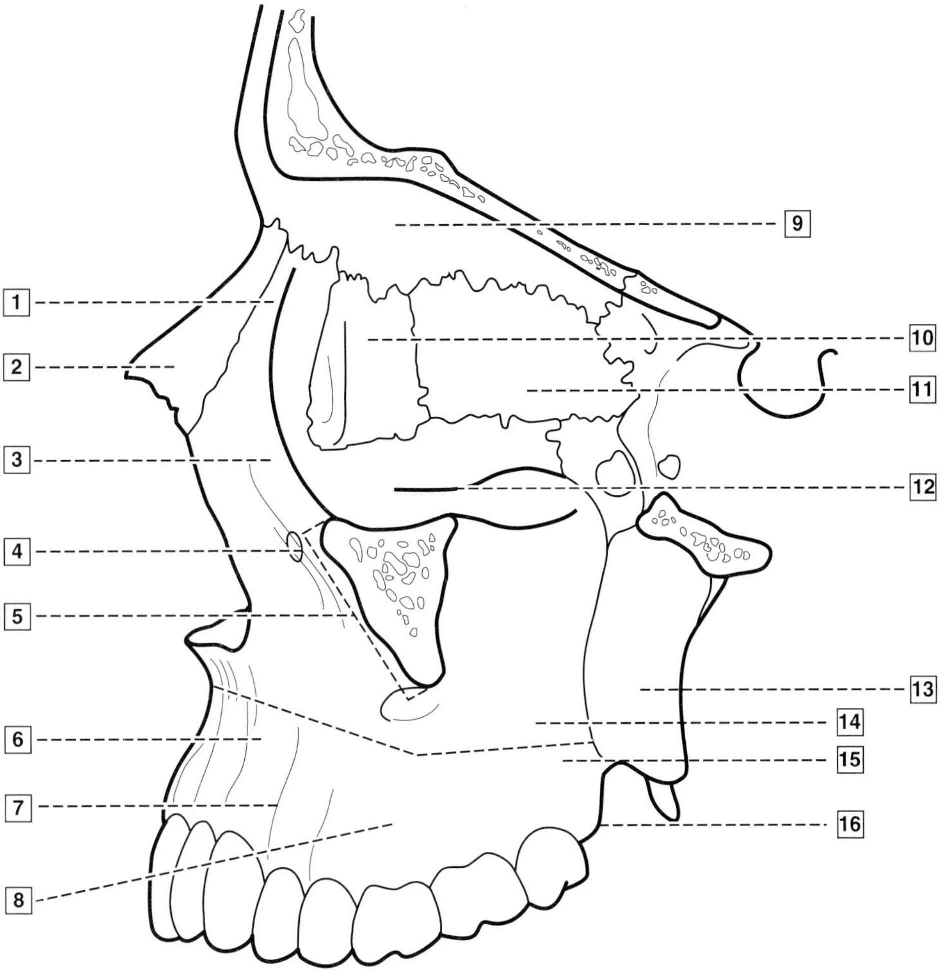

1 Frontal process of maxilla	**8** Alveolar process of maxilla	**15** Posterior superior alveolar foramina
2 Nasal bone	**9** Frontal bone	**16** Maxillary tuberosity
3 Infraorbital rim	**10** Lacrimal bone	
4 Infraorbital foramen	**11** Ethmoid bone	
5 Zygomatic process of maxilla	**12** Infraorbital sulcus	
6 Canine fossa	**13** Sphenoid bone	
7 Canine eminence	**14** Body of maxilla	

REVIEW QUESTIONS: Maxilla

Fill in the blanks by choosing the appropriate terms from the list below.

1. The facial ridge over each of the maxillary canines, the _____, is especially prominent, serving as a landmark for the administration of the anterior superior alveolar nerve block.

2. The _____ of the maxilla inferior to the temple is convex.

3. From the lateral view, each _____ of the maxilla articulates at the zygomaticomaxillary suture with the maxillary process of the zygomatic bone laterally, completing the medial part of the infraorbital rim.

4. On the posterior part of the body of the maxilla is a rounded roughened elevation, the _____, just posterior to the most distal molar of the maxillary arch of the dentition, which is a landmark for an analysis of radiographs and also serves as one of the borders of the infratemporal fossae of the skull.

5. The posterosuperior part of the maxillary tuberosity is perforated multiple times by the _____, where the posterior superior alveolar nerve and blood vessel branches enter the bone from the posterior, serving as a landmark for the administration of the posterior superior alveolar nerve block.

6. Each maxilla articulates with the frontal, lacrimal, nasal, inferior nasal concha, vomer, sphenoid, ethmoid, palatine, and _____.

7. An elongated depression, the canine fossa, is posterosuperior to each of the roots of the _____ canines in the alveolar process of the maxilla.

8. The body of the maxilla has orbital, nasal, infratemporal, and _____ surfaces.

9. The groove in the floor of the orbital surface of each maxilla is the _____.

10. The infraorbital sulcus becomes the infraorbital canal and then terminates on the facial surface of each maxilla as the _____.

maxillary tuberosity	infraorbital foramen	zygomatic bone
zygomatic process	infraorbital sulcus	maxillary
posterior superior alveolar foramina	canine eminence	facial
infratemporal surface		

Reference   Chapter 3, Skeletal system. In Fehrenbach MJ, Herring SW: *Illustrated anatomy of the head and neck,* ed 6, St. Louis, 2021, Saunders.

FIGURE 4.21   Mandible with landmarks (anterolateral view with internal view)

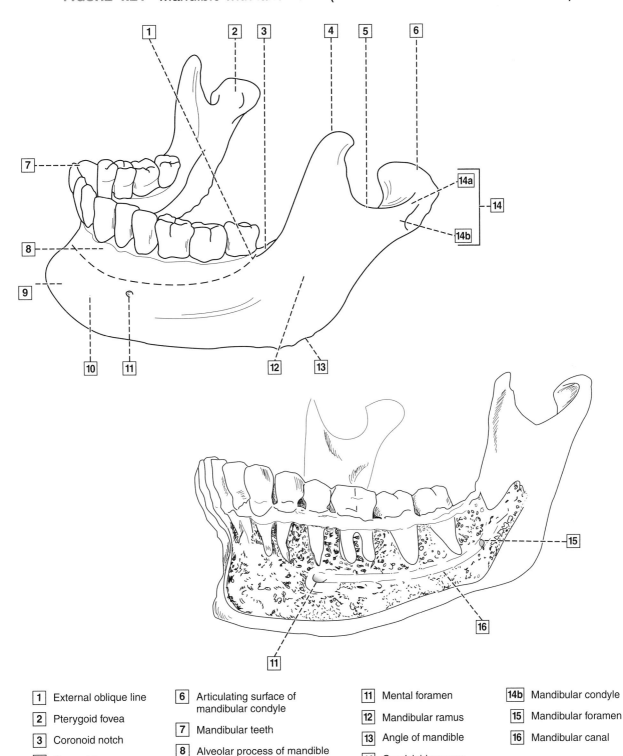

1 External oblique line	**6** Articulating surface of mandibular condyle	**11** Mental foramen	**14b** Mandibular condyle
2 Pterygoid fovea		**12** Mandibular ramus	**15** Mandibular foramen
3 Coronoid notch	**7** Mandibular teeth	**13** Angle of mandible	**16** Mandibular canal
4 Coronoid process	**8** Alveolar process of mandible	**14** Condyloid process	
5 Mandibular notch	**9** Mental protuberance	**14a** Neck of mandibular condyle	
	10 Body of mandible		

REVIEW QUESTIONS: Mandible

Fill in the blanks by choosing the appropriate terms from the list below.

1. The _____ is a single facial bone that forms the lower jaw and is the only freely movable bone of the skull.

2. The heavy horizontal part of the lower jaw inferior to the mental foramen is the _____ of the mandible or *base*.

3. The _____ is the midline bony prominence of the chin, located inferior to the roots of the mandibular incisors.

4. Farther posteriorly on the lateral surface of the mandible, usually inferior to the apices of the mandibular premolars, is an opening, the _____, which allows the entry of the mental nerve and blood vessels into the mandibular canal to merge with the incisive nerve and blood vessels.

5. Superior to the body of the mandible, the part of the lower jaw that contains the roots of the mandibular teeth within the alveoli is the _____ of the mandible.

6. On the lateral aspect of the mandible, the stout flat plate of the _____ rises from the angle and extends superiorly and posteriorly from the body of the mandible on each side.

7. The posterior border of the mandibular ramus becomes thicker and extends from the angle of the mandible, which is the juncture between the mandibular ramus and the body of the mandible, to a large more posterior projection, the _____.

8. The condyloid process consists of two parts, the mandibular condyle and the constricted part that supports it, its _____.

9. The anterior border of the mandibular ramus has a thin sharp margin that terminates in the
   _____.

10. The main part of the anterior border of the mandibular ramus forms a concave forward curve, the
    _____, which is the greatest depression on the anterior border of the mandibular ramus, serving as a landmark for the administration of the inferior alveolar nerve block.

mental protuberance	alveolar process	mandibular ramus
mental foramen	body	condyloid process
mandible	coronoid notch	neck
coronoid process		

Reference   Chapter 3, Skeletal system. In Fehrenbach MJ, Herring SW: *Illustrated anatomy of the head and neck,* ed 6, St. Louis, 2021, Saunders.

FIGURE 4.22 **Mandible with landmarks (medial view with internal view)**

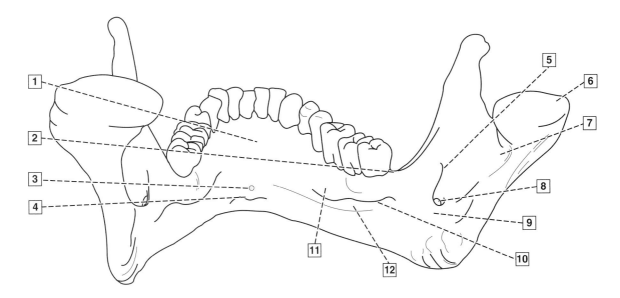

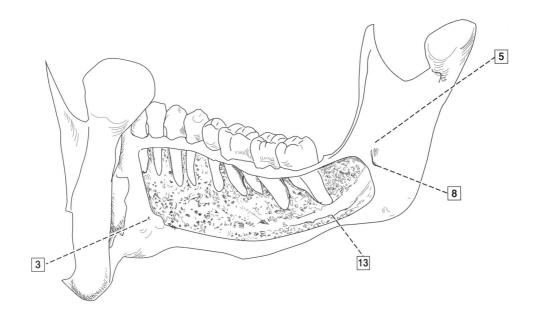

1 Alveolar process of mandible	**6** Articulating surface of condyle	**11** Sublingual fossa
2 Retromolar triangle	**7** Mandibular ramus	**12** Submandibular fossa
3 Lingual foramen	**8** Mandibular foramen	**13** Mandibular canal
4 Genial tubercles	**9** Mylohyoid groove	
5 Lingula	**10** Mylohyoid line	

REVIEW QUESTIONS: Mandible

Fill in the blanks by choosing the appropriate terms from the list below.

1. Near the midline of the mandible on its medial surface are the _____ or *mental spines*, four small projections that serve as a muscle attachment area.

2. At the lateral edge of each mandibular alveolar process is a rounded roughened area, the _____, just posterior to the most distal mandibular molar (if present), which is a bony landmark for the administration of the buccal block, and when covered with soft tissue is seen as the retromolar pad.

3. Along each medial surface of the body of the mandible is the *internal oblique ridge* or _____ that extends posteriorly and superiorly, becoming more prominent as it moves superiorly onto the body of the mandible; this is the point of attachment of the mylohyoid muscle that forms the floor of the mouth.

4. A shallow depression, the _____, which contains the sublingual salivary gland, is located superior to the anterior part of the mylohyoid line on each side.

5. Inferior to the posterior part of the mylohyoid line and inferior to the mandibular posterior teeth is a deeper depression, the _____, which contains the submandibular salivary gland.

6. On the medial surface of the mandibular ramus is the _____, which is the opening of the mandibular canal, with the inferior alveolar nerve and blood vessels exiting the mandible through it.

7. Overhanging the mandibular foramen is a bony spine, the _____, which serves as an attachment for the sphenomandibular ligament associated with the temporomandibular joint.

8. A small groove, the _____, passes anteriorly to and inferiorly from the mandibular foramen, with the mylohyoid nerve and blood vessels traveling in it.

9. The _____ of the condyle is where the mandible articulates with the temporal bone at the temporomandibular joint.

10. Inferior to the articular surface of the condyle on the anterior surface of the neck is a triangular depression, the _____, which serves for the attachment of the lateral pterygoid muscle.

mylohyoid line	mylohyoid groove	sublingual fossa
pterygoid fovea	retromolar triangle	submandibular fossa
articulating surface	genial tubercles	mandibular foramen
lingula		

Reference   Chapter 3, Skeletal system. In Fehrenbach MJ, Herring SW: *Illustrated anatomy of the head and neck,* ed 6, St. Louis, 2021, Saunders.

FIGURE 4.23   Temporomandibular joint: Temporal bone and mandible (lateral, inferolateral of temporal bone, and anterolateral of mandible views)

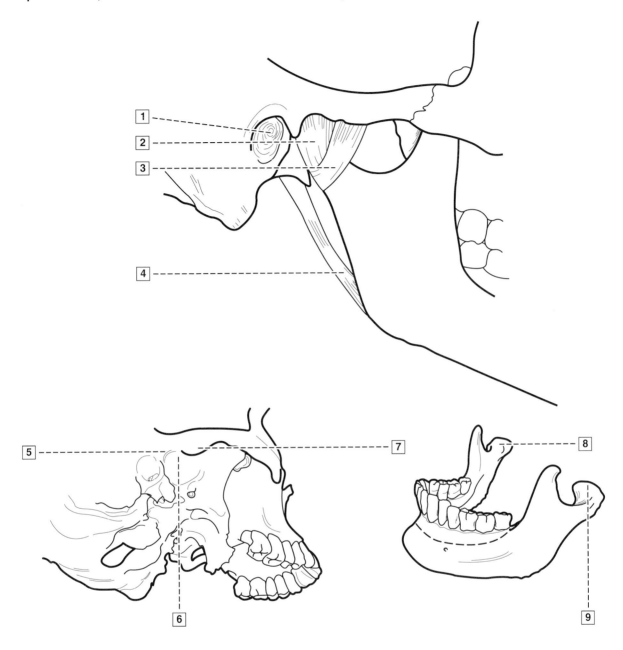

1	External acoustic meatus	**6**	Articular fossa
2	Joint capsule	**7**	Articular eminence
3	Temporomandibular ligament	**8**	Articulating surface of condyle
4	Stylomandibular ligament	**9**	Mandibular condyle
5	Postglenoid process		

REVIEW QUESTIONS: Temporomandibular joint

Fill in the blanks by choosing the appropriate terms from the list below.

1. The _____ is a joint on each side of the head that allows for movement of the mandible for mastication, speech, and respiratory movements.

2. The _____ is a cranial bone of the skull that articulates with the facial skull bone of the mandible at the temporomandibular joint by way of the joint disc.

3. The _____, which is also known as the *mandibular fossa* or *glenoid fossa,* is posterior to the articular eminence and consists of an oval-shaped depression on the temporal bone, which is posterior and medial to the zygomatic process of the temporal bone.

4. Posterior to the articular fossa is a sharper ridge, the _____.

5. The _____ of the condyle is strongly convex in the anteroposterior direction and only slightly convex mediolaterally and is where the mandible articulates with the temporal bone.

6. A fibrous _____ completely encloses the temporomandibular joint, with it superiorly wrapping around the margin of the temporal bone's articular eminence and articular fossa and inferiorly wrapping around the level posteriorly and laterally at the neck, but anteriorly and medially it attaches just to the margin of the articular surface of the condyle.

7. The _____ or *meniscus* is located between the temporal bone and mandibular condyle on each side, allowing articulation between the two bones at the temporomandibular joint.

8. The _____ is a variable ligament formed from the thickened cervical fascia in the area that runs from the styloid process of the temporal bone to the angle of the mandible and separates the parotid and submandibular salivary glands.

9. The _____ is located on the lateral side of each joint forming a reinforcement of the lateral part of the joint capsule of the temporomandibular joint.

10. The joint disc completely divides the temporomandibular joint into two compartments or _____, consisting of an upper and a lower one.

synovial cavities	postglenoid process	articulating surface
temporomandibular ligament	stylomandibular ligament	temporal bone
joint disc	articular fossa	temporomandibular joint
joint capsule		

References Chapter 5, Temporomandibular joint. In Fehrenbach MJ, Herring SW: *Illustrated anatomy of the head and neck,* ed 6, St. Louis, 2021, Saunders; Chapter 19, Temporomandibular joint. In Fehrenbach MJ, Popowics T: *Illustrated dental embryology, histology, and anatomy,* ed 5, St. Louis, 2020, Saunders.

FIGURE 4.24 Temporomandibular joint (medial view)

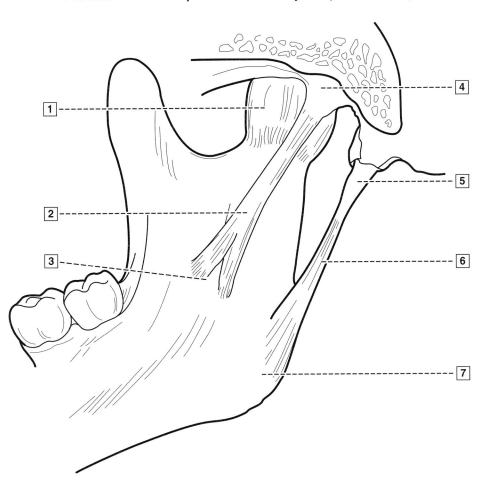

1	Joint capsule
2	Sphenomandibular ligament
3	Lingula over mandibular foramen
4	Spine of sphenoid bone
5	Styloid process of temporal bone
6	Stylomandibular ligament
7	Angle of mandible

REVIEW QUESTIONS: Temporomandibular joint

Fill in the blanks by choosing the appropriate terms from the list below.

1. The mandible is joined to the cranium by ligaments of the _____, which include temporomandibular, stylomandibular, and sphenomandibular ligaments.

2. The _____ is located on the lateral side of each joint, forming a reinforcement of the lateral part of the joint capsule, and is considered the major ligament for the joint since it provides strength to the joint.

3. The triangle-shaped temporomandibular joint ligament has a base that is attached to the zygomatic process of the _____ lateral to the articular eminence; its apex is fixed to the lateral side of the neck of the mandible.

4. The temporomandibular joint ligament prevents excessive _____ or moving backward of the mandible.

5. The _____ runs from the styloid process of the temporal bone to the angle of the mandible, separates the parotid and submandibular salivary glands and becomes taut when the mandible is protruded upon opening of the mouth.

6. The _____ runs from the angular spine of the sphenoid bone to the lingula of the mandibular foramen over the mandibular foramen on the medial aspect of the mandible.

7. The inferior alveolar nerve descends between the sphenomandibular ligament and the mandibular ramus to gain access to the _____, and because of its attachment to the lingula, it overlaps the opening.

8. The sphenomandibular ligament is involved in troubleshooting the inferior alveolar block due to its location; however, it may actually act as an outer barrier to the diffusion of the agent if the medial surface of the _____ is not contacted with the needle at the deeper mandibular foramen with the inferior alveolar nerve.

9. The articular fossa is posterior and _____ to the zygomatic process of the temporal bone.

10. The stylomandibular ligament is a variable ligament formed from thickened cervical _____ in the area.

medial	temporomandibular ligament	mandibular foramen
temporal bone	fascia	mandible
stylomandibular ligament	retraction	sphenomandibular ligament
temporomandibular joint		

References   Chapter 5, Temporomandibular joint. In Fehrenbach MJ, Herring SW: *Illustrated anatomy of the head and neck,* ed 6, St. Louis, 2021, Saunders; Chapter 19, Temporomandibular joint. In Fehrenbach MJ, Popowics T: *Illustrated dental embryology, histology, and anatomy,* ed 5, St. Louis, 2020, Saunders.

FIGURE 4.25 Temporomandibular joint (sagittal section with joint capsule removed)

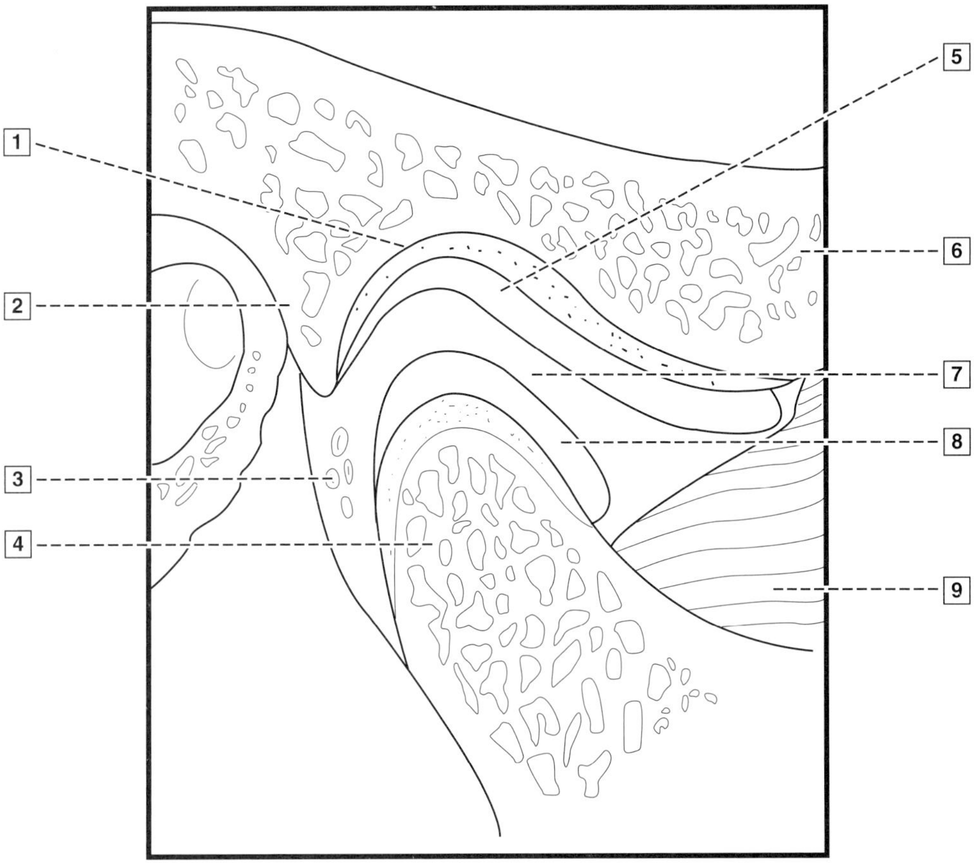

1	Articular fossa	5	Upper synovial cavity	9	Lateral pterygoid muscle
2	Postglenoid process	6	Articular eminence		
3	Blood vessels	7	Joint disc		
4	Mandibular condyle	8	Lower synovial cavity		

REVIEW QUESTIONS: Temporomandibular joint

Fill in the blanks by choosing the appropriate terms from the list below.

1. The shape of the _____ that divides the temporomandibular joint conforms to the shape of the adjacent articulating bones of the joint and is related to joint movements.

2. The central region of the joint disc lacks innervation and _____ (without blood vessels) in contrast to the peripheral region that has both nerves and blood vessels; the central region is also thinner but of denser consistency than the peripheral region.

3. On section, the joint disc appears caplike on the _____, with its superior aspect concavoconvex from anterior to posterior and its inferior aspect concave.

4. The joint disc completely divides the temporomandibular joint into two compartments, the _____ and the lower synovial cavity.

5. The membranes lining the inside of the joint capsule secrete _____, which is a clear viscous liquid that helps lubricate the joint and fills the synovial cavities.

6. The joint disc is not directly attached to the _____ anteriorly, but indirectly through the joint capsule.

7. Posteriorly, the joint disc is divided into two areas or divisions, upper and lower, with the upper division of the posterior part of the disc attached to the _____ of the temporal bone, and the lower division attached to the neck of the condyle.

8. The _____ area of attachment of the joint disc to the joint capsule is one of the locations where nerves and blood vessels enter the joint.

9. The margins of the joint disc are continuous with the _____ or attach into the joint capsule.

10. The joint disc is not free between the two bones but is attached to the _____ and medial poles of the mandibular condyle.

posterior	lateral	joint disc
postglenoid process	mandibular condyle	synovial fluid
temporal bone	avascular	joint capsule
upper synovial cavity		

References   Chapter 5, Temporomandibular joint. In Fehrenbach MJ, Herring SW: *Illustrated anatomy of the head and neck,* ed 6, St. Louis, 2021, Saunders; Chapter 19, Temporomandibular joint. In Fehrenbach MJ, Popowics T: *Illustrated dental embryology, histology, and anatomy,* ed 5, St. Louis, 2020, Saunders.

FIGURE 4.26 Paranasal sinuses (anterior and lateral views)

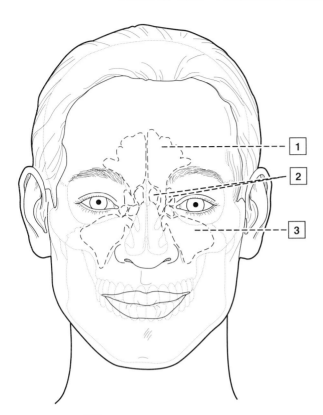

1. Frontal sinus
2. Ethmoidal sinuses
3. Maxillary sinus
4. Sphenoidal sinus

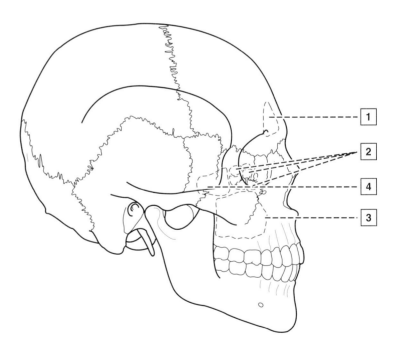

REVIEW QUESTIONS: Paranasal sinuses

Fill in the blanks by choosing the appropriate terms from the list below.

1. The _____ are paired air-filled cavities within the bone of the head that project laterally, superiorly, and posteriorly into the bone surrounding the nasal cavities and are lined with mucous membranes of the respiratory type consisting of ciliated pseudostratified columnar epithelium that is continuous with the epithelial lining of the nasal cavity.

2. The paranasal sinuses communicate with the _____ through ostium or ostia, smaller openings in the lateral nasal wall; these are from the original openings of the outgrowths that persisted.

3. The paired _____ are located in the frontal bone just superior to the nasal cavity, with each one communicating with and draining into the nasal cavity by a constricted canal to the middle nasal meatus, the frontonasal duct; they are not present at birth but at approximately 2 years of age, the two anterior ethmoidal sinuses grow into the frontal bone, forming one on each side that is visible on radiographs of the region by age 7.

4. The paired _____ are located deep within the body of the sphenoid bone and communicate with and drain into the nasal cavity through an opening superior to each superior nasal concha; they are not present at birth but at approximately 2 years of age, the two posterior ethmoidal sinuses grow into the sphenoid bone to form them.

5. The _____ or *ethmoid air cells* are a variable number of small cavities in the lateral mass of each of the ethmoid bones; at birth only a few are present and they do not start to grow until 6 to 8 years of age.

6. The posterior ethmoid air cells open into the _____ of the nasal cavity, and the middle and anterior ethmoid air cells open into the middle nasal meatus.

7. The _____ are paired paranasal sinuses located in each body of the maxillae, just posterior to the maxillary canine and premolars; they are small at birth and grow until puberty and thus are not fully developed until all the permanent teeth have erupted in early adulthood.

8. The maxillary sinuses are the largest of the paranasal sinuses, and each one has a(n) _____, three walls, a roof, and a floor.

9. Each maxillary sinus is further divided into communicating compartments by inner bony walls, or _____.

10. The maxillary sinus drains into the _____ on each side via the ostium.

middle nasal meatus	superior nasal meatus	nasal cavity
septa	sphenoidal sinuses	paranasal sinuses
apex	frontal sinuses	ethmoidal sinuses
maxillary sinuses		

References Chapter 3, Skeletal system. In Fehrenbach MJ, Herring SW: *Illustrated anatomy of the head and neck,* ed 6, St. Louis, 2021, Saunders; Chapter 11, Head and neck structures. In Fehrenbach MJ, Popowics T: *Illustrated dental embryology, histology, and anatomy,* ed 5, St. Louis, 2020, Saunders.

FIGURE 4.27 Temporal fossa with boundaries (lateral view)

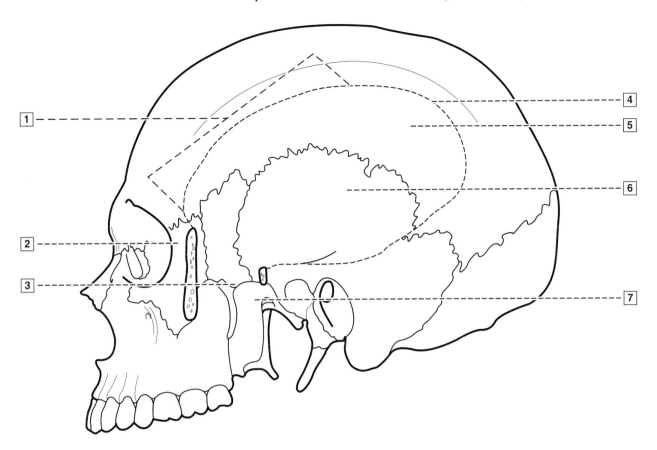

1	Temporal fossa	**5**	Parietal bone
2	Frontal process of zygomatic bone	**6**	Squamous part of temporal bone
3	Infratemporal crest of greater wing of sphenoid bone	**7**	Infratemporal fossa
4	Inferior temporal line		

REVIEW QUESTIONS: Temporal fossa

Fill in the blanks by choosing the appropriate terms from the list below.

1. There are three depressions or fossae present on the skull, _____, infratemporal, and pterygopalatine fossae; two of these fossae are present on the external surface of the skull: the temporal and infratemporal fossae, with the pterygopalatine fossae deep to the infratemporal fossa.

2. The temporal fossa is a flat fan-shaped paired depression on the lateral surface of the _____.

3. The temporal fossa is formed by parts of five different bones, which includes the zygomatic, frontal, greater wing of the sphenoid, temporal, and _____ bones.

4. The borders of the temporal fossa include superiorly and posteriorly, the inferior temporal line; anteriorly, the _____ of the zygomatic bone.

5. Inferiorly, the border between the temporal fossa and the infratemporal fossa is the _____ on the greater wing of the sphenoid bone.

6. The temporal fossa includes a narrow strip of the parietal bone, the _____ of the temporal bone, the temporal surface of the frontal bone, and the temporal surface of the greater wing of the sphenoid bone.

7. The temporal fossa contains the body of the _____.

8. The temporal fossa also contains regional _____ and blood vessels that travel through it.

9. The borders of the temporal fossa include medially, the surface of the _____; laterally, the borders include the zygomatic arch.

10. Inferior to the anterior part of the temporal fossa on the lateral surface of the skull is the depression of the _____.

infratemporal crest	temporalis muscle	infratemporal fossa
squamous part	temporal	nerves
parietal	frontal process	temporal bone
skull		

Reference Chapter 3, Skeletal system. In Fehrenbach MJ, Herring SW: *Illustrated anatomy of the head and neck,* ed 6, St. Louis, 2021, Saunders.

NOTES

FIGURE 4.28   Infratemporal fossae with boundaries (inferior view)

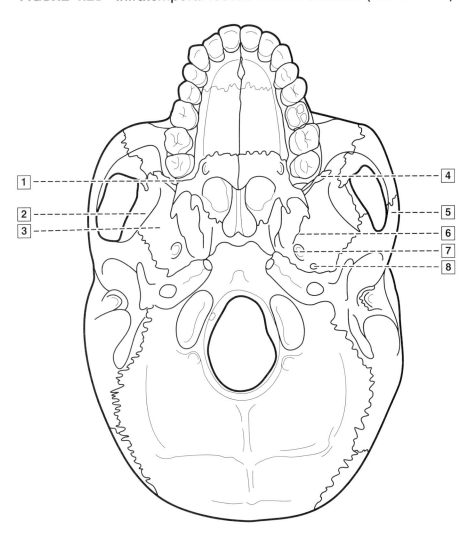

1	Maxillary tuberosity	5	Zygomatic arch
2	Infratemporal crest of great wing of sphenoid bone	6	Lateral pterygoid plate of sphenoid bone
3	Infratemporal fossa	7	Foramen ovale
4	Inferior orbital fissure	8	Foramen spinosum

REVIEW QUESTIONS: Infratemporal fossae

Fill in the blanks by choosing the appropriate terms from the list below.

1. The _____ is a paired depression on the external surface of the skull that is inferior to the anterior part of the temporal fossa.

2. The _____ on the greater wing of the sphenoid bone contributes to the adjoining temporal fossa and infratemporal fossa.

3. The borders of the infratemporal fossa include superiorly, the greater wing of the sphenoid bone; anteriorly, the maxillary tuberosity of the maxilla; medially, the _____ of the sphenoid bone; and laterally, the mandibular ramus and zygomatic arch.

4. No bony inferior or _____ border exists for the infratemporal fossa; only soft tissue.

5. Some structures pass from the infratemporal fossa into the orbit through the _____, which is located at the anterior and superior end of the fossa.

6. Other structures pass into the infratemporal fossa from the _____.

7. The infratemporal fossa contains part of the maxillary artery and its second part branches that begin from here, including the middle meningeal artery, which goes into the cranial cavity through the _____; the inferior alveolar artery, which enters the mandible through the mandibular foramen; and the posterior superior alveolar artery, which enters the maxilla through the posterior superior alveolar foramina on the infratemporal surface of the maxilla.

8. The infratemporal fossa also contains the _____ of veins and the pterygoid muscles.

9. The infratemporal fossa also contains part of the mandibular nerve of the fifth cranial nerve or trigeminal nerve including the inferior alveolar and lingual nerves, which enters the cranial cavity by way of the _____, passing between the cranial and oral cavities.

10. The depression of the _____ is deep to the infratemporal fossa.

pterygopalatine fossa	lateral pterygoid plate	infratemporal fossa
foramen spinosum	inferior orbital fissure	foramen ovale
posterior	infratemporal crest	pterygoid plexus
cranial cavity		

Reference Chapter 3, Skeletal system. In Fehrenbach MJ, Herring SW: *Illustrated anatomy of the head and neck,* ed 6, St. Louis, 2021, Saunders.

NOTES

FIGURE 4.29   Pterygopalatine fossa with boundaries (anterolateral view)

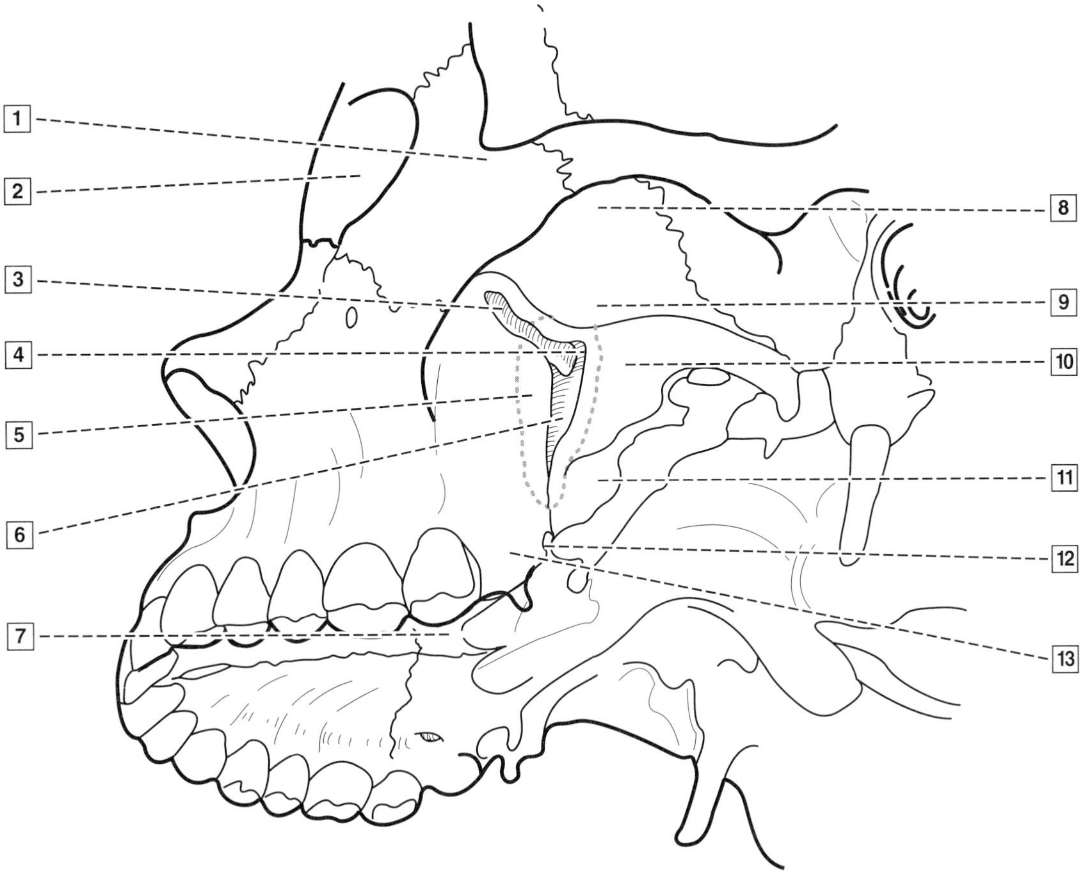

1	Zygomatic arch	8	Temporal fossa
2	Orbit	9	Infratemporal crest of greater wing of sphenoid bone
3	Inferior orbital fissure	10	Infratemporal fossa
4	Sphenopalatine foramen	11	Lateral pterygoid plate of sphenoid bone
5	Pterygopalatine fossa	12	Pterygopalatine canal
6	Pterygomaxillary fissure	13	Maxillary tuberosity
7	Palatine bone		

REVIEW QUESTIONS: Pterygopalatine fossa

Fill in the blanks by choosing the appropriate terms from the list below.

1. The _____ is a cone-shaped paired depression deep to the infratemporal fossa and posterior to the maxilla on each side of the skull.

2. The smaller pterygopalatine fossa is located between the pterygoid process and the _____, close to the apex of the orbit.

3. The pterygopalatine fossa communicates via fissure and foramina in its walls by way of the cranial cavity, the infratemporal fossa, the orbit, the nasal cavity, and the _____.

4. The borders of the pterygopalatine fossa include superiorly, the inferior surface of the body of the sphenoid bone; anteriorly, the maxillary tuberosity of the maxilla; medially, the _____ of the palatine bone.

5. The borders of the pterygopalatine fossa include laterally, the pterygomaxillary fissure; inferiorly, the _____; and posteriorly, the pterygoid process of the sphenoid bone.

6. The pterygopalatine fossa contains part of the _____ and its third part branches that begin here, including the infraorbital and sphenopalatine arteries.

7. The pterygopalatine fossa also contains part of the _____ of the fifth cranial nerve or trigeminal nerve and its branches, as well as the pterygopalatine ganglion.

8. The _____ is the entrance route to the cranial cavity for the maxillary nerve; a second foramen in the pterygoid process, the pterygoid canal, transmits autonomic fibers to the pterygopalatine ganglion.

9. The pterygopalatine canal also connects with the greater and lesser _____ of the palatine bones of the posterior hard palate.

10. The inferior orbital fissure connects the orbit with both the _____ and pterygopalatine fossa.

maxillary nerve	vertical plate	pterygopalatine fossa
infratemporal fossa	oral cavity	pterygopalatine canal
foramen rotundum	maxillary tuberosity	palatine foramina
maxillary artery		

Reference Chapter 3, Skeletal system. In Fehrenbach MJ, Herring SW: *Illustrated anatomy of the head and neck,* ed 6, St. Louis, 2021, Saunders.

FIGURE 4.30 Cervical vertebrae with occipital bone (posterior, superior, and posterosuperior views)

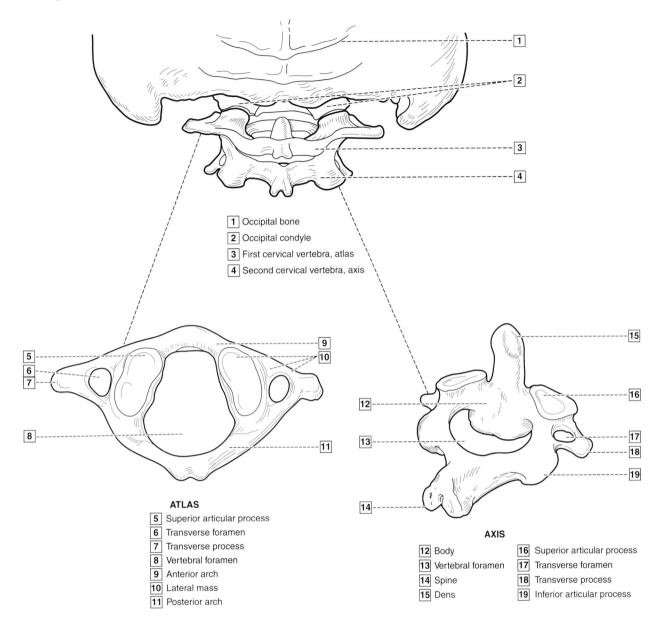

1 Occipital bone
2 Occipital condyle
3 First cervical vertebra, atlas
4 Second cervical vertebra, axis

ATLAS

5 Superior articular process
6 Transverse foramen
7 Transverse process
8 Vertebral foramen
9 Anterior arch
10 Lateral mass
11 Posterior arch

AXIS

12 Body
13 Vertebral foramen
14 Spine
15 Dens
16 Superior articular process
17 Transverse foramen
18 Transverse process
19 Inferior articular process

REVIEW QUESTIONS: Cervical vertebrae with occipital bone

Fill in the blanks by choosing the appropriate terms from the list below.

1. Each _____ of the spine is located in the neck between the base of the skull and the thoracic vertebrae in the trunk.

2. All seven cervical vertebrae are bony rings with a central _____ for the spinal cord and associated tissue.

3. In contrast to most other vertebrae, the cervical vertebrae are characterized by the presence of a _____ in the transverse process on each side of the vertebral foramen, with the vertebral artery running through these structures.

4. The *first cervical vertebra* or _____ articulates with the skull at the occipital condyles of the occipital bone.

5. The atlas has the form of an irregular ring consisting of two _____ of the atlas connected by a shorter anterior arch and a longer posterior arch; it lacks a body and a spine.

6. More medially, the lateral masses of the atlas present large concave _____ for the corresponding convex occipital condyles of the skull.

7. The *second cervical vertebra* or _____ is characterized by having a dens or *odontoid process*.

8. The _____ of the axis articulates anteriorly with the anterior arch of the first cervical vertebra, the atlas.

9. The _____ of the axis is inferior to its dens.

10. The _____ of the axis is located posterior to its body.

atlas	transverse foramen	lateral masses
superior articular processes	body	vertebral foramen
axis	spine	cervical vertebra
dens		

Reference Chapter 3, Skeletal system. In Fehrenbach MJ, Herring SW: *Illustrated anatomy of the head and neck,* ed 6, St. Louis, 2021, Saunders.

NOTES

FIGURE 4.31   Hyoid bone with landmarks (lateral and anterior views)

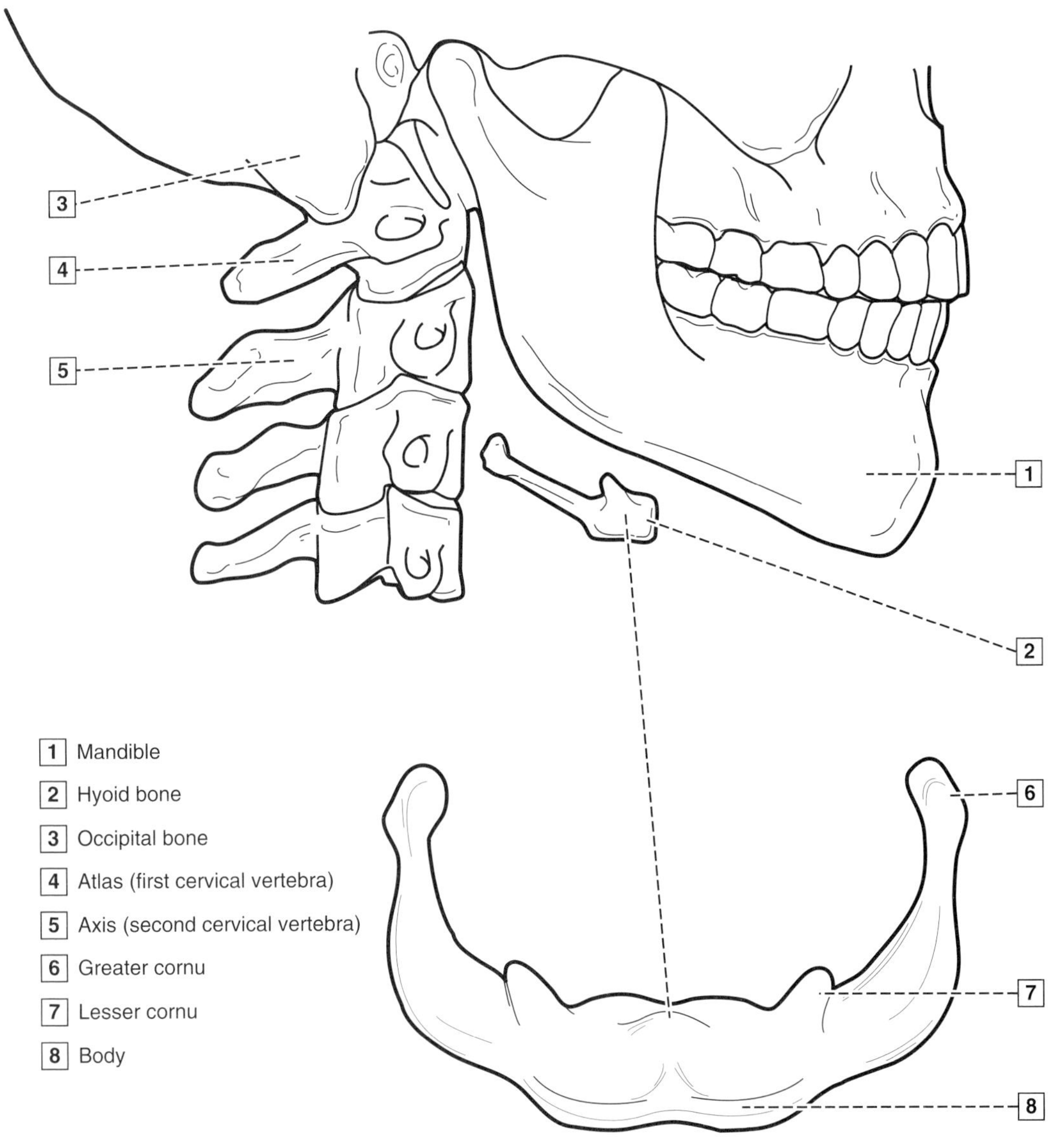

1. Mandible
2. Hyoid bone
3. Occipital bone
4. Atlas (first cervical vertebra)
5. Axis (second cervical vertebra)
6. Greater cornu
7. Lesser cornu
8. Body

275

REVIEW QUESTIONS: Hyoid bone

Fill in the blanks by choosing the appropriate terms from the list below.

1. The _____ is suspended in the neck from the styloid process of the temporal bone by the paired stylohyoid ligaments.

2. The hyoid bone can be palpated by gently feeling inferior to and medial to the angles of the _____.

3. The hyoid bone does not _____ with any other bones, giving it its characteristic mobility, which is necessary for mastication, swallowing, and speech; instead, regional muscles attach to the hyoid bone.

4. It is important to not confuse clinically the hyoid bone with the inferiorly located _____ or "Adam's apple."

5. The hyoid bone is superior and anterior to the thyroid cartilage of the larynx; it is usually at the level of the third _____ but rises during swallowing and other activities.

6. The hyoid bone is lowered after swallowing by the elasticity of its membranous connections, such as the broad _____, a fibrous layer that connects it to the thyroid cartilage.

7. The U-shaped hyoid bone consists of _____ parts as noted from an anterior view.

8. The anterior part of the hyoid bone is the midline _____.

9. A pair of projections is located on each side of the hyoid bone, the _____ cornu and lesser cornu.

10. The projecting horns on the hyoid bone serve as attachments for _____ and ligaments.

thyroid cartilage	hyoid bone	body of the hyoid bone
mandible	greater	thyrohyoid membrane
cervical vertebra	muscles	articulate
five		

Reference   Chapter 3, Skeletal system. In Fehrenbach MJ, Herring SW: *Illustrated anatomy of the head and neck,* ed 6, St. Louis, 2021, Saunders.

NOTES

FIGURE 5.1 Sternocleidomastoid muscle (anterolateral view)

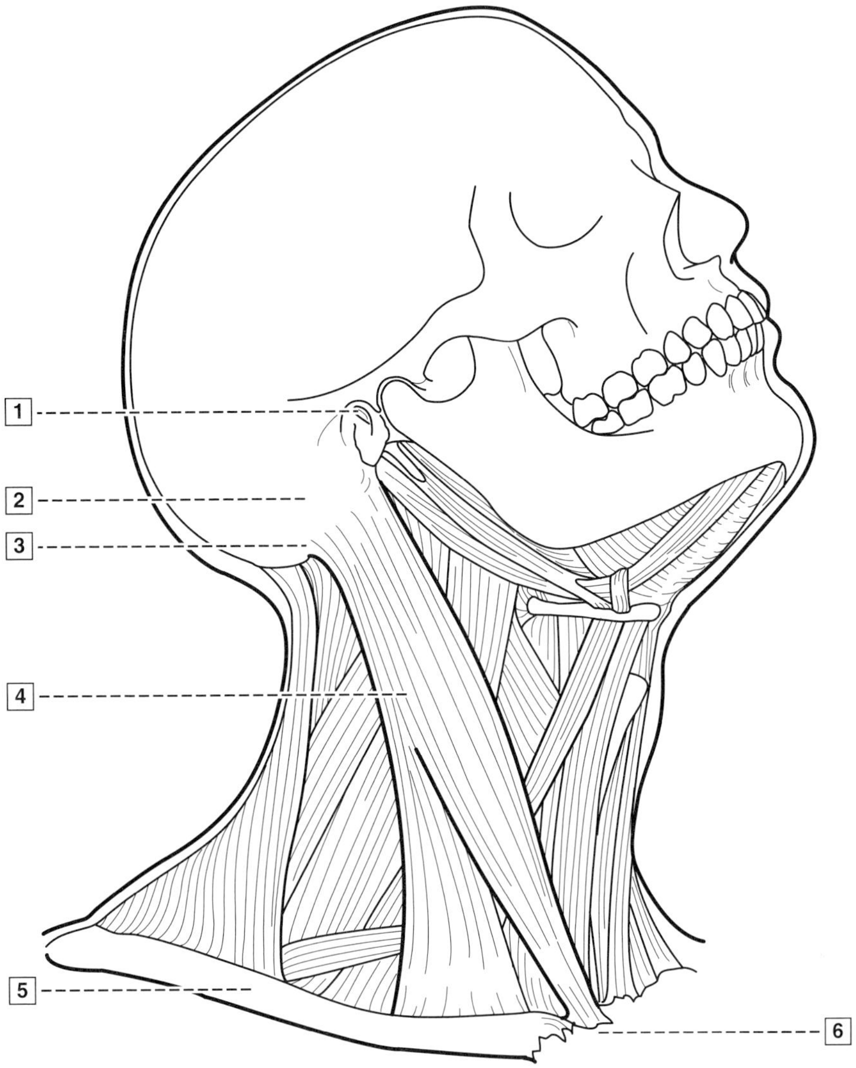

1	External acoustic meatus	5	Clavicle
2	Mastoid process of temporal bone	6	Sternum
3	Superior nuchal line		
4	Sternocleidomastoid		

277

REVIEW QUESTIONS: Sternocleidomastoid muscle

Fill in the blanks by choosing the appropriate terms from the list below.

1. The two _____ include the sternocleidomastoid and trapezius muscles.

2. One of the largest and most superficial cervical muscles is the paired _____.

3. The sternocleidomastoid muscle is a thick muscle of the neck and thus serves as a primary muscular landmark of the _____.

4. The sternocleidomastoid muscle divides the neck region into anterior and posterior _____, which helps define the location of structures, such as the lymph nodes of the head and neck.

5. The sternocleidomastoid muscle _____ from the medial part of the clavicle and the sternum's superior and lateral surfaces.

6. The sternocleidomastoid muscle passes posteriorly and superiorly to _____ on the mastoid process of the temporal bone as well as by a thin aponeurosis or layer of a flat broad tendon into the lateral half of the superior nuchal line of the occipital bone.

7. The insertion of the sternocleidomastoid muscle is just posterior and inferior to the _____ of each ear.

8. If one of the sternocleidomastoid muscles contracts, the head and neck _____ to the ipsilateral side, and the face and anterior part of the neck rotate to the contralateral side.

9. If both sternocleidomastoid muscles contract at the same time, the head will _____ at the neck and extend at the junction between the neck and skull.

10. The sternocleidomastoid muscle is innervated by the eleventh cranial nerve or the _____.

insert	cervical muscles	bend
accessory nerve	originates	external acoustic meatus
flex	sternocleidomastoid muscle	cervical triangles
neck		

Reference Chapter 4, Muscular system. In Fehrenbach MJ, Herring SW: *Illustrated anatomy of the head and neck,* ed 6, St. Louis, 2021, Saunders.

NOTES

FIGURE 5.2 Trapezius muscle (posterolateral view)

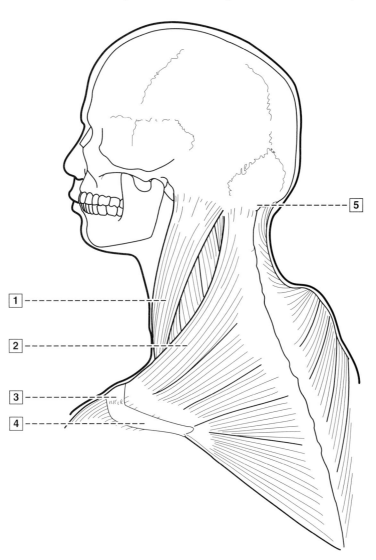

1 Sternocleidomastoid

2 Trapezius

3 Clavicle

4 Scapula

5 Superior nuchal line of occipital bone

REVIEW QUESTIONS: Trapezius muscle

Fill in the blanks by choosing the appropriate terms from the list below.

1. The _____ is a paired superficial cervical muscle that appears as a broad flat triangular muscle that is superficial to both the lateral and posterior surfaces of the neck.

2. The trapezius muscle _____ from the external surface of the occipital bone at the superior nuchal line and the posterior midline of the cervical and thoracic regions.

3. The trapezius muscle _____ on the lateral third of the clavicle and parts of the scapula.

4. The cervical fibers of the trapezius muscle act to _____ the clavicle and scapula, as when the shoulders are shrugged.

5. The trapezius muscle is innervated by the eleventh cranial nerve or the _____ as well as the third and fourth cervical nerves.

6. The curved ridges on the external surface of the occipital bone serve as sites for muscle attachments such as for the origination of both the sternocleidomastoid and trapezius muscles from the

   _____.

7. The descending branches of the _____ supply the trapezius muscle.

8. For those lymph nodes near the _____ such as the inferior deep cervical, accessory, and supraclavicular lymph nodes, it is important to use the trapezius muscle as a base during palpation.

9. The _____ is the fascia that surrounds the neck, continuing onto the masseteric-parotid fascia; this fascia also splits around two salivary glands, the submandibular and parotid salivary glands, and two muscles, the sternocleidomastoid and trapezius, enclosing them completely.

10. Specifically, the _____ is supplied by the eleventh cranial or accessory nerve (CN XI); sensation, including pain and proprioception, travel via the ventral rami of the third (C3) and fourth (C4) cervical nerves.

occipital artery	clavicle	investing fascia
lift	trapezius muscle	motor function
originates	inserts	
accessory nerve	superior nuchal line	

References Chapter 4, Muscular system. In Fehrenbach MJ, Herring SW: *Illustrated anatomy of the head and neck,* ed 6, St. Louis, 2021, Saunders; Chapter 8, Head and neck. In Drake R, Vogl AW, Mitchell AWM: *Gray's anatomy for students,* ed 4, Philadelphia, 2020, Churchill Livingstone.

NOTES

FIGURE 5.3   Muscles of facial expression (anterior view)

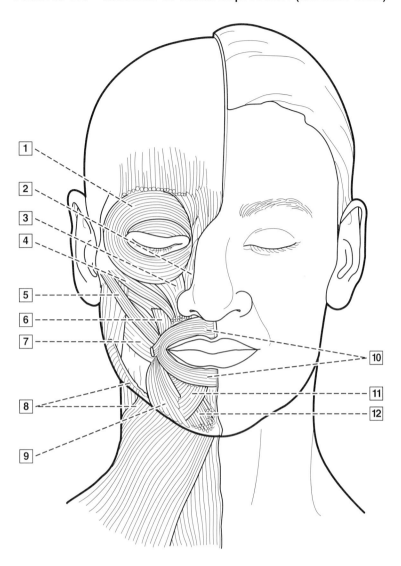

1	Orbicularis oculi	7	Buccinator
2	Levator labii superioris alaeque nasi	8	Platysma
3	Levator labii superioris	9	Depressor anguli oris
4	Zygomaticus minor	10	Orbicularis oris
5	Zygomaticus major	11	Depressor labii inferioris
6	Levator anguli oris	12	Mentalis

REVIEW QUESTIONS: Muscles of facial expression

Fill in the blanks by choosing the appropriate terms from the list below.

1. All the muscles of facial expression are innervated by the seventh cranial nerve or the _____, with each nerve serving the muscles on one side of the face.

2. The _____ or *epicranius* is located in the scalp region where it has two bellies, the frontal belly and occipital belly, that are separated by a large spread-out scalpal tendon, the epicranial aponeurosis or *galea aponeurotica*; the bellies act together to raise the eyebrows and scalp as a muscle of facial expression, such as when a person shows surprise.

3. The _____ encircles the orbit to close the eyelid as a muscle of facial expression.

4. The _____ is deep to the superior part of the orbicularis oculi muscle, and draws the skin of the eyebrow medially and inferiorly toward the nose as a muscle of facial expression, such as when a person frowns.

5. From the facial modiolus, the _____ has vermilion zone fibers of the muscle that encircle the mouth between the skin and labial mucosa of the lips, with no bony attachment, with all its actions involving the lips as a muscle of facial expression.

6. The _____ forms the anterior part of the cheek or the lateral wall within the buccal region of the oral cavity and pulls each labial commissure laterally, shortening the cheek both vertically and horizontally to compress the cheeks as a muscle of facial expression.

7. The _____ as a muscle of facial expression serves to elevate the upper lip.

8. The _____ elevates the upper lip and ala of the nose, and thus also dilates each naris as a muscle of facial expression, such as with a sneering expression or "snarl."

9. The _____ is lateral to the zygomaticus minor muscle and elevates the ipsilateral labial commissure of the upper lip and pulls it laterally as a muscle of facial expression, such as when a person smiles.

10. The _____ is a small variable muscle of facial expression in the oral region, medial to the zygomaticus major muscle that elevates the upper lip, assisting in smiling.

buccinator muscle
levator labii superioris alaeque nasi muscle
orbicularis oculi muscle
levator labii superioris muscle

zygomaticus major muscle
facial nerve
zygomaticus minor muscle

corrugator supercilii muscle
orbicularis oris muscle
epicranial muscle

Reference Chapter 4, Muscular system. In Fehrenbach MJ, Herring SW: *Illustrated anatomy of the head and neck,* ed 6, St. Louis, 2021, Saunders.

FIGURE 5.4   **Muscles of facial expression (lateral view)**

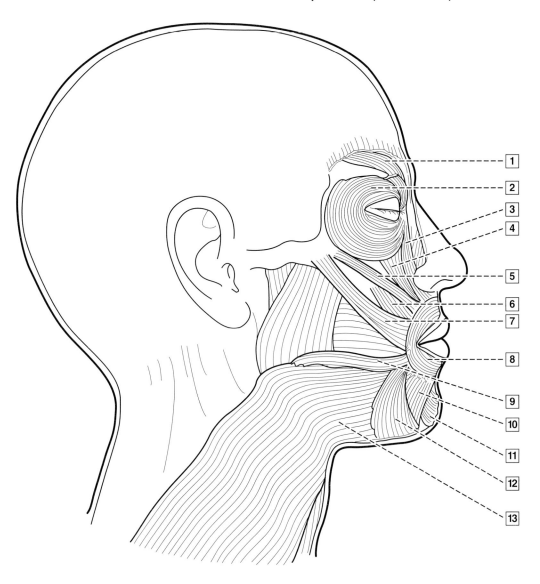

1	Corrugator supercilii	6	Levator anguli oris	11	Mentalis
2	Orbicularis oculi	7	Zygomaticus major	12	Depressor anguli oris
3	Levator labii superioris alaeque nasi	8	Orbicularis oris	13	Platysma
4	Levator labii superioris	9	Risorius		
5	Zygomaticus minor	10	Depressor labii inferioris		

REVIEW QUESTIONS: Muscles of facial expression

Fill in the blanks by choosing the appropriate terms from the list below.

1. The _____ as a muscle of facial expression acts to stretch the lips laterally, retracting the labial commissure and widening the mouth to produce a grimace.

2. The _____ as a muscle of facial expression depresses the ipsilateral labial commissure, such as when a person frowns.

3. Deep to the depressor anguli oris muscle is the _____, which depresses the lower lip as a muscle of facial expression, exposing the mandibular incisors.

4. The _____ as a muscle of facial expression raises the chin, wrinkling its skin, causing the displaced lower lip to protrude, narrowing the oral vestibule as a muscle of facial expression.

5. The _____ as a muscle of facial expression runs from the neck all the way to the mouth superficial to the anterior cervical triangle and external jugular vein that acts to raise the skin of the neck.

6. The platysma muscle directly raises the skin of the neck to form vertical and horizontal ridges and depressions; it can also pull both _____ inferiorly, as when a person grimaces.

7. However, the platysma muscle plays only a minor role in depressing the _____, which instead is mainly depressed instead by the depressor anguli oris and the depressor labii inferioris muscles.

8. The platysma muscle originates in the skin superficial to the clavicle and shoulder; it then passes anteriorly to insert on the _____ of the mandible and into the other muscles surrounding the mouth.

9. Specifically, _____ from the seventh cranial or facial nerve (VIII) emerge from the inferior border of the parotid salivary gland to supply the platysma muscle.

10. Beneath the platysma muscle, the _____ descends from the angle of the mandible to the clavicle.

cervical branches	labial commissures	inferior border
platysma muscle	risorius muscle	external jugular vein
depressor anguli oris muscle	depressor labii inferioris muscle	lower lip
mentalis muscle		

References   Chapter 4, Muscular system. In Fehrenbach MJ, Herring SW: *Illustrated anatomy of the head and neck,* ed 6, St. Louis, 2021, Saunders; Chapter 8, Head and neck. In Drake R, Vogl AW, Mitchell AWM: *Gray's anatomy for students,* ed 4, Philadelphia, 2020, Churchill Livingstone.

NOTES

FIGURE 5.5   Muscles of facial expression: Epicranial (lateral view)

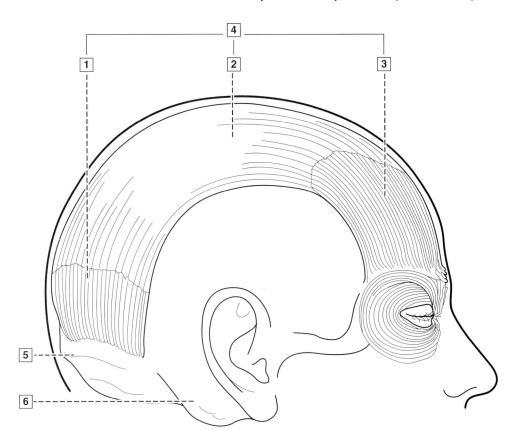

1	Occipital belly	5	Superior nuchal line of occipital bone
2	Epicranial aponeurosis	6	Mastoid process of temporal bone
3	Frontal belly		
4	Epicranial		

REVIEW QUESTIONS: Muscles of facial expression: Epicranial

Fill in the blanks by choosing the appropriate terms from the list below.

1. The epicranial muscle or *epicranius* is a muscle of facial expression where the muscle and its tendon are one of the layers that form the _____.

2. The epicranial muscle has two _____, the frontal and occipital.

3. The two bellies of the epicranial muscle are separated by a large spread-out scalpel tendon, the _____ or *galea aponeurotica*, which is located at the most superior part of the skull.

4. The _____ of the epicranial muscle begins at the epicranial aponeurosis, having no bony attachment.

5. The frontal belly or _____ then inserts into the skin of the eyebrow and root of the nose.

6. The _____ or occipitalis muscle originates from both the superior nuchal line of the occipital bone and the mastoid process of the temporal bone.

7. The occipital belly or _____ then inserts in the epicranial aponeurosis.

8. Both bellies of the epicranial muscle raise the _____ and scalp, as when a person shows surprise.

9. However, the two bellies of the _____ can also act independently of each other during certain facial expressions.

10. The _____ of the seventh cranial or facial nerve (VII) supplies the occipital belly of the epicranial muscle; the temporal branches of the seventh cranial or facial nerve (VII) supply the frontal belly.

epicranial aponeurosis	frontal belly	occipitalis muscle
occipital belly	eyebrows	posterior auricular nerve
bellies	epicranial muscle	
scalp	frontalis muscle	

References Chapter 4, Muscular system. In Fehrenbach MJ, Herring SW: *Illustrated anatomy of the head and neck,* ed 6, St. Louis, 2021, Saunders; Chapter 8, Nervous system. In Fehrenbach MJ, Herring SW: *Illustrated anatomy of the head and neck,* ed 6, St. Louis, 2021, Saunders.

NOTES

FIGURE 5.6 Muscles of facial expression: Buccinator (lateral view)

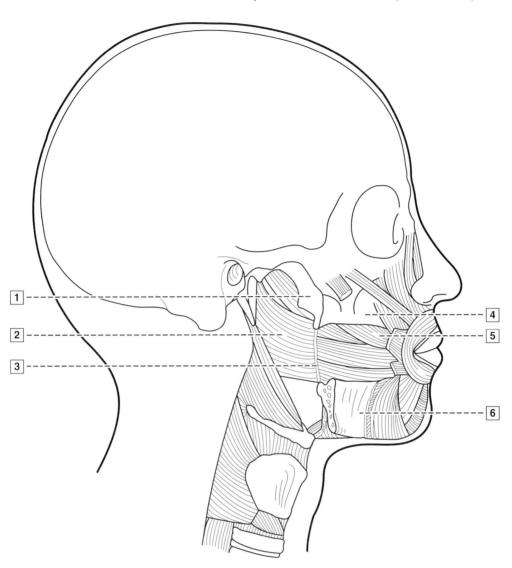

1 Pterygoid plate

2 Superior pharyngeal constrictor

3 Pterygomandibular raphe

4 Maxilla

5 Buccinator

6 Mandible (cut)

REVIEW QUESTIONS: Muscles of facial expression: Buccinator

Fill in the blanks by choosing the appropriate terms from the list below.

1. The _____ is a quadrilateral muscle of facial expression that assists the muscles of mastication.

2. The buccinator muscle forms the anterior part of the _____ or lateral wall within the buccal region of the oral cavity.

3. The buccinator muscle originates from three areas including the alveolar processes of the maxilla and mandible, as well as the tendinous band, the pterygomandibular raphe, which in the oral cavity is noted as the _____ since it becomes accentuated when the mouth opens comfortably wider.

4. The buccinator muscle fibers from the alveolar process of the maxilla and the superior part of the _____ turn inferiorly toward the lower lip, while fibers from the alveolar process of the mandible and inferior part of the same fibrous structure travel turn superiorly toward the upper lip, creating an intersecting pattern at the ipsilateral labial commissure at the facial modiolus.

5. The action of both buccinator muscles causes the muscle to keep food pushed back on the _____ or masticatory surface of the posterior teeth as when a person masticates or chews.

6. By keeping the food in the correct position when chewing, the buccinator muscles assist the _____.

7. In infants, the buccinator muscles provide _____ for nursing.

8. The pterygomandibular fold is a(n) _____ for the administration of the inferior alveolar nerve block.

9. The _____, a branch off the second part of the maxillary artery, passes to the buccal mucosa to supply the buccinator muscle and the buccal region.

10. Nearer to the skull, the visceral fascial layer located posterior and lateral to the pharynx is the _____; this deep cervical fascia encloses the entire superior part of the alimentary canal and is continuous with the fascia covering the buccinator muscle, a location where the buccinator muscle and the superior pharyngeal constrictor muscle come together at the pterygomandibular raphe.

landmark   muscles of mastication   buccal artery
occlusal surface   pterygomandibular fold   buccopharyngeal fascia
cheek   buccinator muscle
pterygomandibular raphe   suction

References   Chapter 4, Muscular system. In Fehrenbach MJ, Herring SW: *Illustrated anatomy of the head and neck,* ed 6, St. Louis, 2021, Saunders; Chapter 6, Vascular system. In Fehrenbach MJ, Herring SW: *Illustrated anatomy of the head and neck,* ed 6, St. Louis, 2021, Saunders; Chapter 11, Fasciae and spaces. In Fehrenbach MJ, Herring SW: *Illustrated anatomy of the head and neck,* ed 6, St. Louis, 2021, Saunders.

FIGURE 5.7 Muscles of mastication: Masseter (lateral view)

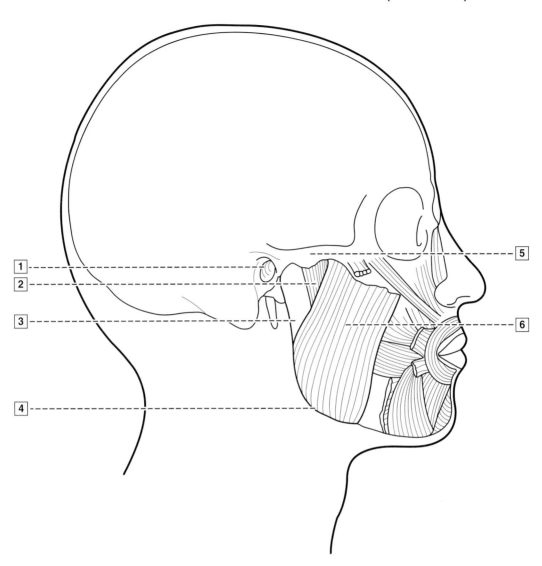

1	External acoustic meatus	5	Zygomatic arch
2	Deep head of masseter	6	Superficial head of masseter
3	Mandibular ramus		
4	Angle of mandible		

289

REVIEW QUESTIONS: Muscles of mastication: Masseter

Fill in the blanks by choosing the appropriate terms from the list below.

1. The _____ are four paired muscles attached in some manner to the mandible and include the masseter, temporalis, medial pterygoid, and lateral pterygoid muscles; these muscles are located deeper within the face than the muscles of facial expression.

2. The muscles of mastication work with the _____ to accomplish movements of the mandible to allow mastication.

3. All the muscles of mastication are innervated by branches of the _____ of the fifth cranial nerve or trigeminal nerve, with each nerve serving one side of the face.

4. The _____ is a broad and thick flat rectangular (almost quadrilateral) muscle of mastication on each side of the face that is anterior to the parotid salivary gland.

5. The masseter muscle has two _____ that differ in depth, the superficial and the deep.

6. The _____ of the masseter muscle originates from the zygomatic process of the maxilla and from the anterior two-thirds of the inferior border of the zygomatic arch.

7. The _____ of the masseter muscle originates from the posterior one-third and the entire medial surface of the zygomatic arch, which is partly concealed by the superficial head of the muscle.

8. Both heads of the masseter muscle pass inferiorly to insert on different parts of the external surface of the _____.

9. The superficial head of the masseter muscle inserts on the lateral surface of the _____ and the deep head of the muscle inserts on the mandibular ramus superior to the angle of the mandible.

10. The action of the masseter muscle during bilateral contraction of the entire muscle is to _____ the mandible, raising the lower jaw; elevation of the mandible occurs during the closing of the jaws.

mandibular nerve	elevate	superficial head
heads	masseter muscle	temporomandibular joint
deep head	mandible	muscles of mastication
angle of the mandible		

Reference Chapter 4, Muscular system. In Fehrenbach MJ, Herring SW: *Illustrated anatomy of the head and neck,* ed 6, St. Louis, 2021, Saunders.

NOTES

FIGURE 5.8   Muscles of mastication: Temporalis (lateral view)

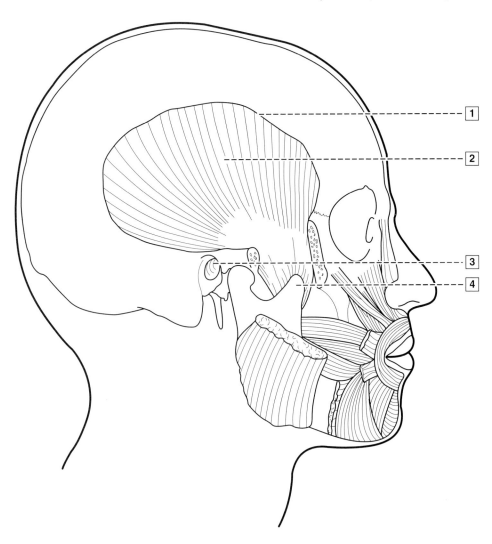

1	Inferior temporal line	4	Coronoid process of mandible
2	Temporalis
3	External acoustic meatus

REVIEW QUESTIONS: Muscles of mastication: Temporalis

Fill in the blanks by choosing the appropriate terms from the list below.

1. The _____ is a broad fan-shaped muscle of mastication on each side of the head that fills the temporal fossa and is located superior to the zygomatic arch.

2. The temporalis muscle originates from the entire _____ on the temporal bone that is bordered superiorly by the inferior temporal line and inferiorly by the infratemporal crest.

3. The temporalis muscle passes inferiorly to insert onto the medial surface, apex, and anterior border of the coronoid process of the _____ at the anteromedial border of the mandibular ramus.

4. If the entire temporalis muscle contracts, the main action is to _____ the lower jaw, raising the mandible.

5. If only the posterior part of the temporalis muscle contracts, the muscle moves the lower jaw _____; moving the lower jaw backward causes retraction of the mandible.

6. The temporalis muscle also maintains the mandible in its physiologic rest position, allowing for _____.

7. The temporalis muscle is innervated by the _____, branches of the mandibular nerve (or third division) of the fifth cranial or trigeminal nerve.

8. The temporal fossa is formed by parts of several bones of the skull and contains the _____ of the temporalis muscle.

9. The _____ muscle lies within the infratemporal fossa, deep to the temporalis muscle.

10. The small _____ supplies the temporalis muscle, which is a branch off the superficial temporal artery from the external carotid artery.

deep temporal nerves	freeway space	lateral pterygoid muscle
temporalis muscle	temporal fossa	middle temporal artery
elevate	backward	
mandible	body	

References   Chapter 3, Skeletal system. In Fehrenbach MJ, Herring SW: *Illustrated anatomy of the head and neck,* ed 6, St. Louis, 2021, Saunders; Chapter 4, Muscular system. In Fehrenbach MJ, Herring SW: *Illustrated anatomy of the head and neck,* ed 6, St. Louis, 2021, Saunders; Chapter 11, Vascular system. In Fehrenbach MJ, Herring SW: *Illustrated anatomy of the head and neck,* ed 6, St. Louis, 2021, Saunders.

NOTES

ANSWER KEY   1. temporalis muscle, 2. temporal fossa, 3. mandible, 4. elevate, 5. backward, 6. freeway space, 7. deep temporal nerves, 8. body, 9. lateral pterygoid muscle, 10. middle temporal artery

FIGURE 5.9   Muscles of mastication: Medial and lateral pterygoid (lateral view)

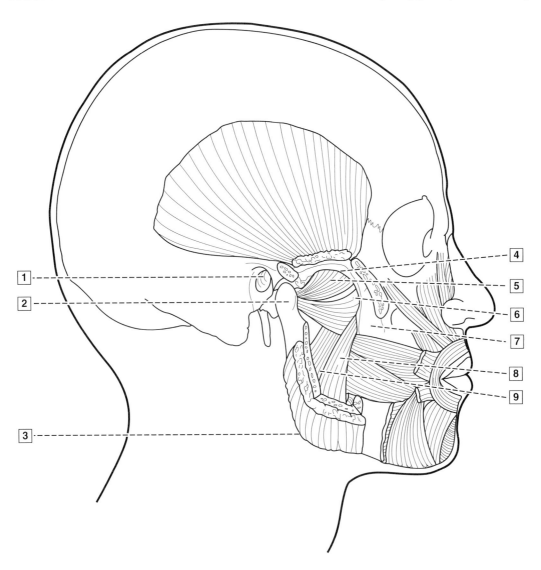

1	External acoustic meatus	**5**	Superior head of lateral pterygoid
2	Mandibular condyle	**6**	Inferior head of lateral pterygoid
3	Angle of mandible	**7**	Maxilla
4	Sphenoid bone	**8**	Superficial head of medial pterygoid
		9	Deep head of medial pterygoid

REVIEW QUESTIONS: Muscles of mastication: Medial and lateral pterygoid

Fill in the blanks by choosing the appropriate terms from the list below.

1. Deeper, yet similar in rectangular form to the more superficial masseter muscle, another muscle of mastication is the _____ or *internal pterygoid muscle*.

2. The medial pterygoid muscle has two _____ of differing depths, the deep and the superficial, similar to the masseter muscle; however, even with these two differing heads, this is the deepest muscle of mastication.

3. The larger _____ of the medial pterygoid muscle originates from the between pterygoid fossa on the medial surface of the lateral pterygoid plate of the sphenoid bone, the adjoining medial side of the lateral pterygoid plate of the sphenoid bone, and often from the lateral side of the medial pterygoid plate.

4. The smaller _____ of the medial pterygoid muscle originates from the lateral surfaces of both the pyramidal process of the palatine bone and maxillary tuberosity of the maxilla.

5. After their point of origin, both heads of the medial pterygoid muscle pass inferiorly, posteriorly, and laterally to insert on the medial surface of the _____ and angle of the mandible, as far superior as the mandibular foramen.

6. The medial pterygoid muscle _____ the mandible, raising the lower jaw with an elevation of the mandible occurring during the closing of the jaws; it parallels the action of the masseter muscle, but the effect is smaller overall.

7. The _____ or *external pterygoid muscle* is a short thick and almost conical muscle of mastication superior to the medial pterygoid muscle and lies entirely within the infratemporal fossa, deep to the temporalis muscle, with the muscle surrounded by the pterygoid plexus of veins.

8. The lateral pterygoid muscle has two separate heads of _____, the superior and the inferior heads; these two heads are separated anteriorly by a slight interval but fused together posteriorly.

9. The superior head of the lateral pterygoid muscle originates from the infratemporal surface and infratemporal crest of the greater wing of the _____ and passes inferiorly to insert on the anterior surface of the neck of the mandibular condyle at the pterygoid fovea of the mandible as well as the anterior margin of the temporomandibular joint disc and capsule; the inferior head originates from the lateral surface of the lateral pterygoid plate of the same bone and also inserts on the anterior surface of the neck of the mandibular condyle at the pterygoid fovea.

10. Unlike the other three muscles of mastication, the lateral pterygoid muscle is the only muscle of mastication that assists in depressing the mandible or lowering the lower jaw as it moves forward or protrudes but the main action when both muscles contract is to bring the lower jaw _____, thus causing the protrusion of the mandible; in contrast, when only one muscle is contracted, the lower jaw shifts to the contralateral side, causing lateral deviation of the mandible.

forward
elevates
mandibular ramus
superficial head
heads
medial pterygoid muscle
deep head
lateral pterygoid muscle
origin
sphenoid bone

Reference Chapter 4, Muscular system. In Fehrenbach MJ, Herring SW: *Illustrated anatomy of the head and neck,* ed 6, St. Louis, 2021, Saunders.

FIGURE 5.10 **Hyoid muscles (anterior view)**

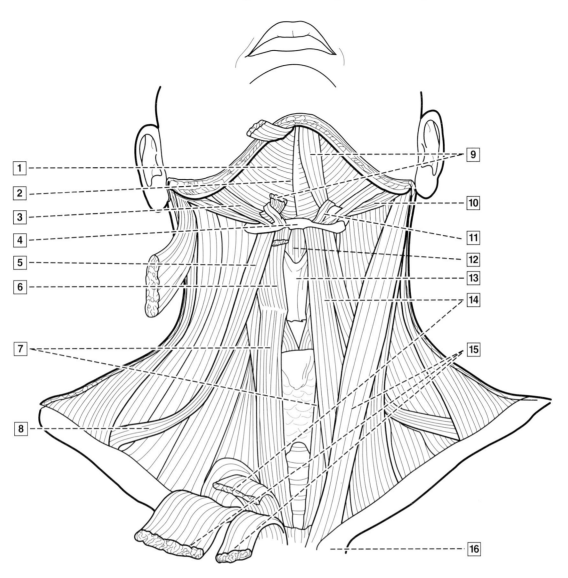

1	Mylohyoid	7	Sternothyroid	13	Thyroid cartilage
2	Mylohoid raphe	8	Inferior belly of omohyoid	14	Sternohyoid
3	Stylohyoid	9	Anterior belly of digastric	15	Sternocleidomastoid
4	Hyoid bone	10	Posterior belly of digastric	16	Sternum
5	Superior belly of omohyoid	11	Intermediate tendon of digastric		
6	Thyrohyoid muscle	12	Thyrohyoid membrane		

REVIEW QUESTIONS: Hyoid muscles

Fill in the blanks by choosing the appropriate terms from the list below.

1. The _____ assist in the actions of mastication and swallowing mainly through their attachment to the hyoid bone; the muscles can be further grouped based on their vertical position in relation to the hyoid bone, the suprahyoid muscles or the infrahyoid muscles.

2. The _____ are superior to the hyoid bone as well as its inferior hyoid muscles; these muscles may be further divided according to their horizontal position in relation to the hyoid bone, being either anterior or posterior.

3. The _____ group includes the anterior belly of the digastric muscle, the mylohyoid muscle, and the geniohyoid muscle.

4. The _____ group includes the posterior belly of the digastric muscle and the stylohyoid muscle.

5. One action of both the anterior and posterior suprahyoid muscles is to cause the hyoid bone and larynx to _____ if the mandible is stabilized by contraction of the muscles of mastication, as occurs during swallowing.

6. The action of anterior suprahyoid muscles causes the mandible to _____ and the jaws to open.

7. The _____ is a suprahyoid muscle that has two separate bellies, anterior belly and posterior belly; the anterior belly is a part of the anterior suprahyoid muscle group and the posterior belly is a part of the posterior suprahyoid muscle group.

8. Each digastric muscle demarcates the superior part of the _____, forming (with the mandible) a submandibular triangle on each side of the neck; the right and left anterior bellies of the muscle also form a single midline submental triangle.

9. The _____ of the digastric muscle originates on the intermediate tendon of the digastric muscle, which is loosely attached to the body and the greater cornu of the hyoid bone, and then passes superiorly and anteriorly to insert onto the digastric fossa on the medial surface of the mandible; its innervation is by the mylohyoid nerve, which is a branch of the mandibular nerve (or third division) of the fifth cranial nerve or trigeminal nerve.

10. The _____ of the digastric muscle begins at the mastoid notch, medial to the mastoid process of the temporal bone, and then passes anteriorly and inferiorly to insert on the intermediate tendon of the muscle; it is innervated by the posterior digastric nerve, which is a branch of the seventh cranial nerve or facial nerve.

anterior belly	anterior suprahyoid muscle	posterior belly
digastric muscle	hyoid muscles	suprahyoid muscles
anterior cervical triangle	posterior suprahyoid muscle	depress
elevate		

Reference Chapter 4, Muscular system. In Fehrenbach MJ, Herring SW: *Illustrated anatomy of the head and neck,* ed 6, St. Louis, 2021, Saunders.

ANSWER KEY 1. hyoid muscles, 2. suprahyoid muscles, 3. anterior suprahyoid muscle, 4. posterior suprahyoid muscle, 5. elevate, 6. depress, 7. digastric muscle, 8. anterior cervical triangle, 9. anterior belly, 10. posterior belly

FIGURE 5.11   Suprahyoid muscles (lateral view without geniohyoid)

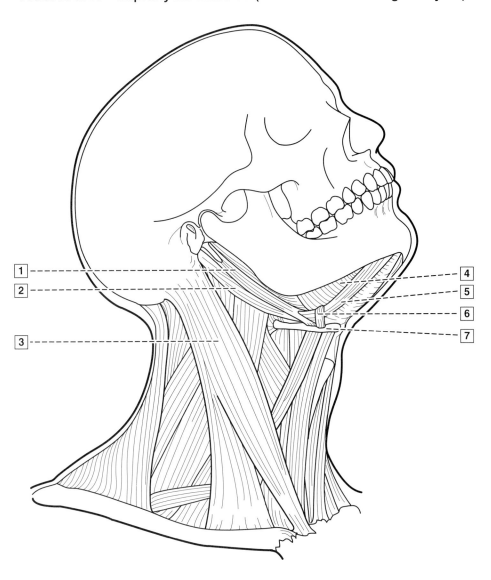

1 Stylohyoid   6 Intermediate tendon of digastric

2 Posterior belly of digastric   7 Hyoid bone

3 Sternocleidomastoid

4 Mylohyoid

5 Anterior belly of digastric

REVIEW QUESTIONS: Suprahyoid muscles

Fill in the blanks by choosing the appropriate terms from the list below.

1. The _____ is an anterior suprahyoid muscle that is deep to the digastric muscle with fibers running transversely between the two mandibular rami.

2. The mylohyoid muscle originates from the mylohyoid line on the medial surface of the _____.

3. The right and left muscles of the mylohyoid muscle pass inferiorly to unite medially at the mylohyoid raphe, a linear midline band of fibrous tissue, forming the _____, with the most posterior fibers of the muscle inserting into the body of the hyoid bone.

4. In addition, the mylohyoid muscle can either elevate the hyoid bone or _____ the mandible.

5. The mylohyoid muscle also helps _____ the tongue.

6. The mylohyoid muscle is innervated by the _____, which is a branch of the mandibular nerve (third division) of the fifth cranial nerve or trigeminal nerve.

7. The _____ is a thin posterior suprahyoid muscle that has two slips, superficial and deep, which are located on either side of the intermediate tendon of the digastric muscle.

8. The stylohyoid muscle originates from the _____ of the temporal bone.

9. The stylohyoid muscle passes anteriorly and inferiorly to insert on the body of the _____.

10. The stylohyoid muscle is innervated by the _____, which is a branch of the seventh cranial nerve or facial nerve.

stylohyoid nerve	floor of the mouth	stylohyoid muscle
mylohyoid muscle	mandible	hyoid bone
elevate	mylohyoid nerve	depress
styloid process		

Reference   Chapter 4, Muscular system. In Fehrenbach MJ, Herring SW: *Illustrated anatomy of the head and neck,* ed 56, St. Louis, 2021, Saunders.

NOTES

FIGURE 5.12   Suprahyoid muscles: Geniohyoid (superior view)

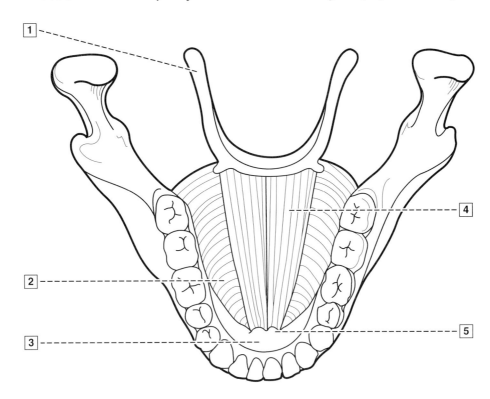

1 Hyoid bone
2 Mylohyoid
3 Medial surface of mandible
4 Geniohyoid
5 Genial tubercles

REVIEW QUESTIONS: Suprahyoid muscles: Geniohyoid

Fill in the blanks by choosing the appropriate terms from the list below.

1. The _____ is an anterior suprahyoid muscle that is superior to the medial border of the mylohyoid muscle.

2. The geniohyoid muscle originates from the medial surface of the mandible, at the _____, near the mandibular symphysis.

3. At the point of origin until insertion, both the right and left geniohyoid muscles are in _____ with each other.

4. The geniohyoid muscle passes posteriorly and inferiorly to insert on the body of the _____.

5. The geniohyoid muscle is innervated by the first cervical nerve, which is conducted by way of the twelfth cranial nerve or _____.

6. The geniohyoid muscle either elevates and protrudes the hyoid bone or depresses the _____.

7. The _____ is a fan-shaped extrinsic tongue muscle superior to the geniohyoid muscle.

8. The geniohyoid muscles from each side are next to each other in the _____.

9. The geniohyoid muscle is superior to the floor of the oral cavity and is not generally considered a muscle of the anterior cervical triangle; however, instead it can be regarded as a(n) _____.

10. The geniohyoid muscle is innervated by the first cervical nerve traveling alongside the twelfth cranial or hypoglossal nerve (XII); these nerve fibers are the _____.

midline	genioglossus muscle	suprahyoid muscle
genial tubercles	geniohyoid muscle	ansa cervicalis
hyoid bone	hypoglossal nerve	
contact	mandible	

References Chapter 4, Muscular system. In Fehrenbach MJ, Herring SW: *Illustrated anatomy of the head and neck,* ed 6, St. Louis, 2021, Saunders; Chapter 8, Head and neck. In Drake R, Vogl AW, Mitchell AWM: *Gray's anatomy for students,* ed 4, Philadelphia, 2020, Churchill Livingstone.

NOTES

ANSWER KEY 1. geniohyoid muscle, 2. genial tubercles, 3. contact, 4. hyoid bone, 5. hypoglossal nerve, 6. mandible, 7. genioglossus muscle, 8. midline, 9. suprahyoid muscle, 10. ansa cervicalis

300

FIGURE 5.13 Infrahyoid muscles (lateral view)

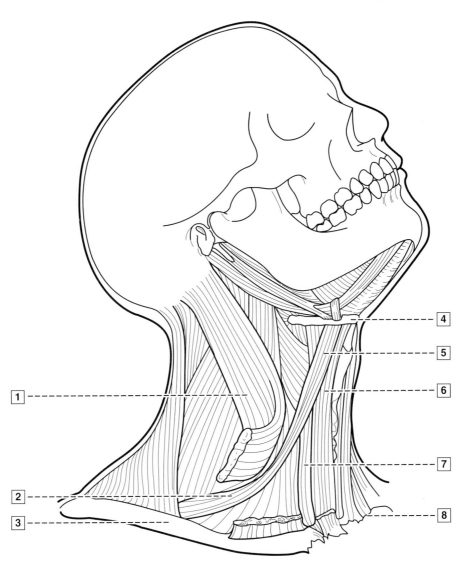

1	Sternocleidomastoid
2	Inferior belly of omohyoid
3	Clavicle
4	Hyoid bone
5	Superior belly of omohyoid
6	Sternohyoid
7	Sternothyroid
8	Sternum

REVIEW QUESTIONS: Infrahyoid muscles

Fill in the blanks by choosing the appropriate terms from the list below.

1. The _____ are four pairs of hyoid muscles inferior to the hyoid bone; they include the omohyoid, sternohyoid, sternothyroid, and thyrohyoid muscles.

2. Most of the infrahyoid muscles _____ the hyoid bone; some of the muscles have additional specific actions and are innervated by the first, second, and third cervical nerves.

3. The _____ is an infrahyoid muscle that is superficial to the thyroid gland and originates from the posterior surface of the sternum, deep and medial to the sternohyoid muscle, at the level of the first rib; it passes superiorly to insert into the thyroid cartilage.

4. The sternothyroid muscle depresses the _____ and larynx but does not directly depress the hyoid bone.

5. The _____ is an infrahyoid muscle that is superficial to the sternothyroid muscle as well as the thyroid cartilage and thyroid gland and that originates from the posterior and superior surfaces of the sternum, near to where the sternum joins each clavicle; it passes superiorly to insert on the body of the hyoid bone to depress the hyoid bone.

6. The _____ is an infrahyoid muscle that is located laterally to both the sternothyroid and thyrohyoid muscles; it has two separate bellies, the superior belly and inferior belly.

7. The _____ of the omohyoid muscle divides the inferior part of the anterior cervical triangle into the carotid and muscular triangles; in the posterior cervical triangle, the inferior belly serves to demarcate the subclavian triangle inferiorly from the occipital triangle superiorly.

8. The _____ of the omohyoid muscle originates from the scapula and then passes anteriorly and superiorly, crossing the internal jugular vein deep to the sternocleidomastoid muscle where it then attaches by a short tendon to the superior belly; the superior belly originates from the short tendon attached to the inferior belly and then inserts on the lateral border of the body of the hyoid bone to depress the hyoid bone.

9. The _____ is located deep in both the omohyoid and sternohyoid muscles; it originates on the thyroid cartilage and inserts on the body and greater cornu of the hyoid bone, appearing as a continuation of the sternothyroid muscle.

10. In addition to depressing the hyoid bone, the thyrohyoid muscle _____ the thyroid cartilage and larynx.

superior belly	sternothyroid muscle	inferior belly
omohyoid muscle	infrahyoid muscles	thyroid cartilage
sternohyoid muscle	raises	thyrohyoid muscle
depress		

Reference   Chapter 4, Muscular system. In Fehrenbach MJ, Herring SW: *Illustrated anatomy of the head and neck,* ed 6, St. Louis, 2021, Saunders.

FIGURE 5.14 Tongue muscles (parasagittal section and frontal section)

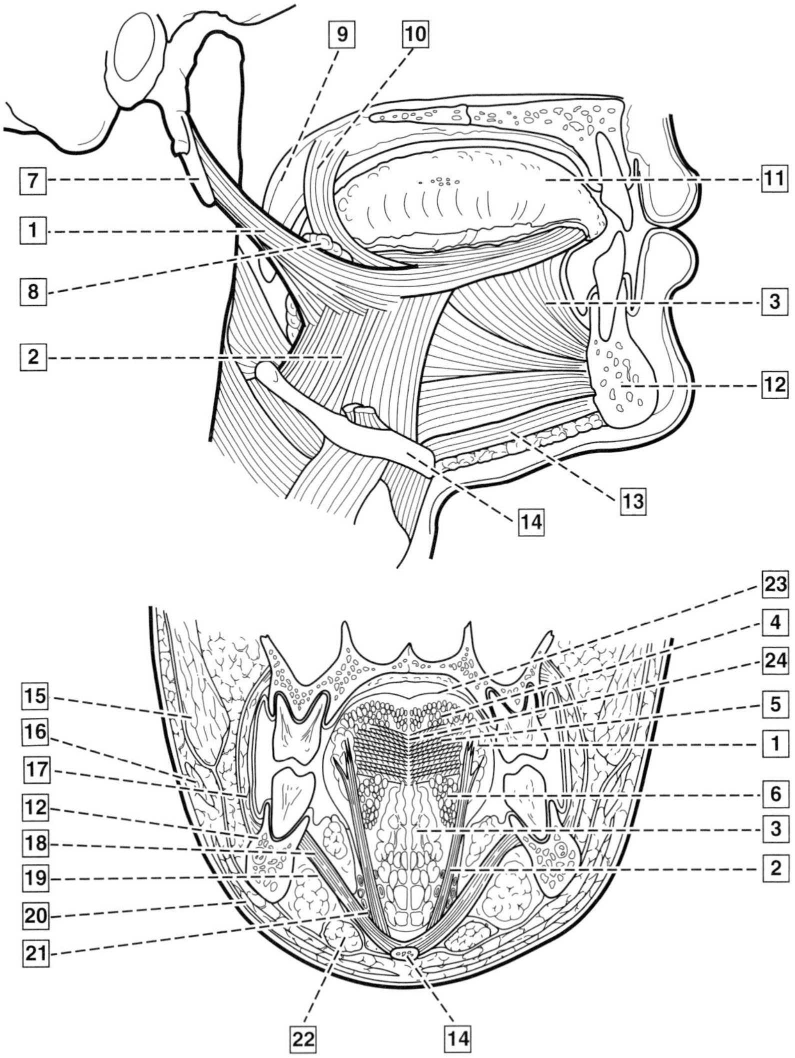

EXTRINSIC

1 Styloglossus
2 Hyoglossus
3 Genioglossus

INTRINSIC

4 Superior longitudinal
5 Transverse and vertical
6 Inferior longitudinal

AREA STRUCTURES

7 Styloid process
8 Palatine tonsil
9 Soft palate
10 Palatoglossus
11 Tongue epithelium overlying intrinsic muscles
12 Mandible
13 Geniohyoid
14 Hyoid bone
15 Masseter

16 Muscles of facial expression
17 Buccinator
18 Mylohyoid
19 Mylohyoid nerve
20 Platysma
21 Hypoglossal nerve (XII)
22 Digastric
23 Tongue epithelium with lingual papillae
24 Median septum

REVIEW QUESTIONS: Tongue muscles

Fill in the blanks by choosing the appropriate terms from the list below.

1. The _____ is a thick vascular mass of voluntary muscle surrounded by a mucous membrane that is anchored to the floor of the mouth by the lingual frenum; it has complex movements during mastication, speaking, and swallowing that are a result of the combined action of its muscles.

2. The muscles of the tongue can be grouped according to their location, intrinsic and extrinsic groups, with both muscle groups intertwining within the structure of the tongue; in addition, each half of the tongue has muscular groups within these two main groups that are separated by the _____, a deep tendinous band located within the midline that corresponds with the median lingual sulcus; all the muscles are innervated by the twelfth cranial or hypoglossal nerve.

3. The _____ are located entirely inside the tongue; these muscles change the shape of the tongue.

4. The _____ is the most superficial of the intrinsic muscles and runs in an oblique and longitudinal direction close to the dorsal surface from the base to the apex; deep to this muscle is the transverse muscle, which runs in a transverse direction from the median septum to pass outward toward the lateral surface.

5. The _____ runs in a vertical direction from the dorsal surface to the ventral surface in the body; in contrast, the inferior longitudinal muscle is close to the ventral surface of the tongue and runs in a longitudinal direction from the base to the apex.

6. The superior and inferior longitudinal muscles act together to change the _____ of the tongue by shortening and thickening it and act singly to help it curl in various directions; the transverse and vertical muscles act together to make the tongue long and narrow.

7. The three pairs of _____ include the styloglossus, genioglossus, and hyoglossus muscles.

8. The _____ is an extrinsic tongue muscle that originates from the styloid process of the temporal bone and then passes inferiorly and anteriorly to insert into two parts of the lateral surface of the tongue including at the apex and at the border between the body and base; it serves to retract the tongue, moving it superiorly and posteriorly.

9. The _____ is a fan-shaped extrinsic tongue muscle superior to the geniohyoid, which begins at the genial tubercles on the medial surface of the mandible; a few of its most inferior fibers insert on the hyoid bone, but most insert into the tongue from its base almost to the apex, with right and left muscles separated by the tongue's median septum so that different parts of the muscle can protrude the tongue out of the oral cavity or depress parts of the tongue surface.

10. The _____ is an extrinsic tongue muscle that originates on both the greater cornu and a part of the body of the hyoid bone to then insert into the lateral surface of the body of the tongue to depress the tongue.

hyoglossus muscle	vertical muscle	median septum
superior longitudinal muscle	extrinsic tongue muscles	shape
tongue	styloglossus muscle	intrinsic tongue muscles
genioglossus muscle		

Reference Chapter 4, Muscular system. In Fehrenbach MJ, Herring SW: *Illustrated anatomy of the head and neck,* ed 6, St. Louis, 2021, Saunders.

FIGURE 5.15 **Muscles of the pharynx (posterior view)**

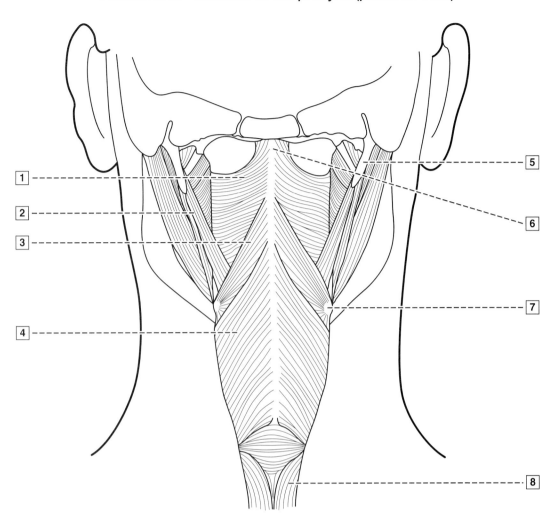

1 Superior pharyngeal constrictor

2 Stylopharyngeus

3 Middle pharyngeal constrictor

4 Inferior pharyngeal constrictor

5 Styloid process of temporal bone

6 Median pharyngeal raphe

7 Hyoid bone

8 Esophagus

REVIEW QUESTIONS: Muscles of the pharynx

Fill in the blanks by choosing the appropriate terms from the list below.

1. The _____ or *throat* is part of both the respiratory and digestive tracts.

2. The pharynx is connected to both the _____ and oral cavity.

3. The pharynx consists of _____ parts including the nasopharynx, oropharynx, and laryngo-pharynx.

4. The _____ are involved in speaking, swallowing, and middle ear function.

5. The muscles of the pharynx are responsible for initiating the _____.

6. The muscles of the pharynx include the stylopharyngeus muscle, the pharyngeal constrictor muscles, and the _____.

7. The _____ is a paired longitudinal muscle of the pharynx that originates from the styloid process of the temporal bone.

8. The stylopharyngeus muscle inserts into the lateral and posterior _____.

9. The stylopharyngeus muscle serves to _____ the pharynx and simultaneously widens the pharynx.

10. The stylopharyngeus muscle is innervated by the ninth cranial nerve or the _____.

pharyngeal walls	elevate	stylopharyngeus muscle
swallowing process	pharynx	three
muscles of the soft palate	muscles of the pharynx	nasal cavity
glossopharyngeal nerve		

References Chapter 2, Surface anatomy. In Fehrenbach MJ, Herring SW: *Illustrated anatomy of the head and neck,* ed 6, St. Louis, 2021, Saunders; Chapter 4, Muscular system. In Fehrenbach MJ, Herring SW: *Illustrated anatomy of the head and neck,* ed 6, St. Louis, 2021, Saunders.

NOTES

FIGURE 5.16 Muscles of the pharynx (lateral view)

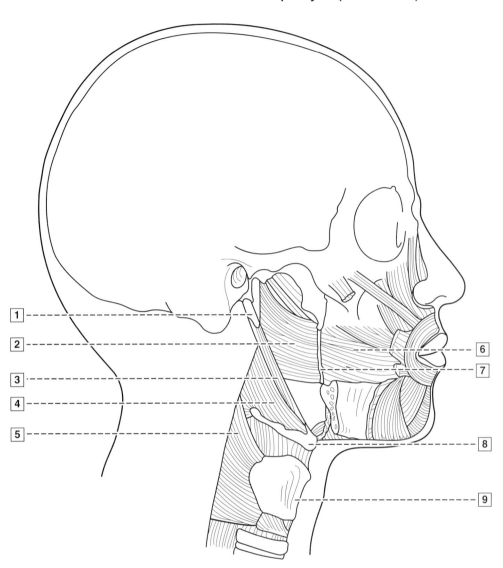

1 Styloid process of temporal bone

2 Superior pharyngeal constrictor

3 Stylopharyngeus

4 Middle pharyngeal constrictor

5 Inferior pharyngeal constrictor

6 Buccinator

7 Pterygomandibular raphe

8 Hyoid bone

9 Thyroid cartilage

REVIEW QUESTIONS: Muscles of the pharynx

Fill in the blanks by choosing the appropriate terms from the list below.

1. The _____ form the lateral and posterior walls of the pharynx.

2. The pharyngeal constrictor muscles consist of _____ paired muscles based on their vertical relationship to the pharynx including the superior, middle, and inferior pharyngeal constrictor muscles.

3. The origin of each pharyngeal constrictor muscle is different, although the muscles overlap each other and also have similar _____.

4. The superior pharyngeal constrictor muscle originates from the hamulus of the medial pterygoid plate, the _____, and the pterygomandibular raphe.

5. The middle pharyngeal constrictor muscle originates on the _____ and stylohyoid ligament.

6. The inferior pharyngeal constrictor muscle originates from both the thyroid cartilage and cricoid cartilage of the _____.

7. When these pharyngeal constrictor muscles overlap each other from the point of insertion, the _____ is the most superficial of the muscles.

8. The pharyngeal constrictor muscles all insert into the _____, a midline tendinous band of the posterior wall of the pharynx that is itself attached to the base of the skull.

9. The pharyngeal constrictor muscles _____ the pharynx and larynx and help drive food inferiorly into the esophagus during swallowing.

10. The pharyngeal constrictor muscles are innervated by the tenth cranial or vagus nerve through the _____.

pharyngeal constrictor muscles	raise	larynx
inferior constrictor muscle	three	hyoid bone
pharyngeal plexus	median pharyngeal raphe	insertions
mandible		

Reference Chapter 4, Muscular system. In Fehrenbach MJ, Herring SW: *Illustrated anatomy of the head and neck,* ed 6, St. Louis, 2021, Saunders.

NOTES

FIGURE 5.17 Muscles of the pharynx: Muscle of the soft palate (posterior views)

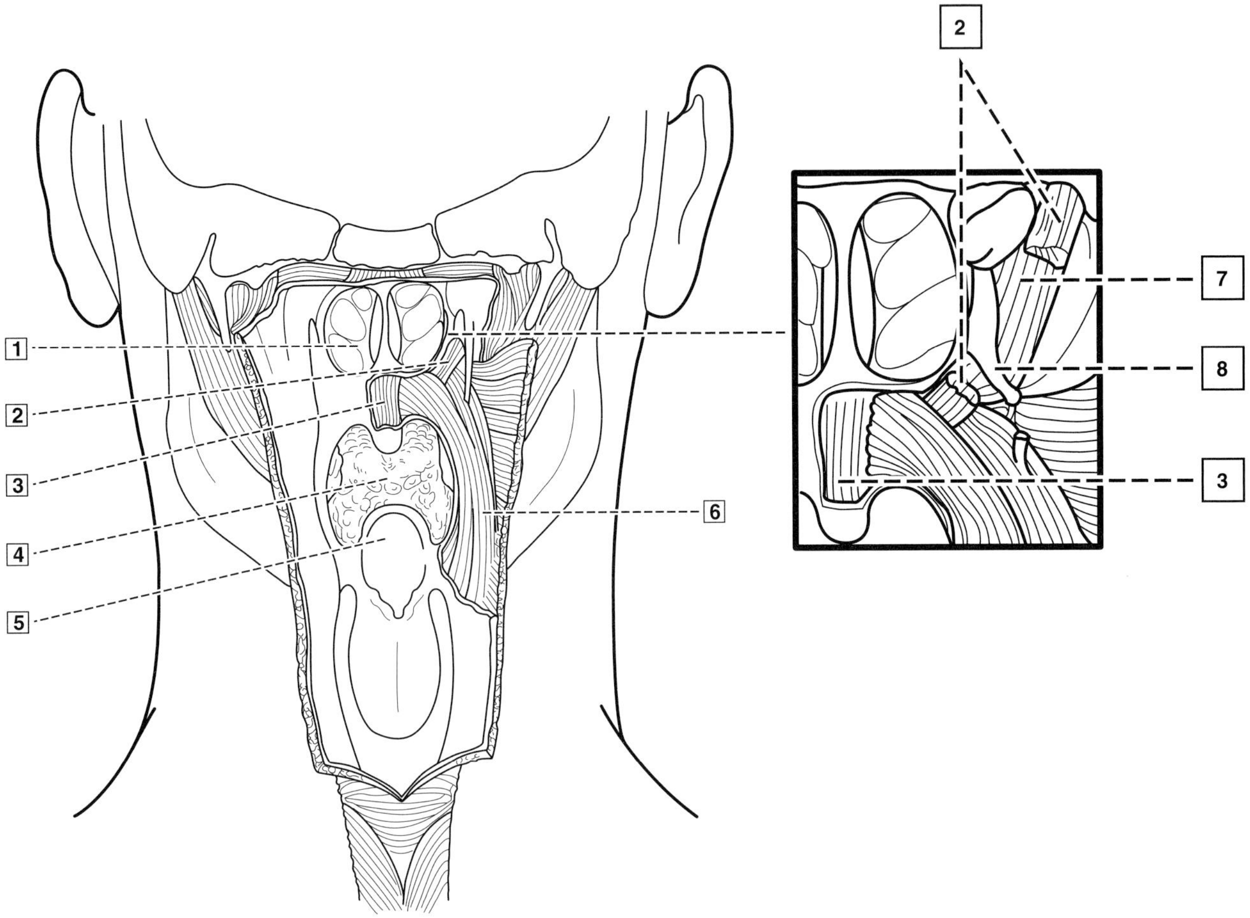

1 Nasal cavity
2 Levator veli palatini
3 Muscle of uvula
4 Dorsal surface of tongue
5 Epiglottis
6 Palatopharyngeus
7 Tensor veli palatini
8 Hamulus of medial pterlygoid plate

Fill in the blanks by choosing the appropriate terms from the list below.

1. The five paired _____ include the palatoglossus muscle, the palatopharyngeus muscle, the levator veli palatini muscle, and the tensor veli palatini muscle, as well as the muscle of the uvula.

2. When the muscles of the soft palate are relaxed, the soft palate extends posteriorly to define the anterior oropharynx, and the combined actions of several muscles of the soft palate move the _____ superiorly and posteriorly to contact the posterior pharyngeal wall that is being moved anteriorly; thus it is the movement of both the soft palate and pharyngeal wall brings a separation between the nasopharynx and oral cavity during swallowing to prevent food from entering the nasal cavity while eating.

3. All the muscles of the soft palate are innervated by the tenth cranial or vagus nerve through the pharyngeal plexus, except the tensor veli palatini muscle, which is supplied by the medial pterygoid nerve, a branch of the _____ (or third division) of the fifth cranial nerve or the trigeminal nerve.

4. The _____ forms the anterior faucial pillar in the oral cavity, a vertical fold anterior to each palatine tonsil that originates from the posterior part of the median palatine raphe and then inserts into the lateral surface of the tongue; it elevates the base of the tongue, arching the tongue against the soft palate, and depresses the soft palate toward the tongue so that the muscles on both sides form a sphincter, separating the oral cavity from the pharynx.

5. The _____ forms the posterior faucial pillar in the oral cavity, a vertical fold posterior to each palatine tonsil that originates in the soft palate and then inserts in the walls of the laryngopharynx and on the thyroid cartilage; it moves the palate posteroinferiorly and the posterior pharyngeal wall anterosuperiorly to help close off the nasopharynx during swallowing.

6. The _____ is located mainly superior to the soft palate, originates from the inferior surface of the temporal bone, and then inserts into the median palatine raphe, a midline tendinous band of the palate.

7. The levator veli palatini muscle _____ the soft palate and helps bring it into contact with the posterior pharyngeal wall to close off the nasopharynx during speech and swallowing.

8. The _____ is a special muscle that tenses and slightly lowers the soft palate, with some of its fibers responsible for opening the auditory (pharyngotympanic) tube to allow air to flow between the pharynx and middle ear cavity.

9. The tensor veli palatine muscle originates from the _____ and the inferior surface of the sphenoid bone and then passes inferiorly between the medial pterygoid muscle and medial pterygoid plate; the muscle forms a tendon near the hamulus of the medial pterygoid plate, a tendon that winds around the hamulus, using it as a pulley, then spreads out to insert into the median palatine raphe.

10. The _____ is a muscle of the soft palate that lies entirely within the uvula of the palate, which is a midline tissue structure that hangs inferiorly from the posterior margin of the soft palate; this muscle shortens and broadens the uvula changing the contour of the posterior part of the soft palate, allowing the soft palate to adapt closely to the posterior pharyngeal wall to help close off the nasopharynx during swallowing.

auditory tube area	soft palate	mandibular nerve
tensor veli palatini muscle	levator veli palatini muscle	palatopharyngeus muscle
raises	muscles of the soft palate	palatoglossus muscle
muscle of the uvula		

Reference Chapter 4, Muscular system. In Fehrenbach MJ, Herring SW: *Illustrated anatomy of the head and neck,* ed 6, St. Louis, 2021, Saunders.

FIGURE 6.1 Pathways to and from the heart: Arteries and veins (frontal view)

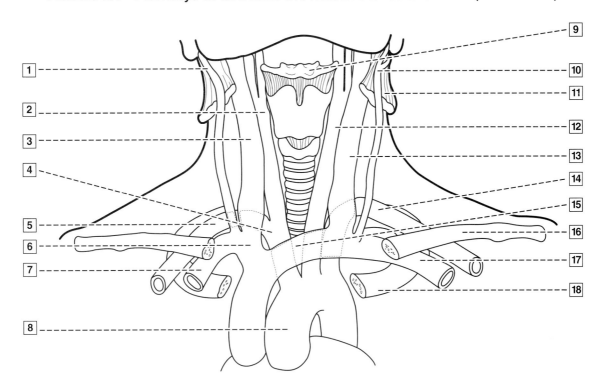

1	Right external jugular vein	**10**	Left external jugular vein
2	Right common carotid artery	**11**	Sternocleidomastoid muscle (cut)
3	Right internal jugular vein	**12**	Left common carotid artery
4	Brachiocephalic artery	**13**	Left internal jugular vein
5	Right subclavian artery	**14**	Left subclavian artery
6	Right brachiocephalic vein	**15**	Left brachiocephalic vein
7	Right subclavian vein	**16**	Clavicle (cut)
8	Aorta	**17**	Left subclavian vein
9	Hyoid bone	**18**	First rib (cut)

REVIEW QUESTIONS: Pathways to and from heart: Arteries and veins

Fill in the blanks by choosing the appropriate terms from the list below.

1. The origins from the _____ of the common carotid arteries and subclavian arteries that supply the head and neck are different for the right and left sides of the body.

2. For the left side of the body, the common carotid artery and subclavian artery begin directly from the _____.

3. For the right side of the body, the common carotid artery and subclavian artery are both branches from the _____, which is a direct branch of the aorta.

4. The _____ is branchless and travels superiorly along the neck in a lateral position to both the trachea and larynx on its way to the superior border of the thyroid cartilage; later it travels in a sheath deep to the sternocleidomastoid muscle that also contains the internal jugular vein and tenth cranial or vagus nerve.

5. The _____ begins lateral to the common carotid artery and gives off branches that supply both intracranial and extracranial structures, but its major destination is the upper extremity (at the arm).

6. The large elastic arteries contain substantial amounts of _____ in the tunica media, allowing expansion and recoil during the cardiac cycle, which helps maintain a constant flow of blood during diastole such as with the aorta, the brachiocephalic trunk, the left common carotid artery, the left subclavian artery, and the pulmonary trunk.

7. The second branch of the arch of the aorta is the left common carotid artery; it begins from the arch immediately to the left and slightly posterior to the brachiocephalic trunk and ascends through the superior mediastinum along the left side of the _____.

8. The left common carotid artery supplies the _____ of the head and neck.

9. The third branch of the _____ of the aorta is the left subclavian artery.

10. Just before the common carotid artery bifurcates into the internal and external carotid arteries, it exhibits a swelling, the _____ ; when the common carotid artery is palpated against the larynx, the most reliable carotid pulse produced can be used for monitoring by qualified emergency medical service personnel.

trachea	elastic fibers	arch
brachiocephalic artery	common carotid artery	carotid sinus
aorta	heart	
subclavian artery	left side	

References Chapter 6, Vascular system. In Fehrenbach MJ, Herring SW: *Illustrated anatomy of the head and neck,* ed 6, St. Louis, 2021, Saunders; Chapter 8, Head and neck. In Drake R, Vogl AW, Mitchell AWM: *Gray's anatomy for students,* ed 4, Philadelphia, 2020, Churchill Livingstone.

ANSWER KEY 1. heart, 2. aorta, 3. brachiocephalic artery, 4. common carotid artery, 5. subclavian artery, 6. elastic fibers, 7. trachea, 8. left side, 9. arch, 10. carotid sinus

FIGURE 6.2   Common carotid artery: Internal and external (lateral view)

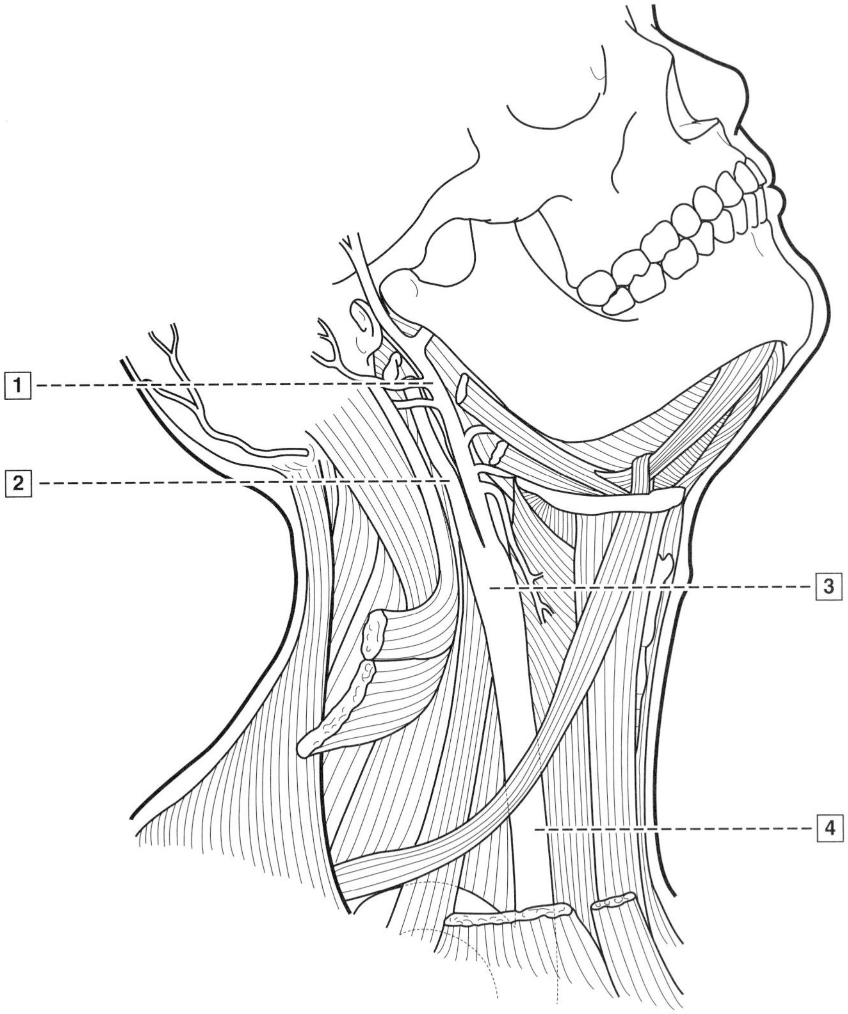

1 External carotid
2 Internal carotid
3 Carotid sinus
4 Common carotid

REVIEW QUESTIONS: Common carotid artery: Internal and external

Fill in the blanks by choosing the appropriate terms from the list below.

1. The _____ is an artery that ends by dividing into the internal and external carotid arteries at approximately the level of the larynx.

2. Just before the common carotid artery bifurcates into the internal and _____ carotid arteries, it exhibits a swelling in the carotid sinus; if the anterior border of the sternocleidomastoid muscle is rolled posteriorly at the level of the thyroid cartilage of the larynx or laryngeal eminence, the carotid pulse produced from the sinus can be felt in the groove of soft tissue.

3. The _____ travels superiorly in a slightly lateral position in relationship to the external carotid artery after leaving the common carotid artery; however, this artery has no branches in the neck but continues adjacent to the internal jugular vein within the carotid sheath to the skull base, where it enters the cranium to supply the intracranial structures and is the source of the ophthalmic artery, which supplies the eye, orbit, and lacrimal gland.

4. As with the internal carotid artery, the _____ begins at the superior border of the thyroid cartilage, at the termination of the common carotid artery and the carotid sheath, and then travels superiorly in a more medial position in relationship to the internal carotid artery after arising from the common carotid artery.

5. The external carotid artery supplies the _____ tissue of the head and neck, including the oral cavity, and has four sets of branches grouped according to their location to the main artery, the anterior, medial, posterior, and terminal branches.

6. The carotid sinus contains receptors that monitor changes in _____.

7. The _____ in the carotid sinus are innervated by a branch of the ninth cranial or glossopharyngeal nerve (IX).

8. As the ninth cranial or glossopharyngeal nerve (IX) passes through the area of the _____, it sends a branch to the carotid sinus.

9. Entering the _____, each internal carotid artery gives off the ophthalmic artery, the posterior communicating artery, the middle cerebral artery, and the anterior cerebral artery.

10. Three small arteries from the internal carotid artery also contribute to the arterial supply of the face; these blood vessels begin from the _____, a branch of the internal carotid artery, after this artery enters the orbit.

receptors	external carotid artery	blood pressure
extracranial	common carotid artery	cranial cavity
internal carotid artery	ophthalmic artery	anterior cervical triangle
external		

References   Chapter 6, Vascular system. In Fehrenbach MJ, Herring SW: *Illustrated anatomy of the head and neck,* ed 6, St. Louis, 2021, Saunders; Chapter 8, Head and neck. In Drake R, Vogl AW, Mitchell AWM: *Gray's anatomy for students,* ed 4, Philadelphia, 2020, Churchill Livingstone.

FIGURE 6.3   Common carotid artery: External carotid (lateral view)

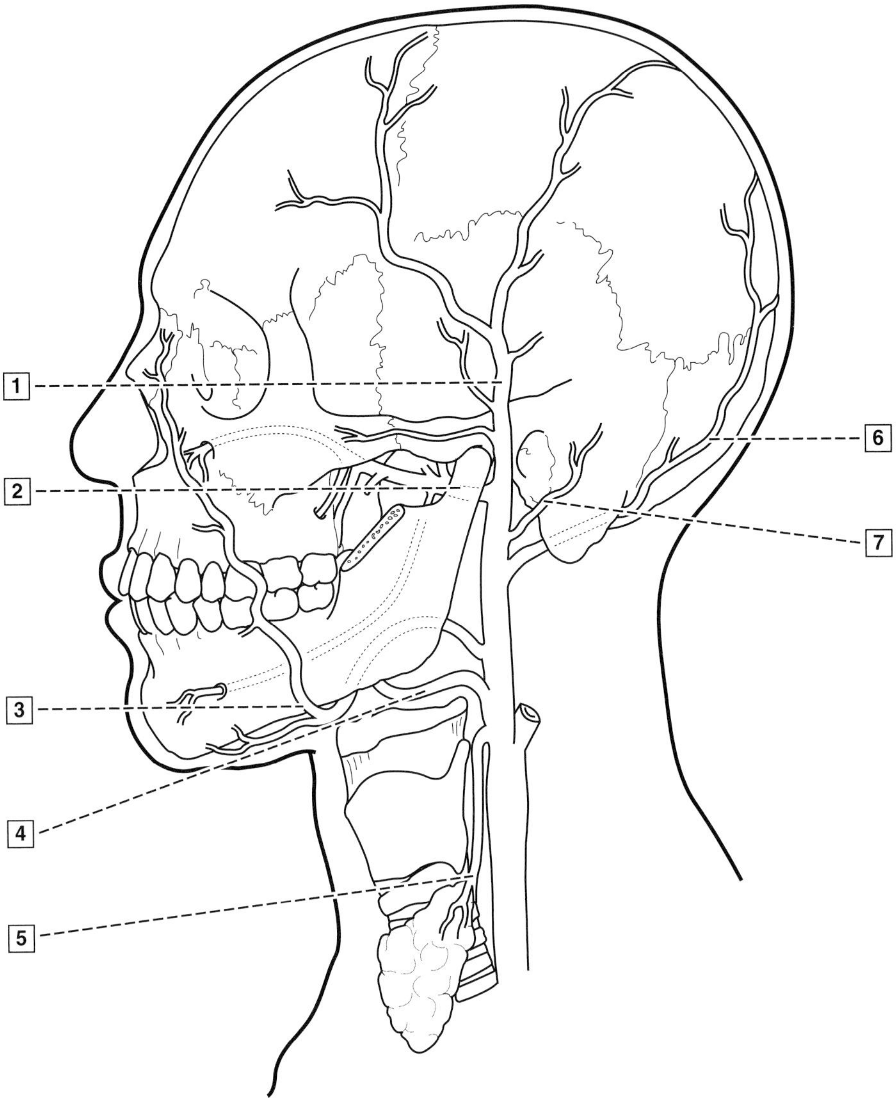

TERMINAL BRANCHES
1 Superficial temporal
2 Maxillary

ANTERIOR BRANCHES
3 Facial
4 Lingual
5 Superior thyroid

POSTERIOR BRANCHES
6 Occipital
7 Posterior auricular

MEDIAL BRANCH
Ascending pharyngeal
(not shown)

REVIEW QUESTIONS: Common carotid artery: External carotid

Fill in the blanks by choosing the appropriate terms from the list below.

1. The _____ travels superiorly in a more medial position in relationship to the internal carotid artery after beginning from the common carotid artery, having four sets of branches grouped according to their location to the main artery including the anterior, medial, posterior, and terminal.

2. The _____ is an anterior branch from the external carotid artery.

3. The superior thyroid artery has _____ branches: the infrahyoid artery, the sternocleidomastoid branch, the superior laryngeal artery, and the cricothyroid branch, which supply the tissue inferior to the hyoid bone, including the infrahyoid muscles, the sternocleidomastoid muscle, the muscles of the larynx, and the thyroid gland.

4. The _____ is an anterior branch from the external carotid artery that begins superior to the superior thyroid artery at the level of the hyoid bone and travels anteriorly to the apex of the tongue by way of its inferior surface to supply the tissue superior to the hyoid bone, including the suprahyoid muscles and floor of the mouth by way of the dorsal lingual, deep lingual, sublingual, and suprahyoid branches.

5. The _____ is an anterior branch from the external carotid artery that begins slightly superior to the lingual artery as it branches off anteriorly; however, in some cases, this artery and the lingual artery share a common trunk.

6. There is only one medial branch from the external carotid artery, the small _____, which begins close to the origin of the external carotid artery.

7. The ascending pharyngeal artery has branches that include the _____ and meningeal branch, which supply the pharyngeal walls (where they anastomose with the ascending palatine artery), soft palate, and meninges, as well as tonsillar branches that supply the pharyngeal tonsils.

8. The _____ is a posterior branch of the external carotid artery that begins from the external carotid artery as it passes superiorly just deep to the ascending mandibular ramus and then travels to the posterior part of the scalp to supply the occipital region and other surrounding region structures.

9. The small _____ is a posterior branch of the external carotid artery that begins superior to the occipital artery and stylohyoid muscle at about the level of the tip of the temporal bone's styloid process to supply the internal ear by its auricular branch and the mastoid process by the stylomastoid artery.

10. The two terminal branches of the external carotid artery include the superficial temporal artery and maxillary artery; the external carotid artery splits into these terminal branches within the _____ on each side of the face; the superficial temporal artery is the smaller branch and can be visible under the skin covering the temporal region in the patient.

posterior auricular artery	pharyngeal branch	parotid salivary gland
four	external carotid artery	superior thyroid artery
occipital artery	facial artery	lingual artery
ascending pharyngeal artery		

Reference Chapter 6, Vascular system. In Fehrenbach MJ, Herring SW: *Illustrated anatomy of the head and neck,* ed 6, St. Louis, 2021, Saunders.

FIGURE 6.4   **External carotid artery: Maxillary (lateral view)**

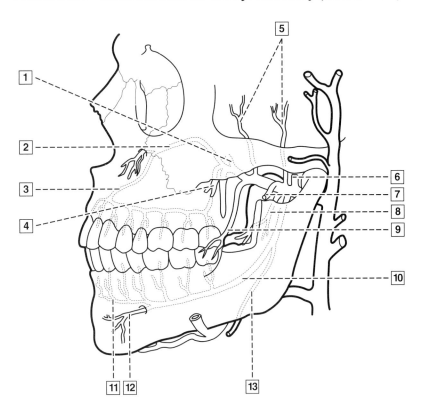

1   Sphenopalatine (cut)

2   Infraorbital

3   Anterior superior alveolar with its dental and alveolar branches (branch of infraorbital)

4   Posterior superior alveolar (part cut)

5   Deep temporals

6   Middle meningeal (cut)

7   Masseteric (cut)

8   Pterygoids

9   Buccal

10   Inferior alveolar

11   Incisive with its dental and alveolar branches

12   Mental

13   Mylohyoid

BRANCHES OF INFERIOR ALVEOLAR

Greater and lesser palatine
Nasal cavity branches
(not shown)

Fill in the blanks by choosing the appropriate terms from the list below.

1. The _____ is the largest terminal branch of the external carotid artery.

2. The _____ supplies the dura mater of the brain and cranial bones by way of the foramen spinosum.

3. The _____ begins from the maxillary artery within the infratemporal fossa and then turns inferiorly to enter the mandibular foramen and then the mandibular canal along with the inferior alveolar nerve and vein; within the canal it gives rise to dental and alveolar branches that supply the pulp of the mandibular posterior teeth by way of each tooth's apical foramen.

4. The _____ begins at the inferior alveolar artery before the main artery enters the mandibular canal by way of the mandibular foramen and then travels with the mylohyoid nerve in the mylohyoid groove on the medial surface of the mandible to supply the floor of the mouth and the mylohyoid muscle.

5. The _____ begins at the inferior alveolar artery and exits the mandibular canal by way of the mental foramen along with the mental nerve, which is located on the lateral surface of the mandible, usually inferior to the apices of the mandibular premolars; after it exits the canal, the artery supplies the chin within the mental region and anastomoses with the inferior labial artery from the facial artery.

6. The _____ branches off the inferior alveolar artery, remaining within the mandibular canal along with the incisive nerve to divide into dental and alveolar branches to supply the pulp of the mandibular anterior teeth by way of each tooth's apical foramen.

7. Just after the maxillary artery leaves the infratemporal fossa and enters the pterygopalatine fossa, it branches off the _____; this artery emerges from the pterygomaxillary fissure and then enters the posterior superior alveolar foramina along with the posterior superior alveolar nerve branches on the outer posterior surface of the maxilla, giving rise to dental branches and alveolar branches to supply the pulp of the maxillary posterior teeth by way of each tooth's apical foramen and anastomoses with the anterior superior alveolar artery.

8. The _____ branches from the maxillary artery in the pterygopalatine fossa but may share a common trunk with the posterior superior alveolar artery; later this artery enters the orbit through the inferior orbital fissure and while in the orbit, the artery travels in the infraorbital canal to provide orbital branches to the orbit as well as giving off the anterior superior alveolar artery that travels nearby to the anterior superior alveolar nerve.

9. After giving off branches in the infraorbital canal, the infraorbital artery emerges onto the face from the infraorbital foramen to supply parts of the infraorbital region of the face by its terminal branches and anastomose with the _____.

10. The _____ branches off from the infraorbital artery and gives rise to dental and alveolar branches that supply the pulp of the maxillary anterior teeth by way of each tooth's apical foramen and anastomoses with the posterior superior alveolar artery.

middle meningeal artery	posterior superior alveolar artery	incisive artery
facial artery	mental artery	inferior alveolar artery
infraorbital artery	maxillary artery	mylohyoid artery
anterior superior alveolar artery		

Reference Chapter 6, Vascular system. In Fehrenbach MJ, Herring SW: *Illustrated anatomy of the head and neck,* ed 6, St. Louis, 2021, Saunders.

FIGURE 6.5 Maxillary artery: Palatal branches (sagittal section of nasal cavity)

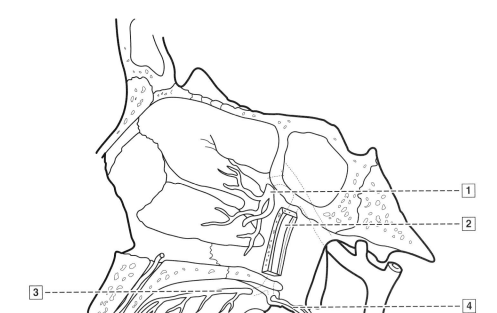

1 Sphenopalatine
2 Descending palatine
3 Greater palatine
4 Lesser palatine

REVIEW QUESTIONS: Maxillary artery: Palatal branches

Fill in the blanks by choosing the appropriate terms from the list below.

1. In the pterygopalatine fossa, the maxillary artery branches off the _____, which travels to the palate through the pterygopalatine canal.

2. The descending palatine artery terminates in both the greater and lesser _____ that travel along with the greater palatine and lesser palatine nerves to exit by way of the greater and lesser palatine foramina to then supply the posterior hard palate with the palatal periodontium and gingiva of the maxillary posterior teeth and soft palate.

3. The maxillary artery ends by becoming the _____, its main terminal branch, which supplies the nasal cavity within the nasal region by way of the sphenopalatine foramen.

4. The sphenopalatine artery gives off the _____ and septal branches.

5. One of the arteries that branches off the sphenopalatine artery includes the _____ that accompanies the nasopalatine nerve through the incisive foramen on the maxillae to supply the anterior hard palate as well as the palatal periodontium and gingiva of the maxillary anterior teeth.

6. The sphenopalatine artery leaves the pterygopalatine fossa medially through the _____ and accompanies the nasal nerves and onto the lateral wall of the nasal cavity.

7. The posterior lateral nasal arteries supply the lateral wall of the _____ and contribute to the supply of the paranasal sinuses to also anastomose anteriorly with branches from the anterior and posterior ethmoidal arteries, and with lateral nasal branches of the facial artery.

8. The septal branches, which travel medially across the roof of the nasal cavity to supply the _____ by its medial wall, have their largest branch pass anteriorly and inferiorly along the nasal septum to anastomose with the terminal part of the greater palatine artery and septal branches of the superior labial artery.

9. Like the sphenopalatine artery, the greater palatine artery begins in the _____ as a branch of the maxillary artery; it passes first onto the roof of the oral cavity by passing inferiorly through the palatine canal and greater palatine foramen to the posterior aspect of the palate, then passes anteriorly on the undersurface of the palate, and superiorly through the incisive fossa and canal to reach the floor of the nasal cavity.

10. The _____ supplies anterior regions of the medial wall and adjacent floor of the nasal cavity and anastomoses with the septal branch of the sphenopalatine artery.

nasal cavity	nasal septum	pterygopalatine fossa
nasopalatine branch	sphenopalatine artery	greater palatine artery
palatine arteries	descending palatine artery	
posterior lateral nasal branches	sphenopalatine foramen	

References   Chapter 6, Vascular system. In Fehrenbach MJ, Herring SW: *Illustrated anatomy of the head and neck,* ed 6, St. Louis, 2021, Saunders; Chapter 8, Head and neck. In Drake R, Vogl AW, Mitchell AWM: *Gray's anatomy for students,* ed 4, Philadelphia, 2020, Churchill Livingstone.

FIGURE 6.6   External carotid artery: Superficial temporal (lateral view)

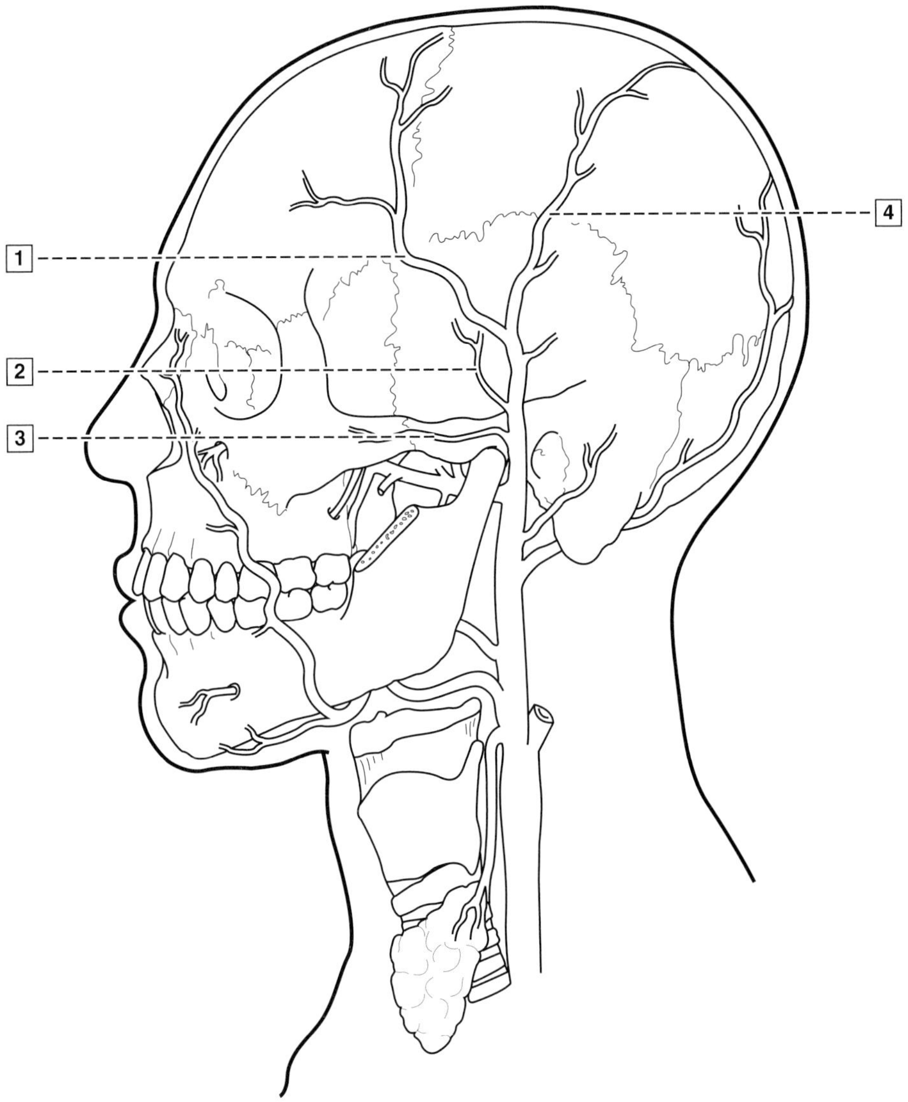

1 Frontal branch
2 Middle temporal
3 Transverse facial
4 Parietal branch

REVIEW QUESTIONS: External carotid artery: Superficial temporal

Fill in the blanks by choosing the appropriate terms from the list below.

1. The _____ is the smaller terminal branch of the external carotid artery that arises within the parotid salivary gland; this artery can be visible under the skin covering the temporal region in the patient.

2. The superficial temporal artery has several branches including the transverse facial artery, the middle temporal artery, the frontal branch, and the _____.

3. The small _____ supplies the parotid salivary gland duct and nearby facial area.

4. The small _____ supplies the temporalis muscle.

5. The _____ and parietal branch supply parts of the scalp in the frontal and parietal regions.

6. The external carotid artery enters into or passes deep to the inferior border of the _____.

7. As the _____ continues in a superior direction, it gives off the posterior auricular artery before dividing into its two terminal branches (the maxillary and superficial temporal arteries) near the inferior border of the ear's auricle; the arterial supply to the auricle is from numerous sources such as the external carotid artery.

8. The superficial temporal artery continues in a superior direction and emerges from the _____ of the parotid salivary gland after giving off the transverse facial artery.

9. Another contributor to the vascular supply of the face is the transverse facial artery, which is a branch of the superficial temporal artery, the smaller of the two _____ branches of the external carotid artery.

10. The transverse facial artery arises from the superficial temporal artery within the substance of the parotid salivary gland, passes through the gland, and crosses the face in a transverse direction; laying on the superficial surface of the _____, being between the zygomatic arch and the parotid duct.

superior border	masseter muscle	external carotid artery
superficial temporal artery	frontal branch	parotid salivary gland
transverse facial artery	middle temporal branch	
parietal branch	terminal	

References   Chapter 6, Vascular system. In Fehrenbach MJ, Herring SW: *Illustrated anatomy of the head and neck,* ed 6, St. Louis, 2021, Saunders; Chapter 8, Head and neck. In Drake R, Vogl AW, Mitchell AWM: *Gray's anatomy for students,* ed 4, Philadelphia, 2020, Churchill Livingstone.

FIGURE 6.7   External carotid artery: Anterior branches (sagittal section)

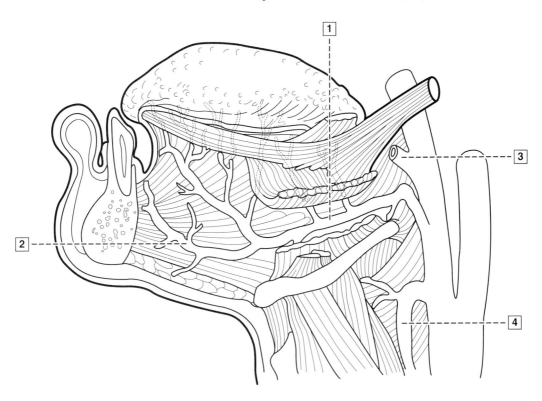

1 Lingual

2 Sublingual

3 Facial (cut)

4 Superior thyroid

REVIEW QUESTIONS: External carotid artery: Anterior branches

Fill in the blanks by choosing the appropriate terms from the list below.

1. There are _____ anterior branches from the external carotid artery including the superior thyroid, the lingual, and the facial arteries.

2. The superior thyroid artery is an anterior branch from the _____.

3. The lingual artery is an anterior branch from the external carotid artery and begins _____ to the superior thyroid artery at the level of the hyoid bone.

4. The lingual artery travels anteriorly to the _____ by way of its inferior surface.

5. The lingual artery supplies the structures superior to the _____ including the suprahyoid muscles and floor of the mouth by the dorsal lingual, deep lingual, sublingual arteries, and suprahyoid branches.

6. The _____ is also supplied by branches of the lingual artery, including several small dorsal lingual branches to the posterior dorsal surface as well as the deep lingual artery, the terminal part of the lingual artery, which courses from the ventral surface to the apex; it also has tonsillar branches to the lingual tonsils and soft palate.

7. The _____ branches off the lingual artery to supply the mylohyoid muscle, sublingual salivary gland, and oral mucosa of the floor of the mouth as well as the lingual periodontium and gingiva of the mandibular teeth in most cases.

8. The small _____ supplies the suprahyoid muscles.

9. The _____ is the final anterior branch from the external carotid artery.

10. The facial artery begins slightly superior to the lingual artery as it branches off anteriorly; however, in some cases this artery and lingual artery share a(n) _____.

facial artery	external carotid artery	sublingual artery
common trunk	tongue	three
hyoid bone	suprahyoid branch	apex of the tongue
superior		

Reference Chapter 6, Vascular system. In Fehrenbach MJ, Herring SW: *Illustrated anatomy of the head and neck,* ed 6, St. Louis, 2021, Saunders.

NOTES

FIGURE 6.8   External carotid artery: Facial (lateral view)

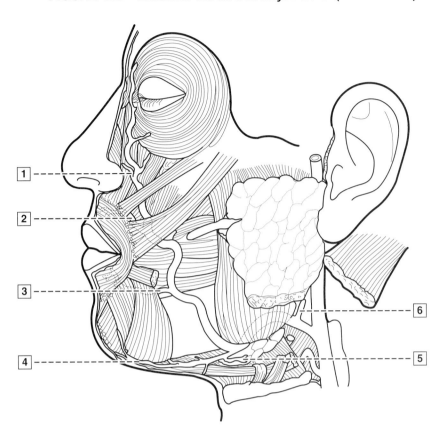

1   Angular

2   Superior labial

3   Inferior labial

4   Submental

5   Glandular branches

6   Ascending palatine

REVIEW QUESTIONS: External carotid artery: Facial

Fill in the blanks by choosing the appropriate terms from the list below.

1. The _____ is an anterior branch from the external carotid artery that begins slightly superior to the lingual artery as it branches off anteriorly; however, in some cases, this artery and lingual artery share a common trunk.

2. The facial artery has a complicated path as it runs medial to the _____, superior to the submandibular salivary gland, and then near the mandible's inferior border at its lateral side.

3. From the inferior border of the mandible, the facial artery runs anteriorly and superiorly near the labial commissure and along the lateral side of the naris of the nose to terminate at the _____ of the eye to supply the face in the oral, buccal, zygomatic, nasal, infraorbital, and orbital regions.

4. The facial artery is mainly parallel to the _____ in the head area, although both blood vessels do not run adjacent to each other.

5. In the neck, the facial artery is separated from the facial vein by the _____, stylohyoid muscle, and submandibular salivary gland.

6. The facial artery's major branches include the ascending palatine branch, glandular branches, submental branch, inferior labial branch, superior labial branch, angular artery, and _____.

7. The _____ is the first branch from the facial artery and supplies the soft palate, palatine muscles, and palatine tonsils by way of tonsillar branches.

8. The _____ supplies the submandibular lymph nodes as well as the mylohyoid and digastric muscles and the glandular branches supply the submandibular salivary gland and nearby muscles; in a lesser number of cases, it also supplies the lingual periodontium and gingiva of the mandibular teeth, either alone or with the sublingual artery.

9. The _____ is a branch from the facial artery that supplies the lower lip area including the area's muscles of facial expression such as the depressor anguli oris muscle; additionally, the superior labial artery is a branch from the facial artery that supplies the upper lip area and similarly the area's muscles of facial expression.

10. The _____ is the terminal branch of the facial artery and supplies the lateral side of the naris of the nose.

ascending palatine artery	angular artery	submental artery
facial artery	posterior belly of the digastric muscle	mandible
facial vein	tonsillar branches	inferior labial artery
medial canthus		

Reference Chapter 6, Vascular system. In Fehrenbach MJ, Herring SW: *Illustrated anatomy of the head and neck,* ed 6, St. Louis, 2021, Saunders.

FIGURE 6.9   External carotid artery: Posterior branches (lateral view)

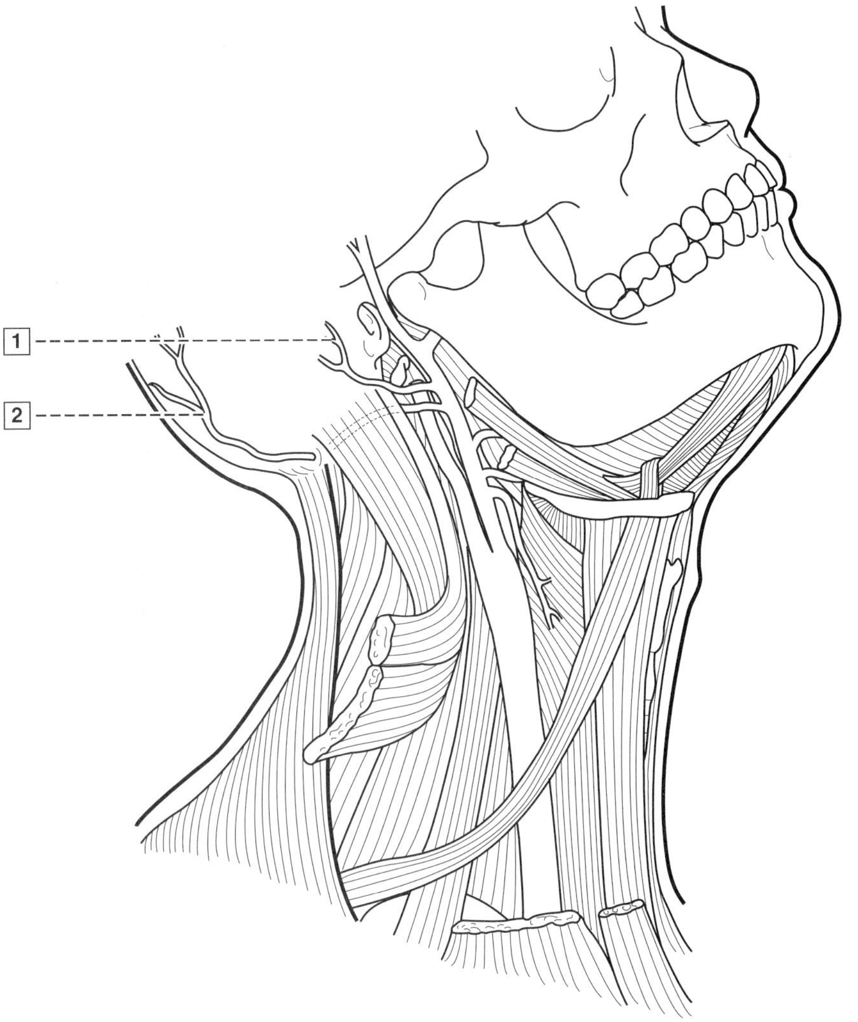

1 Posterior auricular

2 Occipital

REVIEW QUESTIONS: External carotid artery: Posterior branches

Fill in the blanks by choosing the appropriate terms from the list below.

1. There are two posterior branches of the external carotid artery, the occipital and _____ arteries.

2. The occipital artery is a posterior branch of the _____.

3. The occipital artery begins from the external carotid artery as it passes superiorly just deep to the ascending _____ and then travels to the posterior part of the scalp.

4. At its origin, the occipital artery is adjacent to the twelfth cranial nerve or the _____.

5. The occipital artery supplies the suprahyoid and sternocleidomastoid muscles, as well as the scalp and meninges in the _____.

6. The occipital artery supplies the occipital region through the _____, as well as the sternocleidomastoid branches, auricular branches, and meningeal branches.

7. The small posterior auricular artery is also a(n) _____ of the external carotid artery.

8. The posterior auricular artery begins superior to the occipital artery and stylohyoid muscle at approximately the level of the tip of the temporal bone's _____.

9. The posterior auricular artery supplies the internal ear by its _____.

10. The posterior auricular artery supplies the mastoid process by the _____.

stylomastoid artery	auricular branch	external carotid artery
posterior auricular	hypoglossal nerve	occipital region
styloid process	posterior branch	mandibular ramus
muscular branches		

Reference Chapter 6, Vascular system. In Fehrenbach MJ, Herring SW: *Illustrated anatomy of the head and neck,* ed 6, St. Louis, 2021, Saunders.

NOTES

FIGURE 6.10   Internal jugular and facial veins with vessel anastomoses (lateral view)

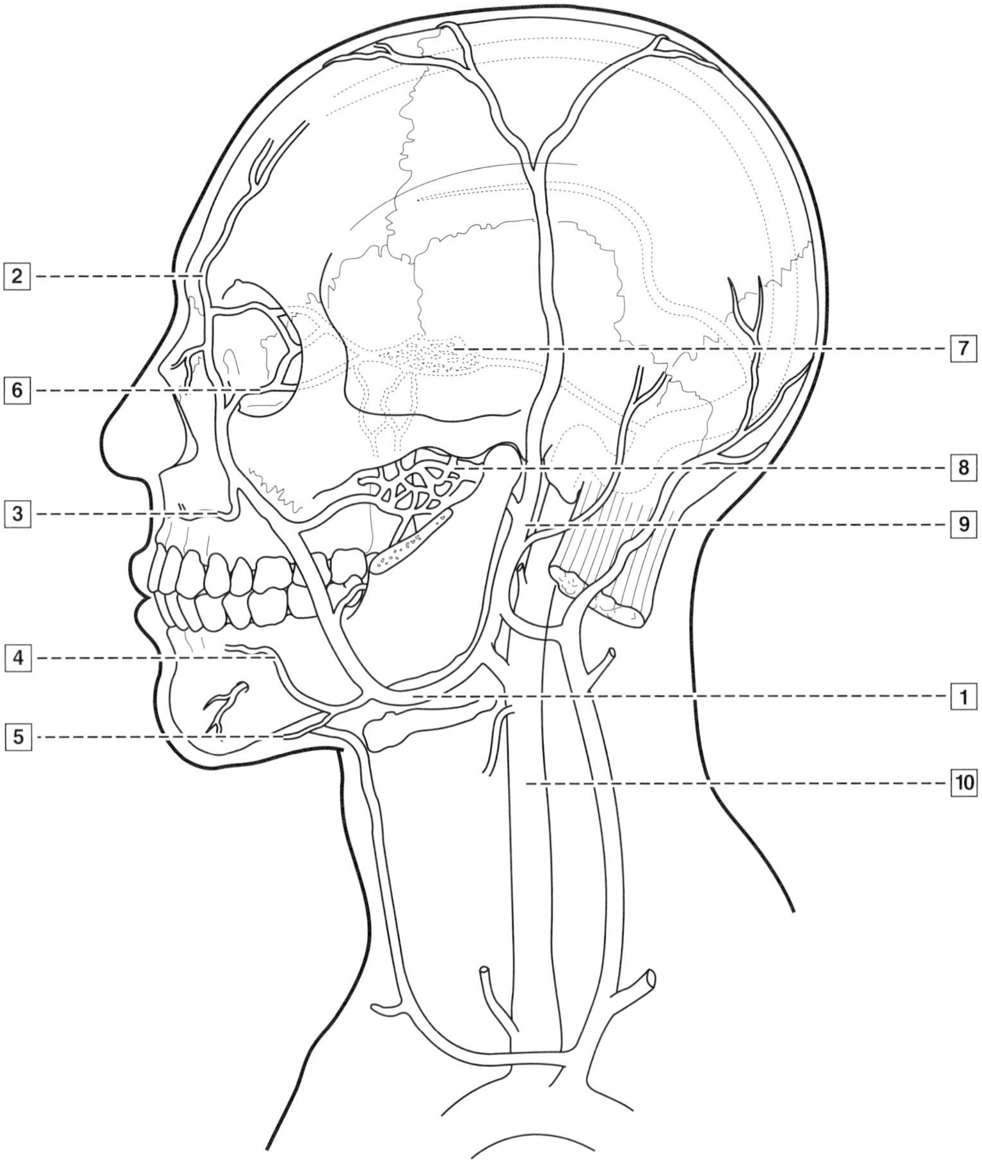

1	Facial		**6**	Ophthalmic
2	Supraorbital		**7**	Cavernous sinus
3	Superior labial	**FACIAL BRANCHES**	**8**	Pterygoid plexus of veins
4	Inferior labial		**9**	Retromandibular
5	Submental		**10**	Internal jugular

REVIEW QUESTIONS: Internal jugular and facial veins with vessel anastomoses

Fill in the blanks by choosing the appropriate terms from the list below.

1. The _____ drains the brain as well as most of the other structures of the head and neck, whereas the external jugular vein drains only a small part of the extracranial tissue; however, the two veins have many anastomoses.

2. The internal jugular vein originates within the cranial cavity and leaves the skull through the _____; it receives many tributaries including the veins from the lingual, sublingual, and pharyngeal areas as well as the facial vein.

3. The internal jugular vein runs with the common carotid artery and its branches as well as the tenth cranial or vagus nerve in the _____.

4. The _____ drains into the internal jugular vein after it begins at the medial canthus of the eye with the junction of two veins from the frontal region, the supratrochlear and supraorbital veins.

5. The supraorbital vein also anastomoses with the ophthalmic veins; the ophthalmic veins drain the orbit and this anastomosis provides a communication with the _____.

6. The facial vein receives branches from the same areas of the face that are supplied by the _____.

7. The facial vein anastomoses with the deep veins such as the _____ within the infratemporal fossa and with the large retromandibular vein before joining the internal jugular vein at the level of the hyoid bone.

8. The facial vein has some important tributaries in the oral region, such as the _____ that drains the upper lip area.

9. The _____ drains the lower lip area in the oral region as a tributary of the facial vein.

10. A facial vein tributary, the _____, drains the tissue of the mental region including the chin as well as the submandibular region.

inferior labial vein	internal jugular vein	cavernous sinus
jugular foramen	carotid sheath	facial artery
submental vein	facial vein	pterygoid plexus of veins
superior labial vein		

Reference   Chapter 6, Vascular system. In Fehrenbach MJ, Herring SW: *Illustrated anatomy of the head and neck,* ed 6, St. Louis, 2021, Saunders.

FIGURE 6.11   External jugular and retromandibular veins with vessel anastomoses (lateral view)

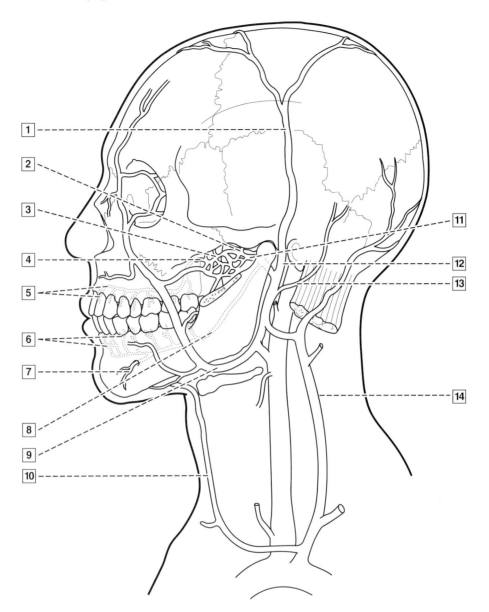

1	Superficial temporal	8	Inferior alveolar
2	Middle meningeal	9	Facial
3	Pterygoid plexus of veins	10	Anterior jugular
4	Posterior superior alveolar	11	Maxillary
5	Alveolar and dental branches of posterior superior alveolar	12	Retromandibular
6	Alveolar and dental branches of inferior alveolar	13	Posterior auricular
7	Mental branch of inferior alveolar	14	External jugular

Fill in the blanks by choosing the appropriate terms from the list below.

1. The _____ forms the external jugular vein from a part of its route, having been initially formed from the merger of the superficial temporal vein and maxillary vein and having drained those areas similar to those supplied by the superficial temporal and maxillary arteries; the vein then emerges from the parotid salivary gland and courses inferiorly.

2. Inferior to the parotid salivary gland, the retromandibular vein usually divides into two parts, with the anterior division joining the facial vein, and the posterior division continuing its inferior course on the surface of the sternocleidomastoid muscle; the posterior division of the retromandibular vein is later joined by the _____, which drains the lateral scalp posterior to the ear that even later becomes the external jugular vein.

3. Superficially located in the skin covering the temporal region, the _____ drains the lateral scalp and goes on to drain into and form the retromandibular vein, along with the deeper maxillary vein.

4. The _____ is deeper than the superficial temporal vein and begins within the infratemporal fossa by collecting blood from the pterygoid plexus of veins while accompanying the maxillary artery, as well as collecting blood from the middle meningeal, posterior superior alveolar, inferior alveolar veins, and other veins such as those from the nasal cavity and palate; after then receiving these veins, it merges with the superficial temporal vein to drain into and form the retromandibular vein.

5. The _____ is a collection of small anastomosing vessels located around the lateral pterygoid muscle and surrounding the maxillary artery on each side of the face within the infratemporal fossa; this vascular plexus anastomoses with both the facial and retromandibular veins as it drains the veins from the deep parts of the face and then drains into the maxillary vein.

6. The _____ also drains the blood from both the dura mater of the meninges (not the arachnoid or pia mater) and the bones of the cranial vault into the pterygoid plexus of veins.

7. The pterygoid plexus of veins also drains the _____, which is formed by the merging of its dental and alveolar branches of the pulp of the maxillary teeth by way of each tooth's apical foramen.

8. The _____ forms from the merging of its dental branches, alveolar branches, and mental branches within the mandible, where they also drain into the pterygoid plexus with the dental branches draining the pulp of the mandibular teeth by way of each tooth's apical foramen; additionally, the mental branches of this vein enter the mental foramen after draining the mental regions with chin area on the outer surface of the mandible, where they anastomose with branches of the facial vein.

9. The _____ drains into the external jugular vein (or directly into the subclavian vein) before it joins the subclavian vein after its beginning inferior to the chin, communicates with veins in the area, and descends near the midline within the superficial fascia, receiving branches from the superficial cervical structures; only one of these veins may be present, but usually two veins are present, anastomosing with each other through a jugular venous arch.

10. On each side of the body, the external jugular vein joins the subclavian vein from the arm, and then the internal jugular vein merges with the subclavian vein to form the brachiocephalic vein, which then unites to form the superior vena cava to travel ultimately to the _____.

pterygoid plexus of veins	posterior superior alveolar vein	posterior auricular vein
superficial temporal vein	inferior alveolar vein	anterior jugular vein
maxillary vein	retromandibular vein	heart
middle meningeal vein		

Reference Chapter 6, Vascular system. In Fehrenbach MJ, Herring SW: *Illustrated anatomy of the head and neck,* ed 6, St. Louis, 2021, Saunders.

FIGURE 7.1 Lacrimal apparatus (frontal and cutaway views)

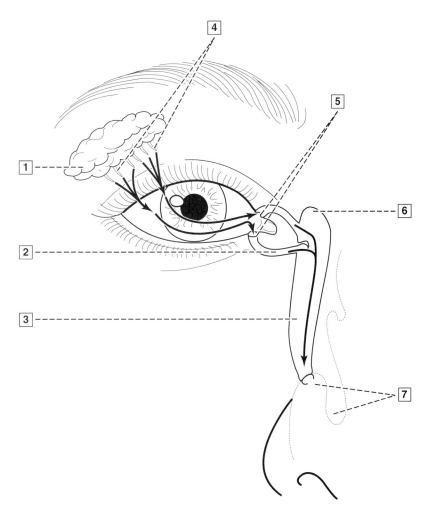

1 Lacrimal gland

2 Lacrimal canal

3 Nasolacrimal duct

4 Lacrimal ducts

5 Lacrimal puncta

6 Lacrimal sac

7 Inferior meatus and turbinate

REVIEW QUESTIONS: Lacrimal apparatus

Fill in the blanks by choosing the appropriate terms from the list below.

1. The _____ are paired almond-shaped exocrine glands that secrete lacrimal fluid or *tears*, which is a watery fluid that lubricates the conjunctiva lining the inside of the eyelids and the front of the eyeball.

2. Each lacrimal gland is located within the depression of the _____ formed from the frontal bone, which is located just inside the lateral part of the supraorbital rim within the orbit.

3. The larger orbital part of the lacrimal gland contains the _____ that drains the gland, because it is an exocrine gland.

4. The lacrimal fluid or *tears* secreted from the lacrimal gland collect in the fornix conjunctiva, folds of the conjunctiva, and pass over the eye surface to the _____, which is a small opening on the surface of the eyelid margin near the medial canthus of both the upper and lower eyelids.

5. Any _____ or *tears* secreted from the lacrimal gland that passes over the eye surface will end up in the lacrimal sac, a thin-walled structure behind each medial canthus within the lacrimal fossa that forms the bulbous beginning of the nasolacrimal duct.

6. From the lacrimal sac, the excess lacrimal fluid secreted by the lacrimal gland continues into the nasolacrimal duct as part of a partial mucosal fold, ultimately draining into the _____ within the nasal cavity; any remaining lacrimal fluid is finally absorbed in the nasopharynx after draining into the inferior nasal meatus.

7. The nasolacrimal duct or *tear duct* begins in the orbit between the _____ and lacrimal bone, from where it passes inferiorly and posteriorly.

8. The lacrimal glands are innervated by parasympathetic fibers from the _____, a branch of the seventh cranial nerve or facial nerve with the preganglionic fibers synapsing at the pterygopalatine ganglion and postganglionic fibers reaching the gland through branches of the fifth cranial or trigeminal nerve and their connections with the lacrimal nerve, an ophthalmic branch of the trigeminal nerve; the lacrimal nerve also serves as an afferent nerve for the gland.

9. The lacrimal gland drains into the _____ of the lymphatic system.

10. The lacrimal gland is supplied by the _____, a branch of the ophthalmic artery of the internal carotid artery; venous blood returns by way of the superior ophthalmic vein.

lacrimal artery	lacrimal fossa	lacrimal puncta
superficial parotid lymph nodes	lacrimal ducts	lacrimal fluid
lacrimal glands	greater petrosal nerve	maxilla
inferior nasal meatus		

Reference Chapter 7, Glandular tissue. In Fehrenbach MJ, Herring SW: *Illustrated anatomy of the head and neck,* ed 6, St. Louis, 2021, Saunders.

FIGURE 7.2 Major salivary glands and ducts (ventral and frontal aspects with internal views)

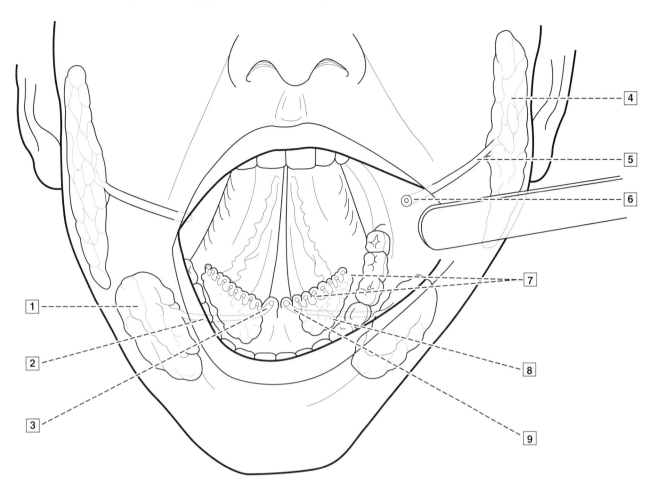

1	Submandibular gland	**5**	Parotid duct (Stenson duct)
2	Submandibular duct (Wharton duct)	**6**	Parotid papilla
3	Sublingual caruncle with duct openings from submandibular and sublingual glands	**7**	Sublingual ducts
4	Parotid gland	**8**	Sublingual gland
		9	Sublingual duct (Bartholin duct)

REVIEW QUESTIONS: Major salivary glands and ducts

Fill in the blanks by choosing the appropriate terms from the list below.

1. The _____ produce saliva, a secretion that is part of the defenses of the immune system as well as the beginning of breakdown of food products as part of the digestive system; saliva lubricates and cleanses the oral cavity and helps in digestion.

2. The salivary glands are controlled by the _____ nervous system.

3. The salivary glands are divided by size into major and minor glands; however, both the major and minor salivary glands are _____ and thus have ducts associated with them that help drain the saliva directly into the oral cavity where the saliva can function.

4. The _____ are large paired salivary glands that have named ducts associated with them.

5. The _____ is the largest encapsulated major salivary gland.

6. The named duct associated with the parotid salivary gland is the _____ or *Stensen duct* which opens up into the adult oral cavity on the inner surface of the cheek, usually opposite the maxillary second molar as marked by the parotid papilla.

7. The _____ is the second largest encapsulated major salivary gland.

8. The named duct associated with the submandibular salivary gland is the _____ or *Wharton duct* that travels along the anterior floor of the mouth and then opens into the oral cavity at the sublingual caruncle.

9. The _____ is the smallest, most diffuse, and only unencapsulated major salivary gland.

10. The named large accessory duct associated with the sublingual salivary gland is the _____ or *Bartholin duct*; the duct opens directly into the oral cavity through the same opening as the submandibular duct, the sublingual caruncle.

major salivary glands	submandibular duct	parotid salivary gland
sublingual duct	autonomic	salivary glands
submandibular salivary gland	sublingual salivary gland	exocrine glands
parotid duct		

References Chapter 7, Glandular tissue. Fehrenbach MJ, Herring SW: *Illustrated anatomy of the head and neck,* ed 6, St. Louis, 2021, Saunders; Chapter 11, Head and neck structures. In Fehrenbach MJ, Popowics T: *Illustrated dental embryology, histology, and anatomy,* ed 5, St. Louis, 2020, Saunders.

NOTES

FIGURE 7.3 Salivary gland (microanatomic view)

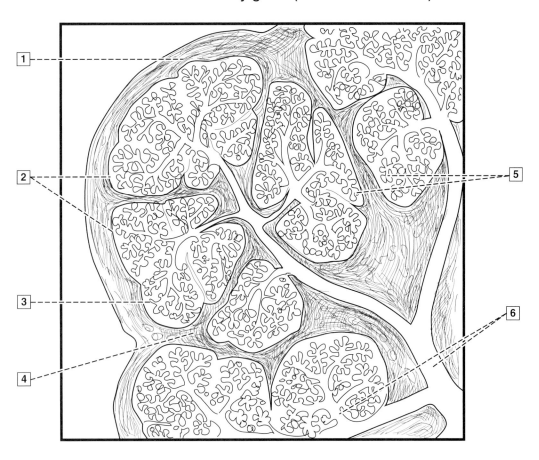

1 Capsule

2 Lobes

3 Lobule

4 Septum

5 Acini

6 Ductal system

REVIEW QUESTIONS: Salivary gland

Fill in the blanks by choosing the appropriate terms from the list below.

1. Connective tissue surrounds each part of the epithelia, protecting and supporting the gland; the connective tissue of the salivary gland is divided into the _____, which surrounds the outer part of the entire gland and the septa.

2. Each _____ helps divide the inner part of the salivary gland into the larger lobes and then smaller lobules; both the capsule and septa also carry nerves and blood vessels that serve the gland.

3. Epithelial cells both line the ducts and produce the saliva; the epithelial cells of the salivary gland that produce saliva are the _____.

4. The secretory cells of the salivary gland are found in a group or a(n) _____; each group is located at the terminal part of the gland connected to the ductal system with many groups within each lobule of the gland.

5. The _____ of salivary glands consists of hollow tubes connected initially with the acinus and then with other ducts as the ducts progressively grow larger from the inner to the outer parts of the salivary gland.

6. The _____ are much smaller than the larger major salivary glands but are more numerous.

7. The minor salivary glands are scattered in the tissue of the buccal, labial, and lingual mucosa, as well as the soft palate, the lateral zones of the hard palate, and the _____.

8. The minor salivary glands, the _____, are associated with the base of the larger circumvallate lingual papillae on the posterior part of the dorsal surface of the tongue; they flush out the trough surrounding the circumvallate lingual papillae with their salivary flow for new taste sensations when eating.

9. Most minor salivary glands secrete a predominantly viscous _____ type of salivary product with slight watery serous influence, because they have mostly mucous acini, with a few having serous demilunes as well as also having a few serous acini; however, the von Ebner salivary glands secrete only a watery serous type of salivary product because these glands contain only serous acini.

10. The minor salivary glands are also _____ like the major salivary glands, but their unnamed ducts are shorter than those of the major ones and open directly onto the oral mucosa surface.

exocrine glands	von Ebner salivary glands	septum
floor of the mouth	mucous	ductal system
secretory cells	acinus	minor salivary glands
capsule		

References   Chapter 7, Glandular tissue. In Fehrenbach MJ, Herring SW: *Illustrated anatomy of the head and neck,* ed 6, St. Louis, 2021, Saunders; Chapter 11, Head and neck structures. In Fehrenbach MJ, Popowics T: *Illustrated dental embryology, histology, and anatomy,* ed 5, St. Louis, 2020, Saunders.

FIGURE 7.4 Salivary glands: Acini and ducts (microanatomic view)

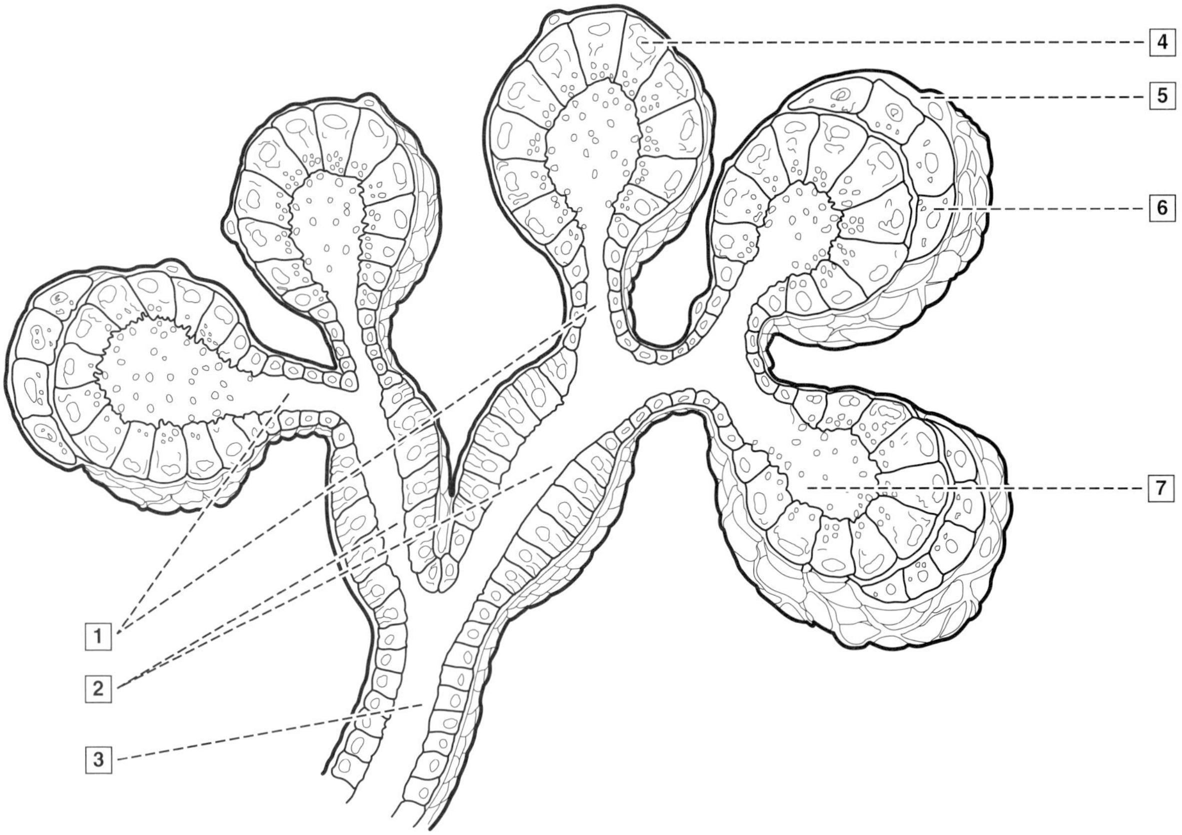

1 Intercalated ducts		**5** Myoepithelial cell
2 Striated ducts		**6** Serous demilune
3 Excretory duct		**7** Lumen of acinus
4 Mucous cell		

REVIEW QUESTIONS: Salivary glands: Acini and ducts

Fill in the blanks by choosing the appropriate terms from the list below.

1. The two main types of _____ within the salivary glands are classified as either mucous or serous cells, depending on the type of secretion produced.

2. Each _____ of the salivary gland consists of a single layer of cuboidal epithelial cells surrounding a lumen, which is a central opening where the saliva is deposited after being produced by the secretory cells.

3. The _____ produce a mucous secretory product with mostly mucins; the mucous acini are composed of these cells that produce a viscous mucous secretory product with flatter nuclei and wider lumens.

4. The _____ produce a serous secretory product with proteins and glycoproteins; the serous acini are composed of these cells that produce a watery serous secretory product with rounder nuclei and narrower lumens.

5. The *mucoserous* or *seromucous* acini have a(n) _____ that consists of a cap of serous cells superficial to the group of mucous secretory cells; the mucous acini with a serous demilune contain both types of secretory cells, therefore they produce a mixed secretory product.

6. To facilitate the flow of saliva out of each lumen of the salivary gland into the connecting ducts, _____ are located on the surface of some of the acini as well as on their connection to the ductal system, the intercalated ducts; each one consists of a cell body with four to eight cytoplasmic processes radiating outward.

7. The duct associated with an acinus or terminal part of the salivary gland is the _____, which is attached to the acinus and consists of a hollow tube lined with a single layer of cuboidal epithelial cells; many of these types of ducts are found in each lobule of the gland.

8. The larger _____ is a part of the ductal system that is connected to the intercalated ducts in the lobules of the salivary gland; it consists of a hollow tube lined with a single layer of columnar epithelial cells characterized by what appear to be *basal striations*.

9. The final part of the salivary gland ductal system is the very large _____ (or secretory duct), which is located in the septum of the salivary gland and is the duct whereby saliva exits into the oral cavity; this duct consists of a hollow tube lined with a variety of epithelial cells.

10. The cells lining the excretory duct initially consist of _____, which then undergoes a transition to stratified cuboidal epithelium as the duct moves to the outer part of the salivary gland: on the outer part of the ductal system that empties into the oral cavity, the excretory duct lining becomes stratified squamous epithelium, blending with surrounding oral mucosa at the ductal opening.

striated duct	mucous cells	acinus
excretory duct	pseudostratified columnar epithelium	intercalated duct
myoepithelial cells	demilune	secretory cells
serous cells		

Reference Chapter 11, Head and neck structures. In Fehrenbach MJ, Popowics T: *Illustrated dental embryology, histology, and anatomy,* ed 5, St. Louis, 2020, Saunders.

ANSWER KEY 1. secretory cells, 2. acinus, 3. mucous cells, 4. serous cells, 5. demilune, 6. myoepithelial cells, 7. intercalated duct, 8. striated duct, 9. excretory duct, 10. pseudostratified columnar epithelium

FIGURE 7.5   Major salivary glands: Parotid gland (lateral view)

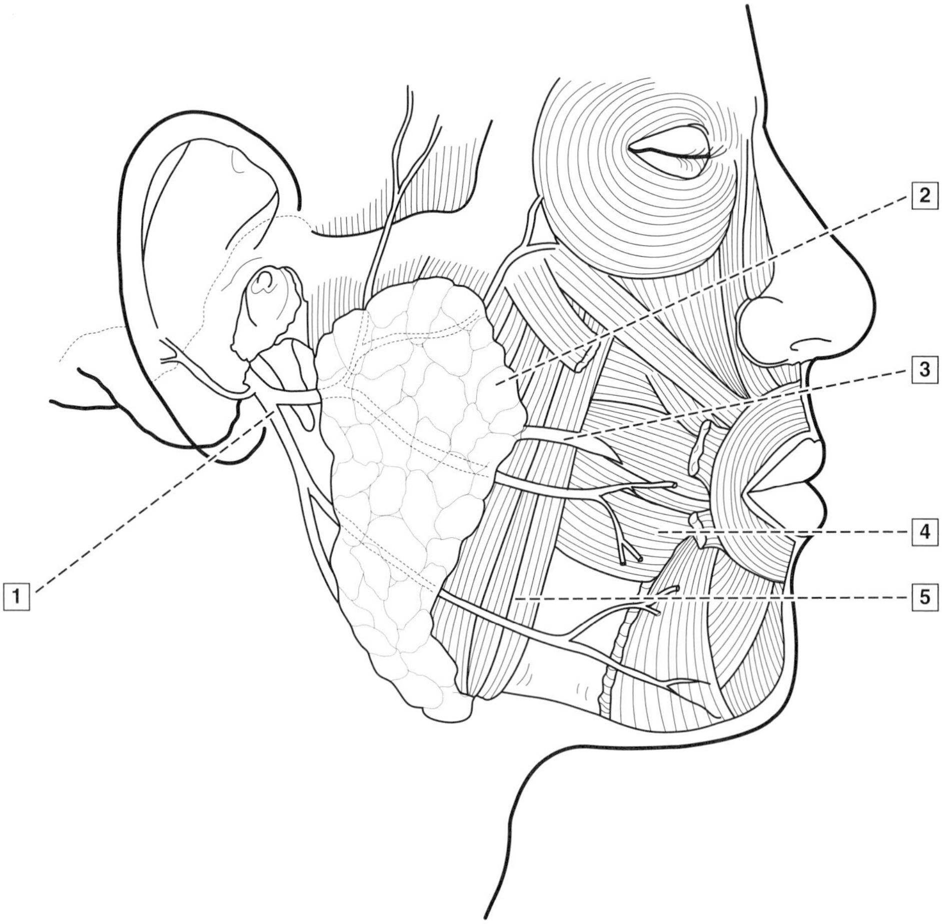

1 Facial nerve (VII)

2 Parotid gland

3 Parotid duct (Stenson duct)

4 Buccinator muscle

5 Masseter muscle

REVIEW QUESTIONS: Major salivary glands: Parotid gland

Fill in the blanks by choosing the appropriate terms from the list below.

1. The _____ is the largest encapsulated major salivary gland.

2. The salivary product from the parotid salivary gland is a only watery _____ type of secretion from having only serous acini.

3. The parotid salivary gland is divided into two _____ by the facial or seventh cranial nerve: the larger superficial and the smaller deep ones.

4. The parotid salivary gland occupies the _____ created inside the investing fascial layer of the deep cervical fascia as it envelops the gland, an area posterior to the mandibular ramus as well as anterior and inferior to the ear.

5. The parotid salivary gland extends irregularly from the _____ to the angle of the mandible.

6. The named duct associated with the parotid salivary gland is the _____ or *Stensen duct*, with it being associated with long intercalated ducts and short striated ducts; this named duct emerges from the anterior border of the parotid salivary gland, superficial to the masseter muscle but at the muscle's anterior border takes a sharp turn medially to then pierce the buccinator muscle to open up into the oral cavity on the inner surface of the cheek, usually opposite the maxillary second molar.

7. The _____ is a small elevation of tissue that marks the opening of the parotid duct on the inner surface of the cheek.

8. The parotid salivary gland is innervated by efferent (parasympathetic) nerves of the _____ of the ninth cranial nerve or glossopharyngeal nerve by way of the lesser petrosal nerve, with these efferent fibers synapsing in it; the postganglionic nerve fibers are carried to the gland by the auriculotemporal nerve of the mandibular nerve of the fifth cranial or trigeminal nerve, which also provides afferent innervation of the area; however, the seventh cranial nerve or facial nerve and its terminal branches travel through the gland between its superficial and deep lobes to serve as a divider but are not involved in its innervation.

9. The parotid salivary gland drains into the _____ of the lymphatic system.

10. The parotid salivary gland is supplied by a branch off the _____ of the vascular system, the transverse facial artery; venous return is by the retromandibular vein.

otic ganglion	parotid fascial space	external carotid artery
parotid papilla	lobes	deep parotid lymph nodes
serous	parotid duct	zygomatic arch
parotid salivary gland		

References Chapter 7, Glandular tissue. In Fehrenbach MJ, Herring SW: *Illustrated anatomy of the head and neck,* ed 6, St. Louis, 2021, Saunders; Chapter 11, Head and neck structures. In Fehrenbach MJ, Popowics T: *Illustrated dental embryology, histology, and anatomy,* ed 5, St. Louis, 2020, Saunders.

ANSWER KEY 1. parotid salivary gland, 2. serous, 3. lobes, 4. parotid fascial space, 5. zygomatic arch, 6. parotid duct, 7. parotid papilla, 8. otic ganglion, 9. deep parotid lymph nodes, 10. external carotid artery

FIGURE 7.6   Major salivary glands: Submandibular gland (lateral view)

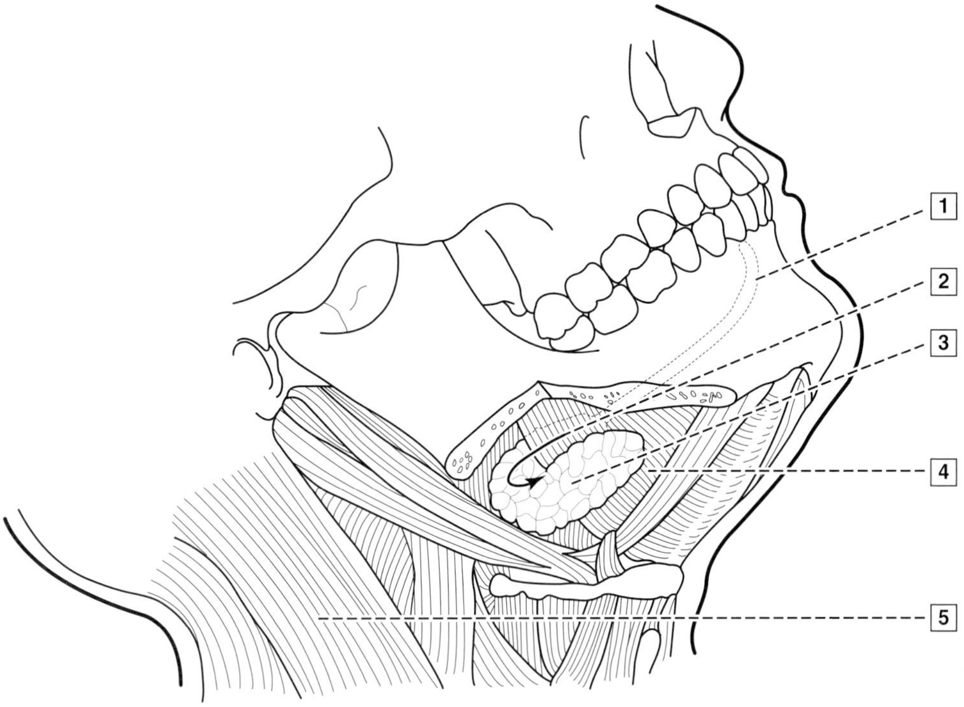

1 Submandibular duct (Wharton duct)

2 Deep lobe, submandibular gland

3 Superficial lobe, submandibular gland

4 Mylohyoid muscle

5 Sternocleidomastoid muscle

343

REVIEW QUESTIONS: Major salivary glands: Submandibular gland

Fill in the blanks by choosing the appropriate terms from the list below.

1. The _____ is the second largest encapsulated major salivary gland.

2. The saliva from the submandibular salivary gland is a _____ salivary product that has both serous and mucous secretions from both serous and mucoserous acini; the gland also contains serous demilunes.

3. The submandibular salivary gland occupies the _____ in the submandibular space, mainly in its posterior part.

4. Most of the submandibular salivary gland comprises the larger lobe superficial to the _____, but the smaller and deeper lobe wraps around the posterior border of the muscle to sit on its superior surface.

5. The submandibular salivary gland is located _____ to the sublingual salivary gland; the gland is contained in the submandibular fascial space located lateral and posterior to the submental space on each side of the jaws as part of the submandibular triangle.

6. The named duct associated with the submandibular salivary gland is the _____ or *Wharton duct*; the gland is associated with short intercalated ducts and long striated ducts.

7. The long submandibular duct travels from the deeper lobe anteromedially along the anterior floor of the mouth between the mylohyoid, hypoglossus, and genioglossus muscles; the duct then ascends into the oral cavity at the _____ with its one to three openings, a small papilla near the midline of the floor of the mouth on each side and at the base of the lingual frenum.

8. The submandibular salivary gland is innervated by the efferent (parasympathetic) fibers of the _____ of the seventh cranial or facial nerve that synapse in the submandibular ganglion; the postganglionic fibers are delivered to the sublingual salivary gland by the lingual nerve, a branch of the mandibular division (or third division) of the fifth cranial or trigeminal nerve.

9. The submandibular salivary gland drains into the _____ of the lymphatic system.

10. The submandibular salivary gland is supplied by glandular branches of the _____; venous return of the gland is mainly by the facial vein.

facial artery
submandibular salivary gland
mixed
chorda tympani

submandibular fossa
submandibular duct
mylohyoid muscle

posterior
submandibular lymph nodes
sublingual caruncle

References   Chapter 7, Glandular tissue. In Fehrenbach MJ, Herring SW: *Illustrated anatomy of the head and neck,* ed 6, St. Louis, 2021, Saunders; Chapter 11, Head and neck structures. In Fehrenbach MJ, Popowics T: *Illustrated dental embryology, histology, and anatomy,* ed 5, St. Louis, 2021, Saunders.

ANSWER KEY 1. submandibular salivary gland, 2. mixed, 3. submandibular fossa, 4. mylohyoid muscle, 5. posterior, 6. submandibular duct, 7. sublingual caruncle, 8. chorda tympani, 9. submandibular lymph nodes, 10. facial artery

FIGURE 7.7 Major salivary glands: Sublingual gland (superior and ventral aspects with internal view)

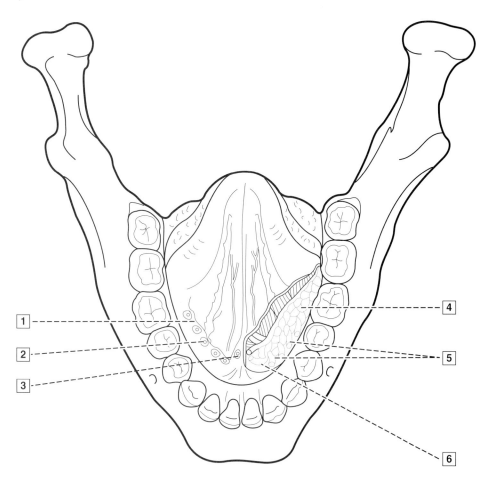

1 | Sublingual fold

2 | Sublingual duct opening

3 | Sublingual carnucle with duct openings from submandibular and sublingual glands

4 | Sublingual gland

5 | Sublingual ducts

6 | Sublingual duct (Bartholin duct)

REVIEW QUESTIONS: Major salivary glands: Sublingual gland

Fill in the blanks by choosing the appropriate terms from the list below.

1. The _____ is the smallest, most diffuse, and only unencapsulated major salivary gland.

2. The saliva from the sublingual salivary gland is a(n) _____ salivary product, but with the mucous secretion predominating; the gland has mostly mucous acini with some mucous acini having serous demilunes.

3. The almond-shaped sublingual salivary gland occupies the _____ in the sublingual space at the floor of the mouth deep to the sublingual fold.

4. The sublingual salivary gland is located _____ to the mylohyoid muscle and medial to the body of the mandible.

5. The sublingual salivary gland is located _____ to the submandibular salivary gland.

6. The named main duct associated with the sublingual salivary gland is the _____ or *Bartholin duct*; the gland is associated with absent intercalated ducts and rare or absent striated ducts.

7. The sublingual duct opens directly into the oral cavity through the same opening as the _____, the sublingual caruncle; other smaller ducts of the gland open along the sublingual fold and are collectively called the *ducts of Rivinus*.

8. The sublingual salivary gland has the same innervation as the _____ .

9. The sublingual salivary gland drains into the _____ of the lymphatic system.

10. The sublingual salivary gland is supplied by the _____ of the vascular system off the lingual artery, with venous return parallel the arterial supply.

sublingual fossa	submandibular lymph nodes	sublingual salivary gland
anterior	submandibular duct	submandibular salivary gland
sublingual duct	superior	sublingual artery
mixed		

References Chapter 7, Glandular tissue. In Fehrenbach MJ, Herring SW: *Illustrated anatomy of the head and neck,* ed 6, St. Louis, 2021, Saunders; Chapter 11, Head and neck structures. In Fehrenbach MJ, Popowics T: *Illustrated dental embryology, histology, and anatomy,* ed 5, St. Louis, 2020, Saunders.

NOTES

FIGURE 7.8   Thyroid and parathyroid glands (anterior and posterior views)

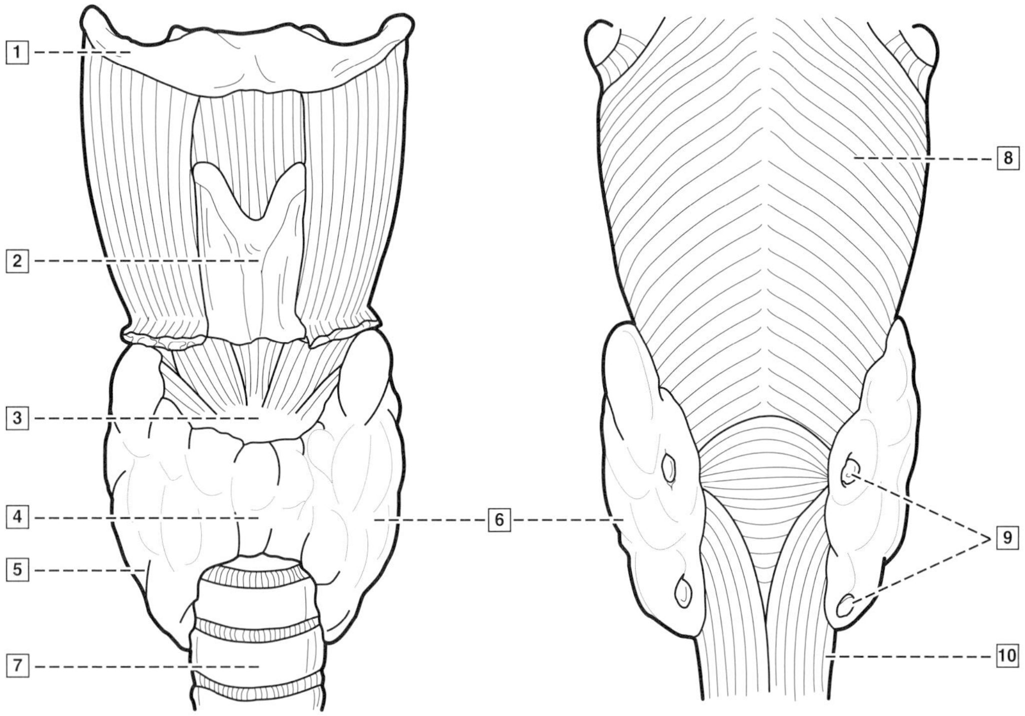

1	Hyoid bone	**6**	Left lobe of thyroid gland
2	Thyroid cartilage	**7**	Trachea
3	Cricoid cartilage	**8**	Interior pharyngeal constrictor muscle
4	Isthmus	**9**	Parathyroid glands
5	Right lobe of thyroid gland	**10**	Esophagus

REVIEW QUESTIONS: Thyroid and parathyroid glands

Fill in the blanks by choosing the appropriate terms from the list below.

1. The _____ is the largest endocrine gland; because it is ductless, the gland produces and secretes its hormones directly into the vascular system, such as thyroxine, which stimulates the metabolic rate.

2. The thyroid gland consists of two _____, right and left, connected anteriorly by a midline isthmus within a visceral compartment of the neck, along with the hyoid bone, larynx, trachea, esophagus, and pharynx.

3. The thyroid gland is located in the anterolateral regions of the _____, inferior to the thyroid cartilage, which is at the junction between the larynx and trachea; the gland is also within the visceral compartment of the neck, along with the hyoid bone, larynx, trachea, esophagus, and pharynx.

4. The thyroid gland is _____ when swallowing occurs because of its fascial encasement; thus, when a person swallows, the gland moves superiorly, as does the whole larynx.

5. The thyroid gland is supplied by the _____ of the vascular system.

6. The parathyroid glands usually consist of two small _____, with two on each side; because the glands are ductless, they produce and secrete parathyroid hormone directly into the vascular system to regulate calcium and phosphorus levels.

7. The parathyroid glands are usually adjacent to or within the thyroid gland on its _____.

8. Both the thyroid gland and parathyroid glands are innervated by _____ through the cervical ganglia; however, these nerves do not control endocrine secretion since the release of hormones by the thyroid gland is regulated by the pituitary gland.

9. Both the thyroid gland and parathyroid glands drain into the _____ of the lymphatic system.

10. The parathyroid glands are primarily supplied by the _____, as is the surrounding thyroid gland, with the former by way of its cricothyroid branch or by the thyroid ima artery in a small number of cases; venous return is by the superior, middle, and inferior thyroid veins, which form a venous plexus.

thyroid gland	sympathetic nerves	lateral lobes
superior and inferior thyroid arteries	neck	inferior thyroid arteries
endocrine glands	posterior surface	superior deep cervical lymph nodes
mobile		

References   Chapter 7, Glandular tissue. In Fehrenbach MJ, Herring SW: *Illustrated anatomy of the head and neck,* ed 6, St. Louis, 2021, Saunders; Chapter 11, Head and neck structures. In Fehrenbach MJ, Popowics T: *Illustrated dental embryology, histology, and anatomy,* ed 5, St. Louis, 2020, Saunders.

FIGURE 7.9   **Thyroid gland (microanatomic view)**

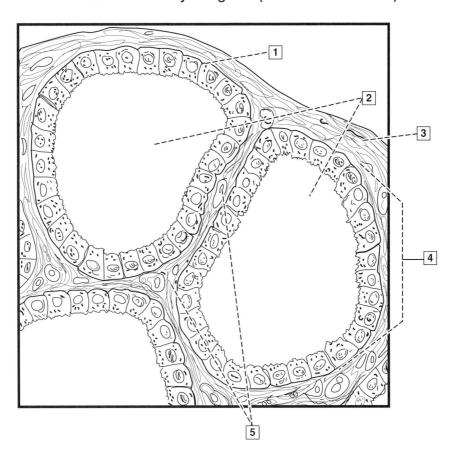

1	Thyroid epithelium
2	Colloid
3	Capsule
4	Follicle
5	Septum

REVIEW QUESTIONS: Thyroid gland

Fill in the blanks by choosing the appropriate terms from the list below.

1. The thyroid gland is covered by the _____ composed of connective tissue that then extends into the gland by way of septa.

2. The _____ divides the thyroid gland into larger lobes and smaller lobules.

3. Each _____ is composed of follicles in the thyroid gland, irregularly-shaped spheroidal masses that are embedded in a meshwork of reticular fibers.

4. Each _____ consists of a layer of simple cuboidal epithelium enclosing a cavity that is usually filled with colloid in the thyroid gland.

5. The _____ is a stiff material that is reserved for the future production of thyroxine by the thyroid gland.

6. The thyroid gland is covered by the _____ capsule that then extends into the gland by way of septa.

7. The septa divide the thyroid gland into larger _____ and then smaller lobules.

8. Each lobule is composed of follicles in the thyroid gland, irregularly-shaped spheroidal masses that are embedded in a meshwork of _____.

9. Each follicle in the thyroid gland consists of a layer of simple _____ enclosing a cavity that is usually filled with colloid.

10. Colloid in the thyroid gland is a stiff material, which is reserved for the future production of _____.

lobule	septa	reticular fibers
colloid	connective tissue	cuboidal epithelium
follicle	lobes	thyroxine
capsule		

Reference   Chapter 11, Head and neck structures. In Fehrenbach MJ, Popowics T: *Illustrated dental embryology, histology, and anatomy,* ed 5, St. Louis, 2020, Saunders.

NOTES

ANSWER KEY   1. capsule, 2. septa, 3. lobule, 4. follicle, 5. colloid, 6. connective tissue, 7. lobes, 8. reticular fibers, 9. cuboidal epithelium, 10. thyroxine

350   Copyright © 2023 Elsevier Inc. All Rights Reserved.

FIGURE 7.10   **Thyroid gland development**

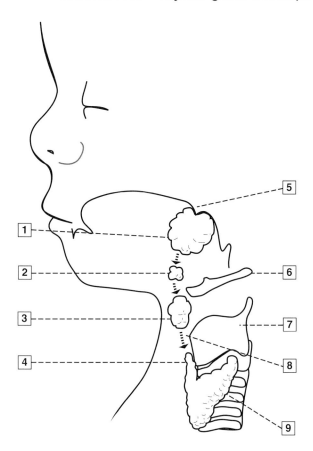

1	Lingual thyroid	6	Hyoid bone
2	Accessory thyroid tissue	7	Thyroid cartilage
3	Cervical thyroid	8	Tract of thyroglossal duct
4	Pyramidal thyroid	9	Normal position of thyroid
5	Foramen cecum		

REVIEW QUESTIONS: Thyroid gland development

Fill in the blanks by choosing the appropriate terms from the list below.

1. The thyroid gland is the first _____ to appear in embryonic development and develops from endoderm invaded by mesenchyme.

2. The thyroid gland develops during _____.

3. The thyroid gland forms from a median downgrowth at the _____, connected by a thyroglossal duct, a narrow tube that later closes off and becomes obliterated.

4. The _____ shows the origin of the thyroid gland and the migration pathway of the thyroid gland into the neck region.

5. The _____, which is the opening of the thyroglossal duct associated with the development of the thyroid gland, is a small pitlike depression located at the apex of the sulcus terminalis where it points backward toward the oropharynx.

6. The thyroglossal duct usually _____ early in development.

7. The tissue descends as the thyroglossal duct from the foramen cecum in the posterior aspect of the tongue to pass adjacent to the anterior aspect of the center of the _____.

8. The thyroid tissue continues to migrate inferiorly and eventually comes to rest at the anterior aspect of the _____ in the root of the neck.

9. There may also be a functional thyroid gland associated with the tongue, a lingual thyroid, anywhere along the path of _____ within the thyroid gland, or extending upward from the gland along the path of the thyroglossal duct, a pyramidal lobe.

10. The _____ is derived from the third (inferior parathyroid glands) and fourth (superior parathyroid glands) pharyngeal pouches, these paired structures migrate to their final positions and are named accordingly.

migration	parathyroid gland	trachea
endocrine gland	base of the tongue	pharynx
thyroglossal duct	prenatal development	hyoid bone
foramen cecum	disappears	

References   Chapter 11, Head and neck structures. In Fehrenbach MJ, Popowics T: *Illustrated dental embryology, histology, and anatomy,* ed 5, St. Louis, 2020, Saunders; Chapter 8, Head and neck. In Drake R, Vogl AW, Mitchell AWM: *Gray's anatomy for students,* ed 4, Philadelphia, 2020, Churchill Livingstone.

FIGURE 7.11 Thymus gland (anterior view)

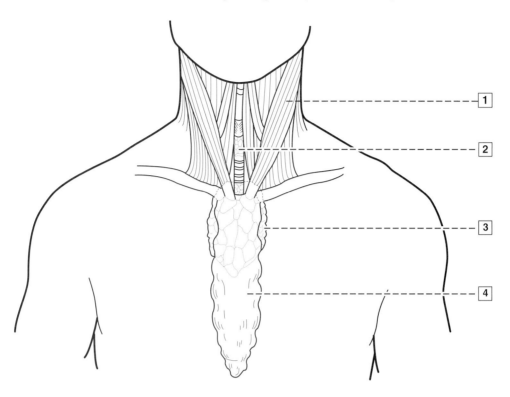

1	Sternocleidomastoid muscle
2	Thyroid gland
3	Thymus gland
4	Sternum

REVIEW QUESTIONS: Thymus gland

Fill in the blanks by choosing the appropriate terms from the list below.

1. The thymus gland is a(n) _____ and therefore ductless; the gland is made of many lobules, with each lobule having an outer cortex and an inner medulla and separated by connective tissue septa.

2. The thymus gland is part of the _____ that fights disease processes; within the gland the T-cell lymphocytes, white blood cells of the immune system, mature in the gland in response to stimulation by thymus hormones.

3. The gland grows from birth to puberty as part of the immune system; after puberty, the thymus gland stops growing and starts to shrink, undergoing thymic _____ through the process of atrophy.

4. In adulthood, the thymus gland has almost _____ and returns to its low birth weight, making it mainly a temporary structure.

5. The adult thymus gland consists of two _____, right and left, connected by a midline isthmus; other associated lobular structures may also be present.

6. The thymus gland is located in the thorax (chest) and the anterior region of the base of the neck, _____ to the thyroid gland.

7. The thymus gland is _____ and lateral to the trachea and deep to the sternum and the origins of the sternohyoid and sternothyroid muscles.

8. The thymus gland is innervated by branches of the tenth cranial nerve or the _____ and cervical nerves.

9. The lymphatic system of the thymus gland begins within the substance of the gland and terminates in the _____; thus the gland does not have any afferent vessels.

10. The thymus gland is supplied by the _____ and the internal thoracic artery; the main venous return is by veins in the posterior surface of the gland that run directly into the brachiocephalic veins that are formed by the union of the internal jugular and subclavian veins.

immune system	involution	disappeared
superficial	vagus nerve	endocrine gland
inferior thyroid artery	inferior	internal jugular vein
lateral lobes		

References Chapter 7, Glandular tissue. In Fehrenbach MJ, Herring SW: *Illustrated anatomy of the head and neck,* ed 6, St. Louis, 2021, Saunders; Chapter 8, Head and neck. In Drake R, Vogl AW, Mitchell AWM: *Gray's anatomy for students,* ed 4, Philadelphia, 2020, Churchill Livingstone.

ANSWER KEY 1. endocrine gland, 2. immune system, 3. involution, 4. disappeared, 5. lateral lobes, 6. inferior, 7. superficial, 8. vagus nerve, 9. internal jugular vein, 10. inferior thyroid artery

FIGURE 8.1 Brain (ventral view)

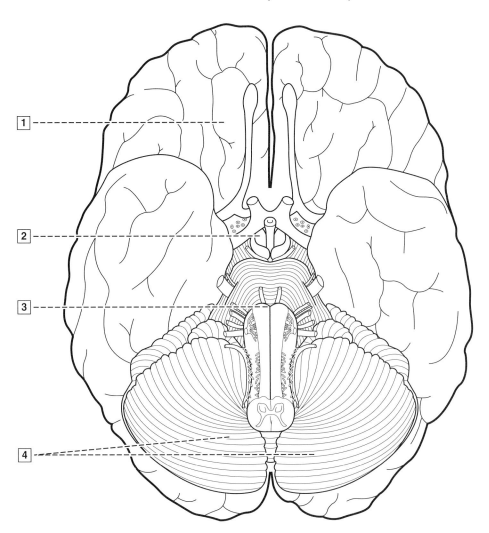

1 Cerebral hemisphere

2 Diencephalon

3 Brainstem

4 Cerebellum

REVIEW QUESTIONS: Brain

Fill in the blanks by choosing the appropriate terms from the list below.

1. The _____ is an extensive and intricate network of neural structures that activates, co-ordinates, and controls all functions of the body; it has two major divisions, the central nervous system and the peripheral nervous systems.

2. One of the major divisions of the nervous system, the _____ consists of the brain and spinal cord.

3. The central nervous system is surrounded by bone, either the skull or vertebrae, and a layering of _____.

4. Both the bones of the skull and vertebrae and the layering of membranes serve to _____ the central nervous system.

5. The major divisions of the _____ of the central nervous system include the cerebrum, cerebellum, brainstem, and diencephalon.

6. The _____ is the largest division of the brain.

7. The cerebrum of the brain consists of two _____.

8. The cerebrum of the brain _____ sensory data and motor functions and governs many aspects of intelligence and reasoning, learning, and memory.

9. The _____ is the second largest division of the brain after the cerebrum.

10. The cerebellum of the brain functions to _____ muscle coordination and maintains usual level of muscle tone and posture as well as coordinates balance.

brain	cerebellum	cerebrum
produce	protect	coordinates
central nervous system	membranes	cerebral hemispheres
nervous system		

Reference   Chapter 8, Nervous system. In Fehrenbach MJ, Herring SW: *Illustrated anatomy of the head and neck,* ed 6, St. Louis, 2021, Saunders.

NOTES

FIGURE 8.2   Brain and spinal cord (sagittal section)

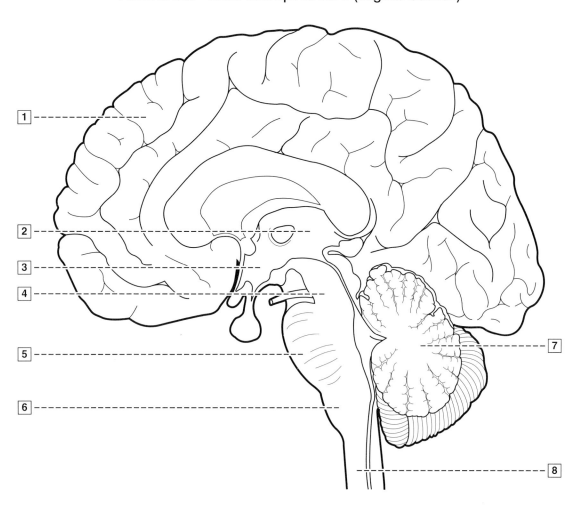

1	**CEREBRAL HEMISPHERE**	**BRAINSTEM**	7	**CEREBELLUM**
DIENCEPHALON		4 Midbrain	8	**SPINAL CORD**
2 Thalamus		5 Pons		
3 Hypothalamus		6 Medulla		

REVIEW QUESTIONS: Brain and spinal cord

Fill in the blanks by choosing the appropriate terms from the list below.

1. The _____ of the brain has a number of divisions that include the medulla, pons, and midbrain.

2. The _____ of the brainstem is closest to the spinal cord and is involved in the regulation of heartbeat, breathing, vasoconstriction (blood pressure), and reflex centers for vomiting, coughing, sneezing, swallowing, and hiccupping; the cell bodies of the motor neurons for the tongue are located there.

3. The _____ of the brainstem connects the medulla with the cerebellum and with higher brain centers; the cell bodies for fifth (trigeminal) and seventh (facial) cranial nerves are found there.

4. The _____ of the brainstem includes relay stations for hearing, vision, and motor pathways.

5. Superior to the brainstem, the _____ of the brain mainly includes the thalamus and hypothalamus.

6. The _____ of the diencephalon serves as a central relay point for incoming nerve impulses.

7. The _____ of the diencephalon regulates homeostasis; it has specific regulatory areas for thirst, hunger, body temperature, water balance, and blood pressure; all these regulatory areas help to link the nervous system to the endocrine system.

8. The other component of the central nervous system besides the brain, the _____, runs along the dorsal side of the body and links the brain to the rest of the body; it consists of two components of brain substance, gray matter and white matter, and in adults is encased in a series of bony vertebrae that comprise the vertebral column.

9. The inner _____ of the spinal cord consists mostly of unmyelinated cell bodies and dendrites, with the surrounding white matter made up of tracts of axons, insulated in sheaths of myelin formed from a combination of lipids and proteins.

10. Some tracts are _____ (charged with carrying messages to the brain), and others are descending (charged with carrying messages from the brain); the spinal cord is also involved in reflexes that do not immediately involve the brain.

pons	hypothalamus	midbrain
diencephalon	ascending	medulla
gray matter	brainstem	thalamus
spinal cord		

Reference   Chapter 8, Nervous system. In Fehrenbach MJ, Herring SW: *Illustrated anatomy of the head and neck,* ed 6, St. Louis, 2021, Saunders.

FIGURE 8.3   Meninges of the brain (cutaway sagittal section)

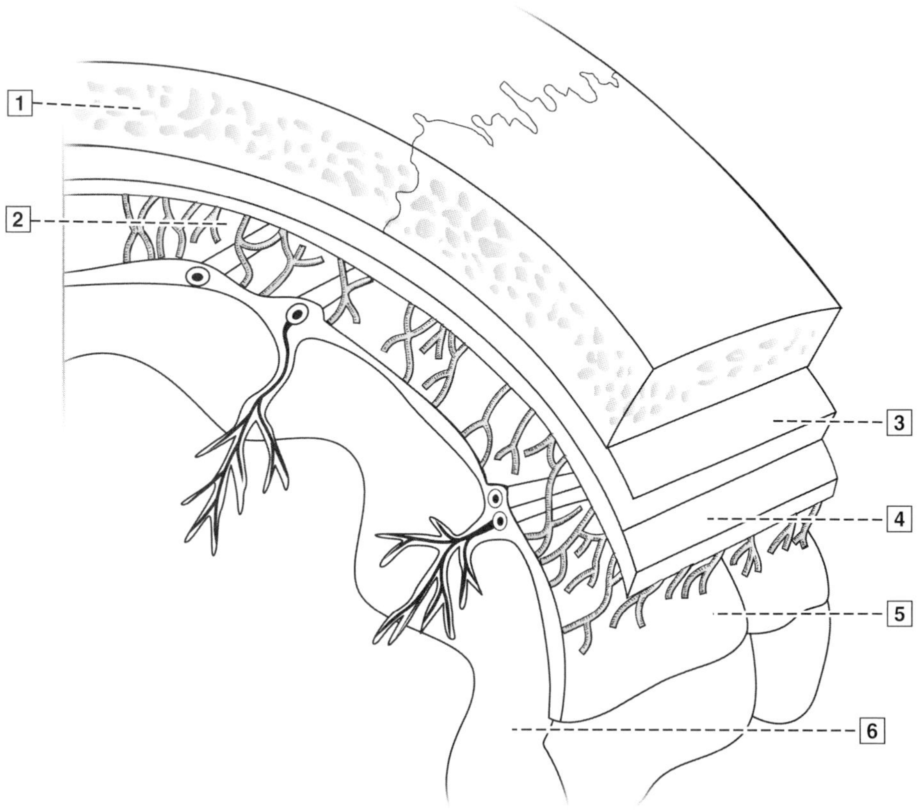

1 Skull

2 Subarachnoid space

3 Dura mater

4 Arachnoid mater

5 Pia mater

6 Cerebral cortex

REVIEW QUESTIONS: Meninges of brain

Fill in the blanks by choosing the appropriate terms from the list below.

1. The central nervous system is surrounded by bone, either the skull or vertebrae, and a layering of
_____; both the bone and membranes serve to protect it.

2. The membranes of the brain are _____.

3. The meninges of the central nervous system have _____ layers including the dura mater, arachnoid mater, and pia mater; the cranial meninges are continuous with, and similar to, the spinal meninges through the foramen magnum, with only a difference in the layering of the dura mater.

4. The tough outermost layer of the meninges, the _____, surrounds and supports the brain and spinal cord of the central nervous system as well as lining the inner surface of the skull; the dura mater consists of two layers, an outer periosteal layer and an inner meningeal layer.

5. The delicate middle layer of the meninges is the _____; it lines, but is not adherent to, the inner surface of the dura mater.

6. Underneath the arachnoid mater is the subarachnoid space that contains _____, which acts to cushion the brain.

7. From the inner surface of arachnoid mater of the meninges, thin processes or _____ extend downward, cross the subarachnoid space, and become continuous with the pia mater; unlike the pia mater, the arachnoid mater does not enter the grooves or fissures of the brain, except for the longitudinal fissure between the two cerebral hemispheres.

8. The inner layer of the meninges that is firmly attached to the surface of the brain is the
_____; it closely invests the surface of the brain.

9. The pia mater of the meninges is a thin delicate innermost membrane that follows the contours of the brain, entering the grooves and fissures on its surface, and is closely applied to the roots of the
_____ at their origins.

10. The dura mater of the meninges also surrounds and supports the large _____ (dural sinuses) carrying blood from the brain toward the heart; thus, the dural venous sinuses are endothelial-lined spaces between the outer periosteal and the inner meningeal layers of the dura mater, which eventually lead to the internal jugular veins.

cranial nerves	dura mater	meninges
pia mater	membranes	three
venous channels	arachnoid mater	cerebrospinal fluid
trabeculae		

References Chapter 8, Nervous system. In Fehrenbach MJ, Herring SW: *Illustrated anatomy of the head and neck,* ed 6, St. Louis, 2021, Saunders; Chapter 8, Head and neck. In Drake R, Vogl AW, Mitchell AWM: *Gray's anatomy for students,* ed 4, Philadelphia, 2020, Churchill Livingstone.

ANSWER KEY 1. membranes, 2. meninges, 3. three, 4. dura mater, 5. arachnoid mater, 6. trabeculae, 7. cerebrospinal fluid, 8. pia mater, 9. cranial nerves, 10. venous channels.

FIGURE 8.4   Brain and cranial nerves with structural innervations (ventral surface showing nerve attachments)

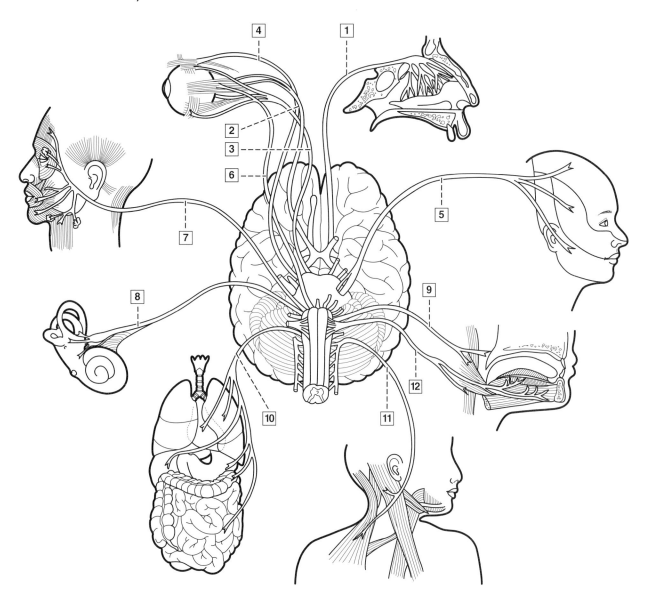

1	Olfactory nerve (I)	**7**	Facial nerve (VII)
2	Optic nerve (II)	**8**	Vestibulocochlear nerve (VIII)
3	Oculomotor nerve (III)	**9**	Glossopharyngeal nerve (IX)
4	Trochlear nerve (IV)	**10**	Vagus nerve (X)
5	Trigeminal nerve (V)	**11**	Accessory nerve (XI)
6	Abducens nerve (VI)	**12**	Hypoglossal nerve (XII)

REVIEW QUESTIONS: Brain and cranial nerves with structural innervations

Fill in the blanks by choosing the appropriate terms from the list below.

1. The _____ are an important part of the peripheral nervous system; the paired 12 are connected to the brain at its base and pass through the skull by way of fissures or foramina.

2. The first cranial nerve (I) or _____ transmits smell from the nasal mucosa to the brain and thus functions as an afferent nerve; the nerve enters the skull through the perforations in the cribriform plate of the ethmoid bone to join the olfactory bulb in the brain.

3. The second cranial nerve (II) or _____ transmits sight from the retina of the eye to the brain and thus functions as an afferent nerve; the nerve enters the skull through the optic canal of the sphenoid bone on its way from the retina.

4. In the skull, both the right and left optic nerves join at the _____, where many of the fibers cross to the contralateral side before continuing into the brain as the optic tracts.

5. The third cranial nerve (III) or _____ serves as an efferent nerve to some of the eye muscles that move the eyeball; the nerve also carries preganglionic parasympathetic fibers to the ciliary ganglion near the eyeball, and the postganglionic fibers innervate small muscles inside the eyeball.

6. The oculomotor nerve lies within the lateral wall of the cavernous sinus and exits the skull through the superior orbital fissure of the _____ on its way to the orbit.

7. The small fourth cranial nerve (IV) or _____ serves as an efferent nerve for one eye muscle, as well as proprioception, similar to the oculomotor nerve but without any parasympathetic fibers.

8. Similar to the oculomotor nerve, the trochlear nerve lies within the lateral wall of the cavernous sinus and exits the skull through the _____ of the sphenoid bone on its way to the orbit.

9. The fifth cranial nerve (V) or _____ has both an efferent component for the muscles of mastication (as well as some other cranial muscles) and an afferent component for the teeth, tongue, and oral cavity, as well as most of the skin of the face and head; additionally, it has no preganglionic parasympathetic fibers, although many postganglionic parasympathetic fibers travel along with its branches.

10. The trigeminal nerve is the largest cranial nerve and has two _____, sensory and motor.

trigeminal nerve	optic chiasma	olfactory nerve
cranial nerves	oculomotor nerve	superior orbital fissure
trochlear nerve	sphenoid bone	roots
optic nerve		

Reference Chapter 8, Nervous system. In Fehrenbach MJ, Herring SW: *Illustrated anatomy of the head and neck,* ed 6, St. Louis, 2021, Saunders.

FIGURE 8.5 Cranial nerves within skull and associated structures (superior view of internal skull)

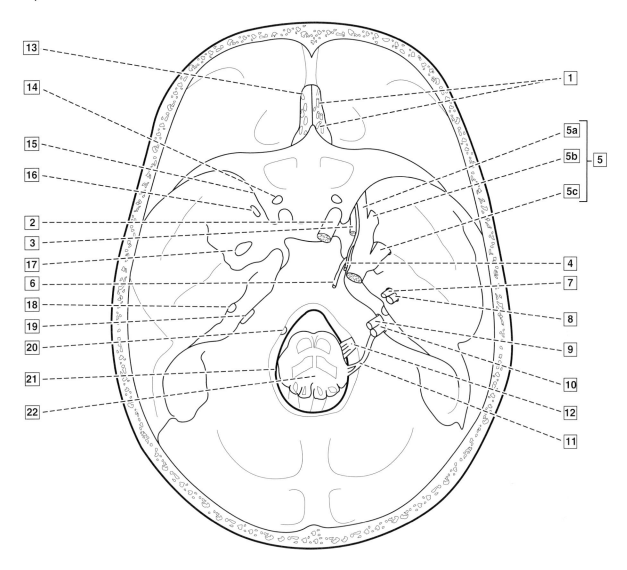

CRANIAL NERVES (many are cut)

1 Olfactory nerve (I)	**6** Abducens nerve (VI)
2 Optic nerve (II)	**7** Facial nerve (VII)
3 Oculomotor nerve (III)	**8** Vestibulocochlear nerve (VIII)
4 Trochlear nerve (IV)	**9** Glossopharyngeal nerve (IX)
5 **Trigeminal nerve (V)**	**10** Vagus nerve (X)
5a Ophthalmic nerve (V$_1$)	**11** Accessory nerve (XI)
5b Maxillary nerve (V$_2$)	**12** Hypoglossal nerve (XII)
5c Mandibular nerve (V$_3$)	

ASSOCIATED STRUCTURES

13 Cribriform plate
14 Optic canal
15 Superior orbital fissure
16 Foramen rotundum
17 Foramen ovale
18 Internal acoustic meatus
19 Jugular foramen
20 Hypoglossal canal
21 Foramen magnum
22 Spinal cord

REVIEW QUESTIONS: Cranial nerves within skull and associated structures

Fill in the blanks by choosing the appropriate terms from the list below.

1. The sixth cranial nerve (VI) or _____ or abducent nerve serves as an efferent nerve to one of the muscles that moves the eyeball, similar to the oculomotor and trochlear nerves; similar to both of those cranial nerves, the nerve exits the skull through the superior orbital fissure of the sphenoid bone on its way to the orbit but before the nerve runs through the sinus rather than lying within the wall of the cavernous sinus.

2. The seventh cranial nerve (VII) or _____ carries both efferent and afferent components; the nerve carries an efferent component for the muscles of facial expression and the posterior suprahyoid muscles, as well as for the preganglionic parasympathetic innervation of the lacrimal gland (relaying in the pterygopalatine ganglion) and the submandibular and sublingual salivary glands (relaying in the submandibular ganglion).

3. The facial nerve's afferent component serves as a tiny patch of skin behind the ear and taste sensation with the taste buds of certain lingual papillae from the anterior two-thirds of the tongue; then the nerve leaves the cranial cavity by passing through the _____, which leads to the facial canal inside the temporal bone to finally exit the skull by way of the stylomastoid foramen of the temporal bone.

4. The eighth cranial nerve (VIII) or _____ serves as an afferent nerve for hearing and balance because it conveys signals from the inner ear of the temporal bone to the brain; it then enters the cranial cavity through the internal acoustic meatus of the temporal bone and supplies the two major parts of the inner ear, the cochlea and semicircular canals.

5. The ninth cranial nerve (IX) or _____ carries an efferent component for the pharyngeal muscle and the stylopharyngeus muscle and also provides preganglionic gland parasympathetic innervation for the parotid salivary gland (relaying the otic ganglion); the nerve also carries an afferent component for the oropharynx and for taste and general sensation from the base of the tongue, and thus is the afferent limb of the gag reflex.

6. The glossopharyngeal nerve passes through the skull by way of the _____, between the occipital and temporal bones; the tympanic branch, with sensory fibers for the middle ear and preganglionic parasympathetic fibers for the parotid salivary gland, begins here and reenters the skull.

7. After supplying the ear, parasympathetic fibers of the glossopharyngeal nerve leave the skull through the _____ of the sphenoid bone as the lesser petrosal nerve; its preganglionic fibers then terminate in the otic ganglion, which is located near the medial surface of the mandibular nerve of the trigeminal nerve, just inferior to the foramen ovale, to supply the inferior branches of the nerve supply the carotid artery, oropharynx, and base of the tongue (afferent component), as well as the stylopharyngeus muscle.

8. The tenth cranial nerve (X) or _____ carries a large somatic efferent component for the muscles of the soft palate, pharynx, larynx, and a large autonomic (parasympathetic) component (and associated visceral afferent fibers) to organs in the thorax and abdomen including the thymus gland, heart, and stomach; it also carries a smaller afferent component for a small amount of skin around the ear and for taste sensation for the epiglottis; the nerve passes through the skull by way of the jugular foramen, between the occipital and temporal bones.

9. The eleventh cranial nerve (XI) or _____ functions as an efferent nerve for the trapezius and sternocleidomastoid muscles as well as assisting the tenth cranial nerve or vagus nerve in the innervation of muscles of the soft palate and pharynx and while exiting the skull through the jugular foramen, between the occipital and temporal bones; the nerve is only partly a cranial nerve and consists of two roots, one from the brain and one from the spinal cord.

10. The twelfth cranial nerve (XII) or _____ functions as a somatic efferent nerve for both the intrinsic and extrinsic muscles of the tongue; the nerve exits the skull through the hypoglossal canal in the occipital bone.

facial nerve   vagus nerve   accessory nerve
abducens nerve   glossopharyngeal nerve   internal acoustic meatus
hypoglossal nerve   vestibulocochlear nerve   jugular foramen
foramen ovale

Reference Chapter 8, Nervous system. In Fehrenbach MJ, Herring SW: *Illustrated anatomy of the head and neck,* ed 6, St. Louis, 2021, Saunders.

ANSWER KEY 1. abducens nerve, 2. facial nerve, 3. internal acoustic meatus, 4. vestibulocochlear nerve, 5. glossopharyngeal nerve, 6. jugular foramen, 7. foramen ovale, 8. vagus nerve, 9. accessory nerve, 10. hypoglossal nerve

FIGURE 8.6   Cranial nerves significant to dental professionals (superior view of internal skull)

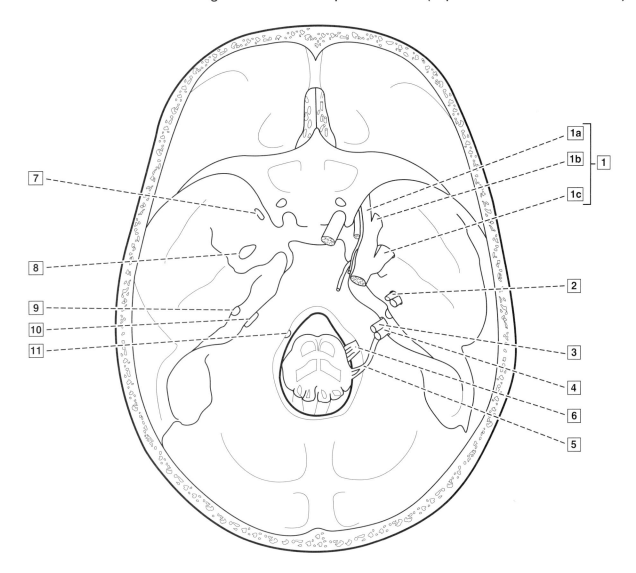

CRANIAL NERVES (many are cut)

1	Trigeminal nerve (V)
1a	Ophthalmic nerve (V_1)
1b	Maxillary nerve (V_2)
1c	Mandibular nerve (V_3)
2	Facial nerve (VII)
3	Glossopharyngeal nerve (IX)
4	Vagus nerve (X)
5	Accessory nerve (XI)
6	Hypoglossal nerve (XII)

ASSOCIATED STRUCTURES

7	Foramen rotundum
8	Foramen ovale
9	Internal acoustic meatus
10	Jugular foramen
11	Hypoglossal canal

REVIEW QUESTIONS: Cranial nerves significant to dental professionals

Fill in the blanks by choosing the appropriate terms from the list below.

1. The fifth cranial nerve (V) or _____ has an afferent component for the teeth, tongue, and oral cavity.

2. The seventh cranial nerve (VII) or _____ carries an efferent component for the preganglionic parasympathetic innervation of both the submandibular and sublingual salivary glands (relaying in the submandibular ganglion) as well as the anterior two-thirds of the tongue.

3. The ninth cranial nerve (IX) or _____ carries an efferent component for the preganglionic gland parasympathetic innervation for the parotid salivary gland (relaying the otic ganglion); the nerve also carries an afferent component for the oropharynx and for taste by way of the circumvallate lingual papillae and general sensation from the base of the tongue and thus is the afferent limb of the gag reflex.

4. The _____ of the glossopharyngeal nerve has preganglionic parasympathetic fibers for the parotid salivary gland; these preganglionic fibers then terminate in the otic ganglion.

5. The tenth cranial nerve (X) or _____ carries a large somatic efferent component for the muscles of the soft palate.

6. The tenth cranial (X) or vagus nerve descends through the _____ and into the thorax (chest) and abdomen where it innervates internal organs.

7. The eleventh cranial (XI) or _____ functions as an efferent nerve for the trapezius and sternocleidomastoid muscles as well as for muscles of the soft palate.

8. Certain cranial nerves are either afferent or efferent, and others have both types of _____.

9. The _____ serve to innervate structures in the head or neck.

10. The cranial nerves are numbered according to their location in regard to the brain, going from the _____ of the brain to its posterior.

neck	cranial nerves
glossopharyngeal nerve	trigeminal nerve
vagus nerve	tympanic branch
facial nerve	accessory nerve
neural processes	anterior

References   Chapter 8, Nervous system. In Fehrenbach MJ, Herring SW: *Illustrated anatomy of the head and neck,* ed 6, St. Louis, 2020, Saunders; Chapter 8, Head and neck. In Drake R, Vogl AW, Mitchell AWM: *Gray's anatomy for students,* ed 4, Philadelphia, 2020, Churchill Livingstone.

FIGURE 8.7   Trigeminal nerve (V): Ganglion and divisions with innervation coverage (cutaway lateral view)

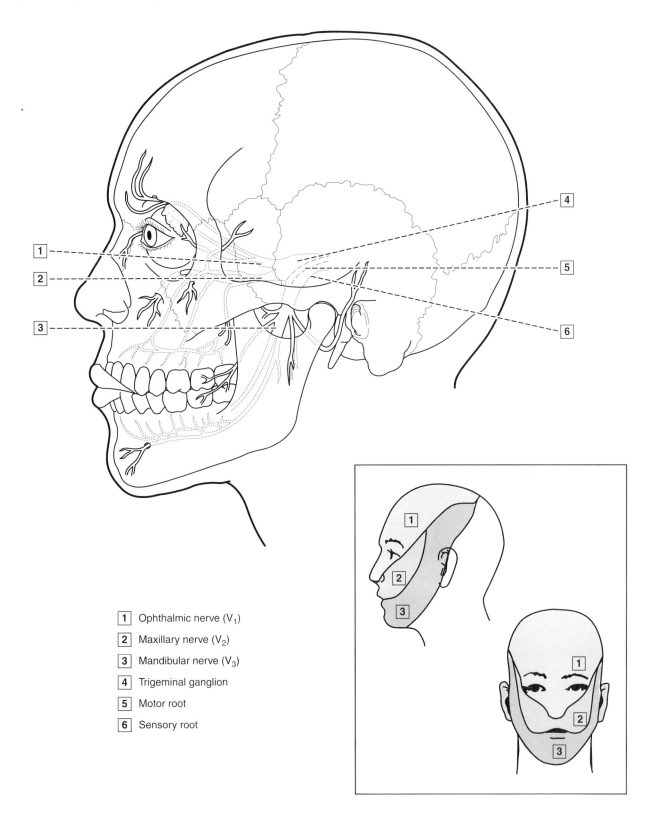

1   Ophthalmic nerve (V_1)
2   Maxillary nerve (V_2)
3   Mandibular nerve (V_3)
4   Trigeminal ganglion
5   Motor root
6   Sensory root

367

REVIEW QUESTIONS: Trigeminal nerve (V): Ganglion and divisions with innervation coverage

Fill in the blanks by choosing the appropriate terms from the list below.

1. Within the skull, a bulge can be noted in the sensory root of the trigeminal nerve; the bulge is the _____ (or semilunar or gasserian ganglion), which is located on the anterior surface of the petrous part of the temporal bone.

2. Anterior to the trigeminal ganglion, the _____ begins from three nerves or divisions that pass into the skull by way of three different fissures or foramina in the sphenoid bone.

3. The sensory root's three nerves or _____ include the ophthalmic, maxillary, and mandibular nerves.

4. The _____ of the sensory root provides sensation to the upper face and scalp.

5. The _____ of the sensory root provides sensation to the middle face and its deeper regions such as the oral cavity.

6. The _____ of the sensory root provides sensation to the lower face and its deeper regions such as the oral cavity.

7. The ophthalmic nerve and maxillary nerve of the sensory root carry only _____.

8. In contrast, the mandibular nerve of the sensory root runs together with the motor root and thus carries both afferent nerve fibers and _____.

9. Each of the three nerves of the thicker sensory root of the trigeminal nerve enters the skull in one of three different locations in the _____; the ophthalmic nerve enters through the superior orbital fissure; the maxillary nerve enters by way of the foramen rotundum; and the mandibular nerve passes through the skull by way of the foramen ovale.

10. As part of the mandibular nerve, the _____ of the trigeminal nerve exits the skull at the foramen ovale of the sphenoid bone and then travels with the mandibular nerve of the sensory root of the trigeminal nerve to supply the efferent nerves for the muscles of mastication.

afferent nerve fibers	sphenoid bone	efferent nerve fibers
trigeminal ganglion	sensory root	maxillary nerve
motor root	divisions	ophthalmic nerve
mandibular nerve		

References   Chapter 8, Nervous system. In Fehrenbach MJ, Herring SW: *Illustrated anatomy of the head and neck,* ed 6, St. Louis, 2021, Saunders; Chapter 8, Head and neck. In Drake R, Vogl AW, Mitchell AWM: *Gray's anatomy for students,* ed 4, Philadelphia, 2020, Churchill Livingstone.

NOTES

ANSWER KEY   1. trigeminal ganglion, 2. sensory root, 3. divisions, 4. ophthalmic nerve, 5. maxillary nerve, 6. mandibular nerve, 7. afferent nerve fibers, 8. efferent nerve fibers, 9. sphenoid bone, 10. motor root

FIGURE 8.8   Trigeminal nerve (V): Ophthalmic (V$_1$) and associated structures with innervation coverage (lateral view of cutaway orbital region)

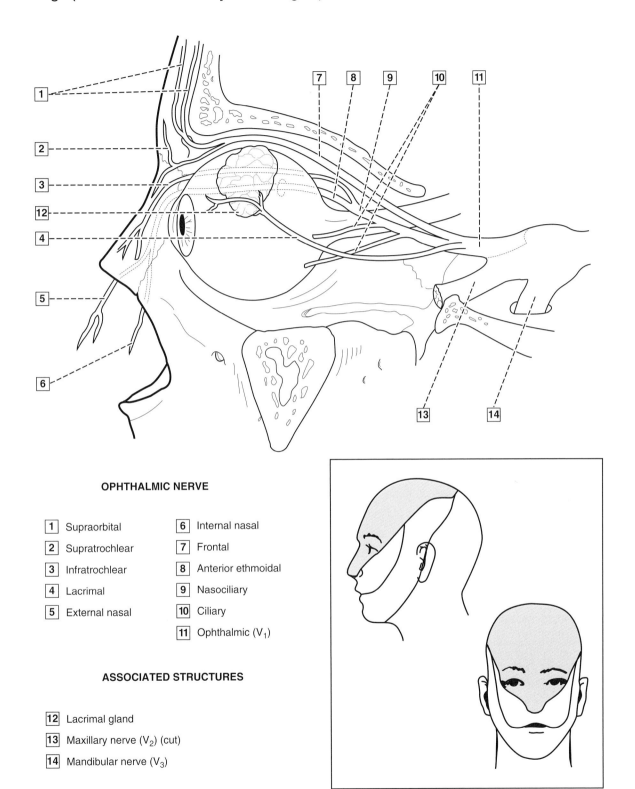

OPHTHALMIC NERVE

1	Supraorbital	6	Internal nasal
2	Supratrochlear	7	Frontal
3	Infratrochlear	8	Anterior ethmoidal
4	Lacrimal	9	Nasociliary
5	External nasal	10	Ciliary
		11	Ophthalmic (V$_1$)

ASSOCIATED STRUCTURES

12 Lacrimal gland
13 Maxillary nerve (V$_2$) (cut)
14 Mandibular nerve (V$_3$)

REVIEW QUESTIONS: Trigeminal nerve (V): Ophthalmic (V₁) and associated structures with innervation coverage

Fill in the blanks by choosing the appropriate terms from the list below.

1. The first nerve division or V_1 of the sensory root of the trigeminal nerve is the _____.

2. The ophthalmic nerve is the smallest division of the _____ of the trigeminal nerve and serves as an afferent nerve for the conjunctiva, cornea, eyeball, orbit, forehead, and ethmoidal and frontal sinuses, plus a part of the dura mater and parts of the nasal cavity and nose.

3. The ophthalmic nerve carries sensory information toward the brain by way of the _____ of the sphenoid bone; other nerves that traverse this passageway include the third, fourth, and sixth cranial nerves.

4. The ophthalmic nerve begins from _____ major nerves: the frontal, lacrimal, and naso-ciliary nerves.

5. The _____ is an afferent nerve located in the orbit and is composed of a merger of the supraorbital nerve from the forehead and anterior scalp and the supratrochlear nerve from the bridge of the nose and medial parts of the upper eyelid and forehead.

6. The frontal nerve courses along the roof of the _____ toward the superior orbital fissure of the sphenoid bone where it is joined by the lacrimal and nasociliary nerves to form V_1.

7. The _____ serves as an afferent nerve for the lateral part of the upper eyelid, conjunctiva, and lacrimal gland, as well as delivering postganglionic parasympathetic nerves to the lacrimal gland because these latter fibers are responsible for the production of lacrimal fluid or tears.

8. The lacrimal nerve runs posteriorly along the lateral roof of the orbit and then joins the frontal and nasociliary nerves near the superior orbital fissure of the _____ to form V_1.

9. Several afferent nerve branches converge to form the _____, including the infratrochlear nerve from the skin of the medial part of the eyelids and the side of the nose, ciliary nerves to and from the eyeball, and anterior or posterior ethmoidal nerve from the nasal cavity and paranasal sinuses; additionally, the anterior ethmoidal nerve is formed by the external nasal nerve from the skin of the ala and apex of the nose and the internal nasal nerves from the anterior part of the nasal septum and lateral wall of the nasal cavity.

10. The nasociliary nerve is a(n) _____ that runs within the orbit, superior to the second cranial nerve or optic nerve, to join the frontal and lacrimal nerves near the superior orbital fissure of the sphenoid bone to form V_1.

lacrimal nerve	nasociliary nerve	ophthalmic nerve
sphenoid bone	superior orbital fissure	sensory root
frontal nerve	orbit	afferent nerve
three		

Reference Chapter 8, Nervous system. In Fehrenbach MJ, Herring SW: *Illustrated anatomy of the head and neck,* ed 6, St. Louis, 2021, Saunders.

FIGURE 8.9 Trigeminal nerve (V): Maxillary (V₂) with innervation coverage (cutaway lateral view)

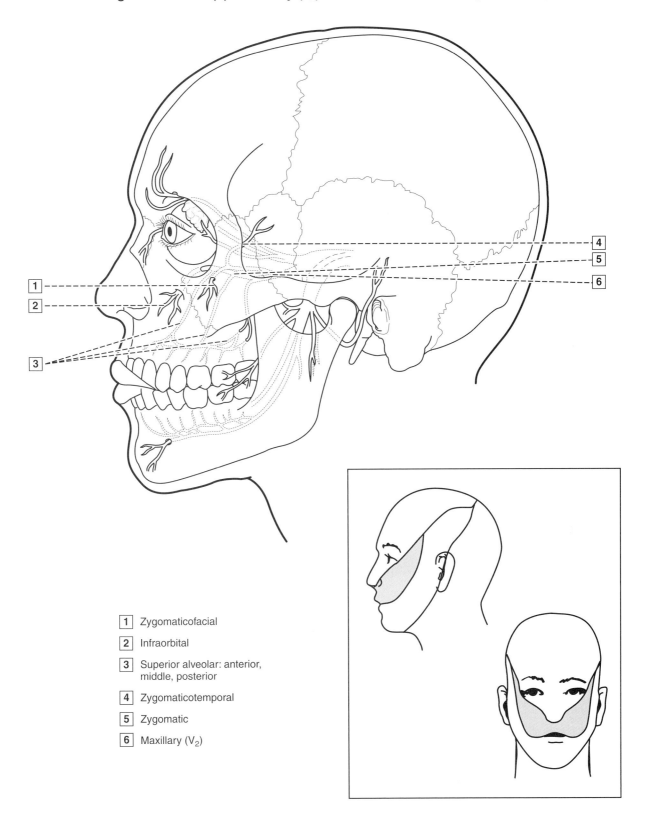

1 Zygomaticofacial

2 Infraorbital

3 Superior alveolar: anterior, middle, posterior

4 Zygomaticotemporal

5 Zygomatic

6 Maxillary (V₂)

REVIEW QUESTIONS: Trigeminal nerve (V): Maxillary (V$_2$) with innervation coverage

Fill in the blanks by choosing the appropriate terms from the list below.

1. The second nerve division or V$_2$ from the sensory root of the trigeminal nerve is the _____; the afferent nerve branches of the nerve carry sensory information for the maxillae and overlying skin, oral mucosa, maxillary sinuses, nasal cavity, palate, nasopharynx, and part of the dura mater.

2. The maxillary nerve is a nerve trunk formed within the _____ by the convergence of many nerves; the largest contributor is the infraorbital nerve.

3. Tributaries of the infraorbital or maxillary nerve trunk include the zygomatic, the anterior, middle, and posterior superior alveolar, the greater and lesser palatine, and the nasopalatine nerves; after all these branches come together in the pterygopalatine fossa to form the maxillary nerve, the nerve enters the skull through the _____ of the sphenoid bone.

4. The _____ is an afferent nerve composed of the merger of the zygomaticofacial nerve and the zygomaticotemporal nerve in the orbit nerve and also conveys the postganglionic parasympathetic fibers for the lacrimal gland to the lacrimal nerve; later, the nerve courses posteriorly along the lateral orbit floor and enters the pterygopalatine fossa through the inferior orbital fissure, which between the sphenoid bone and maxilla, to finally join V$_2$.

5. The rather small _____ serves as an afferent nerve for the skin of the cheek as the nerve pierces the frontal process of the zygomatic bone at the zygomaticofacial foramen and enters the orbit through its lateral wall; the nerve then turns posteriorly to join with the zygomaticotemporal nerve.

6. The _____ serves as an afferent nerve for the skin of the temporal region by piercing the temporal surface of the zygomatic bone at the zygomaticotemporal foramen; the nerve then traverses the lateral wall of the orbit to join the zygomaticofacial nerve, forming the zygomatic nerve.

7. The _____ is an afferent nerve formed from the merger of cutaneous branches from the upper lip, the medial part of the cheek, side of the nose, and the lower eyelid.

8. The infraorbital nerve then passes into the infraorbital foramen of the maxilla to travel posteriorly through the infraorbital canal, along with the infraorbital blood vessels where it is joined by the _____; the infraorbital foramen serves as a landmark for the administration of the infraorbital nerve block.

9. From the infraorbital canal and groove, the infraorbital nerve passes into the pterygopalatine fossa through the inferior orbital fissure and after it leaves the infraorbital groove and within the pterygopalatine fossa, the infraorbital nerve receives the _____ and joins with it or directly with the maxillary nerve.

10. The anterior superior alveolar nerve originates from dental branches in the pulp of the maxillary anterior teeth and then ascends along the anterior wall of the maxillary sinus to join the infraorbital nerve within the infraorbital canal, along with the _____ that serves the maxillary premolars through its dental branches, if present.

posterior superior alveolar nerve	pterygopalatine fossa	maxillary nerve
infraorbital nerve	zygomaticofacial nerve	zygomaticotemporal nerve
zygomatic nerve	foramen rotundum	middle superior alveolar nerve
anterior superior alveolar nerve		

References Chapter 8, Nervous system. In Fehrenbach MJ, Herring SW: *Illustrated anatomy of the head and neck,* ed 6, St. Louis, 2021, Saunders; Chapter 9, Anatomy of local anesthesia. In Fehrenbach MJ, Herring SW: *Illustrated anatomy of the head and neck,* ed 6, St. Louis, 2021, Saunders.

FIGURE 8.10   Maxillary nerve (V₂): Major branches with associated structures (cutaway skull with lateral wall of orbit partially removed)

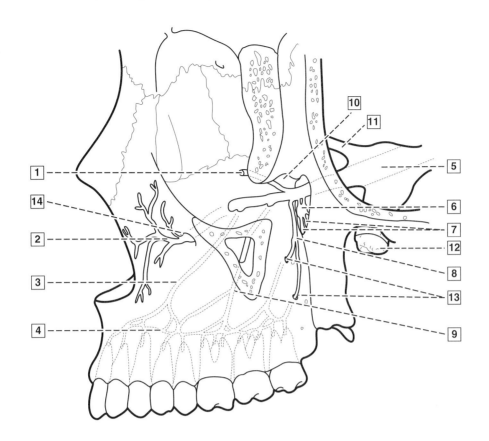

MAXILLARY NERVE

1 Zygomatic (cut)
2 Infraorbital
3 Anterior superior alveolar
4 Superior dental plexus
5 Maxillary (V₂)

6 Pterygopalatine ganglion
7 Greater and lesser palatine
8 Posterior superior alveolar
9 Middle superior alveolar

ASSOCIATED STRUCTURES

10 Inferior orbital fissure
11 Ophthalmic nerve (V₁)
12 Mandibular nerve (V₃)
13 Posterior superior alveolar foramina
14 Infraorbital foramen

Fill in the blanks by choosing the appropriate terms from the list below.

1. The _____ serves as an afferent nerve of sensation for the maxillary central incisors, lateral incisors, and canine, as well as associated labial periodontium and gingiva to the midline.

2. The anterior superior alveolar nerve originates from dental branches in the pulp of the maxillary anterior teeth that exit through the apical foramina; this nerve also receives interdental branches from the surrounding periodontium which together become part of the _____ within the maxillary arch that is a landmark for the administration of the anterior superior alveolar nerve block.

3. The anterior superior alveolar nerve then ascends along the _____ of the maxillary sinus to join the infraorbital nerve within the infraorbital canal.

4. The _____ serves as an afferent nerve for the maxillary premolars and mesiobuccal root of the maxillary first molar and associated buccal periodontium and gingiva, if the nerve is present.

5. The middle superior alveolar nerve when present originates from dental branches in the pulp that exit the maxillary teeth served through the apical foramina, as well as interdental and interradicular branches from the periodontium if present; the nerve, like the posterior superior alveolar and anterior superior alveolar nerves, is part of the superior dental plexus within the _____, which is a landmark for the administration of the middle superior alveolar nerve block.

6. The middle superior alveolar nerve then ascends to join the infraorbital nerve by running within the _____ of the maxillary sinus when present; with it being present, there is communication between the middle superior alveolar nerve and both the anterior superior alveolar nerve and posterior superior alveolar nerve.

7. The middle superior alveolar nerve is not always _____; and if that is what occurs, the area is innervated by both the anterior superior alveolar nerve and posterior superior alveolar nerve, but mainly by the anterior superior alveolar nerve.

8. The _____ joins the infraorbital nerve (or maxillary nerve directly in some cases) within the pterygopalatine fossa; then the nerve serves as an afferent nerve for most parts of the maxillary molars and their periodontium and buccal gingiva as well as the mucous membranes of the maxillary sinus because some afferent nerve branches of the nerve originate from dental branches in the pulp of each of the maxillary molars that exit the teeth by way of the apical foramina, which are later joined by interdental branches and interradicular branches from the periodontium that is part of a superior dental plexus within the maxillary arch.

9. All the internal branches of the posterior superior alveolar nerve enter the multiple _____ on the surface of the maxilla, with the posterior superior alveolar blood vessels also traveling through these same foramina, which are landmarks for the administration of the posterior superior alveolar nerve block.

10. Both the external and internal branches of the posterior superior alveolar nerve move superiorly together along the maxillary tuberosity, which forms the _____ of the maxillary sinus, to join either the infraorbital nerve or maxillary nerve; the posterior superior alveolar foramina are posterosuperior on the maxillary tuberosity as well as superior to the apex of the maxillary second molar.

present	maxillary arch	lateral wall
middle superior alveolar nerve	posterior superior alveolar foramina	posterior superior alveolar nerve
anterior wall	anterior superior alveolar nerve	posterolateral wall
superior dental plexus		

References Chapter 8, Head and neck. In Drake R, Vogl AW, Mitchell AWM: *Gray's anatomy for students,* ed 4, Philadelphia, 2020, Churchill Livingstone; Chapter 8, Nervous system. In Fehrenbach MJ, Herring SW: *Illustrated anatomy of the head and neck,* ed 6, St. Louis, 2021, Saunders; Chapter 9, Anatomy of local anesthesia. In Fehrenbach MJ, Herring SW: *Illustrated anatomy of the head and neck,* ed 6, St. Louis, 2021, Saunders.

ANSWER KEY 1. anterior superior alveolar nerve, 2. superior dental plexus, 3. anterior wall, 4. middle superior alveolar nerve, 5. maxillary arch, 6. lateral wall, 7. present, 8. posterior superior alveolar nerve, 9. posterior superior alveolar foramina, 10. posterolateral wall

FIGURE 8.11 Maxillary nerve (V$_2$): Palatine branches with associated structures (sagittal section of lateral nasal wall, hard palate, opened pterygopalatine canal, and nasal septum removed with oblique lateral view inset)

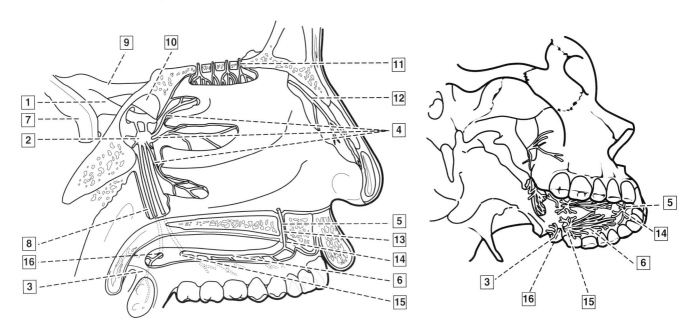

MAXILLARY NERVE

| 1 | Maxillary (V$_2$) | 3 | Lesser palatine | 5 | Nasopalatine |
| 2 | Pterygopalatine ganglion | 4 | Lateral nasal branches | 6 | Greater palatine |

ASSOCIATED STRUCTURES

7	Mandibular nerve (V$_3$)	11	Branches of olfactory nerve (I)	15	Greater palatine foramen
8	Pterygopalatine canal	12	External nasal nerve (V$_1$)	16	Lesser palatine foramen
9	Ophthalmic nerve (V$_1$)	13	Incisive canal		
10	Sphenoidal sinus	14	Incisive foramen		

REVIEW QUESTIONS: Maxillary nerve (V₂): Palatine branches with associated structures

Fill in the blanks by choosing the appropriate terms from the list below.

1. Both palatine nerves join with the _____ from the palate.

2. The _____ (or anterior palatine nerve) with its nerve trunk is located in the deepest part of the mucoperiosteum and bone of the posterior hard palate and its branches closer to the surface; the nerve serves as an afferent nerve for the posterior hard palate and the associated palatal periodontium and gingiva of the ipsilateral maxillary posterior teeth, with communication possibly occurring with the terminal fibers of the nasopalatine nerve in the associated palatal periodontium and gingiva of the maxillary first premolar.

3. Posteriorly, the greater palatine nerve enters the _____ in the horizontal plate of palatine bone superior to the apices of the maxillary second or third molar to travel within the pterygopalatine canal along with the greater palatine blood vessels, serving as a landmark for the administration of the greater palatine nerve block.

4. The _____ (or posterior palatine nerve) serves as an afferent nerve for the soft palate and palatine tonsils.

5. The lesser palatine nerve enters the _____ in the palatine bone near its junction with the pterygoid process of the sphenoid bone along with the lesser palatine blood vessels; the lesser palatine nerve then joins the greater palatine nerve within the pterygopalatine canal.

6. Both palatine nerves move superiorly through the _____ toward the maxillary nerve in the pterygopalatine fossa; on the way, the palatine nerves are joined by lateral nasal branches, which are afferent nerves from the posterior nasal cavity.

7. The _____ originates in the mucosa of the anterior hard palate, palatal to the maxillary central incisors.

8. Both the right and left nasopalatine nerves enter the _____ by way of the incisive foramen, located between the articulating palatine processes of the maxillae and deep to its incisive papilla, thus exiting the oral cavity but serving as landmarks for the administration of the nasopalatine nerve block.

9. After traveling in the incisive canal upon entering by way of the _____, both nasopalatine nerves then travel superiorly and posteriorly along the nasal septum, which they also innervate; each nasopalatine nerve leaves the nasal cavity through the sphenopalatine foramen to enter the pterygopalatine fossa and join the maxillary nerve.

10. The nasopalatine nerve serves as an afferent nerve for the _____ and the associated palatal periodontium and gingiva of the maxillary anterior teeth bilaterally from maxillary canine to canine, as well as the nasal septal tissue; communication also occurs with the terminal fibers of the greater palatine nerve in the associated palatal periodontium and gingiva of the maxillary canine.

greater palatine nerve	incisive foramen	lesser palatine nerve
lesser palatine foramen	anterior hard palate	greater palatine foramen
incisive canal	nasopalatine nerve	pterygopalatine canal
maxillary nerve		

References Chapter 8, Nervous system. In Fehrenbach MJ, Herring SW: *Illustrated anatomy of the head and neck,* ed 6, St. Louis, 2021, Saunders; Chapter 9, Anatomy of local anesthesia. In Fehrenbach MJ, Herring SW: *Illustrated anatomy of the head and neck,* ed 6, St. Louis, 2021, Saunders.

ANSWER KEY 1. maxillary nerve, 2. greater palatine nerve, 3. greater palatine foramen, 4. lesser palatine nerve, 5. lesser palatine foramen, 6. pterygopalatine canal, 7. nasopalatine nerve, 8. incisive canal, 9. incisive foramen, 10. anterior hard palate

FIGURE 8.12   Trigeminal nerve (V): Mandibular (V₃) with innervation coverage (cutaway lateral view of skull)

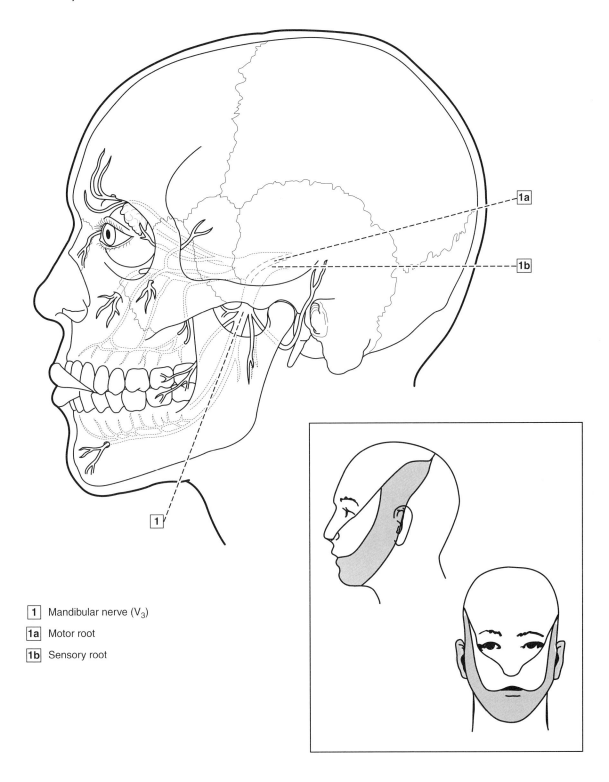

1   Mandibular nerve (V₃)

1a Motor root

1b Sensory root

REVIEW QUESTIONS: Trigeminal nerve (V): Mandibular (V₃) with innervation coverage

Fill in the blanks by choosing the appropriate terms from the list below.

1. The third nerve division or V_3 of the trigeminal nerve is the _____, which is a short main trunk formed by the merger of a smaller anterior trunk and a larger posterior trunk within the infratemporal fossa deep to the base of the skull but before the nerve passes through the foramen ovale of the sphenoid bone; it is derived from both the sensory root and motor root of the cranial nerve.

2. The mandibular nerve then joins with the ophthalmic nerve and maxillary nerve to form the _____ of the trigeminal nerve.

3. The mandibular nerve is a(n) _____ nerve with both afferent nerves and efferent nerves and contains the entire efferent part of the trigeminal nerve.

4. A few small branches arise from the V_3 trunk before its separation into anterior and posterior _____; these branches from the undivided mandibular nerve include the meningeal branches, which are afferent nerves for parts of the dura mater.

5. Also from the undivided mandibular nerve is the _____, which is an efferent nerve for the medial pterygoid and tensor tympani muscles as well as a muscle of the middle ear, the tensor veli palatini.

6. The mandibular nerve is the largest of the three nerve divisions that form the _____ or fifth cranial nerve (V).

7. The larger anterior oval opening on the sphenoid bone, the _____, is for the mandibular nerve (or third division) of the fifth cranial or trigeminal nerve (V).

8. The _____ also contains a part of the mandibular nerve (or third division) of the fifth cranial or trigeminal nerve (V) including the inferior alveolar and lingual nerves.

9. The mandibular nerve enters the infratemporal fossa by way of the foramen ovale, passing between the _____ and oral cavity.

10. The _____ of the fifth cranial or trigeminal nerve (V) accompanies the mandibular nerve of the sensory root and also exits the skull through the foramen ovale of the sphenoid bone.

trigeminal nerve	infratemporal fossa	foramen ovale
mixed	mandibular nerve	motor root
trigeminal ganglion	trunks	cranial cavity
medial pterygoid nerve		

Reference Chapter 8, Nervous system. In Fehrenbach MJ, Herring SW: *Illustrated anatomy of the head and neck,* ed 6, St. Louis, 2021, Saunders.

NOTES

FIGURE 8.13 Mandibular nerve (V₃): Anterior trunk (lateral view of cutaway skull)

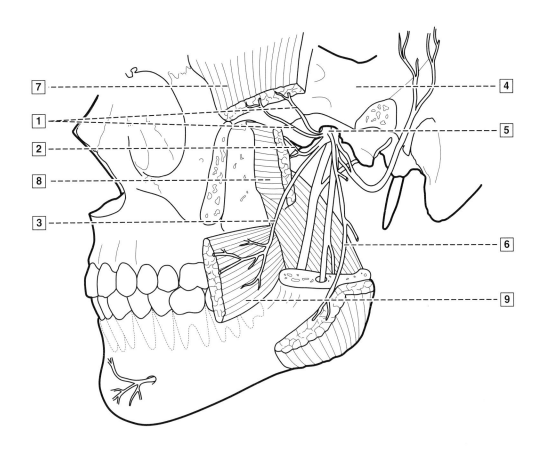

MANDIBULAR NERVE: ANTERIOR TRUNK

1. Anterior and posterior deep temporal
2. Lateral pterygoid
3. Buccal
4. Trigeminal ganglion location
5. Mandibular (V₃)
6. Masseteric

ASSOCIATED STRUCTURES

7. Temporalis muscle (cut)
8. Lateral pterygoid muscle (cut)
9. Masseter muscle (cut)

REVIEW QUESTIONS: Mandibular nerve (V₃): Anterior trunk

Fill in the blanks by choosing the appropriate terms from the list below.

1. The _____ or *anterior division* of the mandibular nerve is formed by the merger of the buccal nerve and additional muscular nerve branches.

2. The anterior trunk of the mandibular nerve has both _____ and efferent nerves.

3. The _____ (or long buccal nerve) serves as an afferent nerve for the skin of the cheek, buccal mucosa, as well as the associated buccal periodontium and gingiva of the mandibular molars.

4. The buccal nerve is initially located on the surface of the _____ and then travels posteriorly in the cheek, deep to the masseter muscle.

5. At the level of the _____ of the most distal molar of the mandibular arch, the buccal nerve crosses anteriorly to the anterior border of the mandibular ramus and goes between the two heads of the lateral pterygoid muscle to join the anterior trunk of V₃, a landmark for the administration of the buccal nerve block.

6. Several _____ are part of the anterior trunk of V₃; they begin off the motor root of the trigeminal nerve.

7. The _____, usually two in number with both anterior and posterior nerves, are efferent nerves that pass between the sphenoid bone and the superior head of the lateral pterygoid muscle and turn around the infratemporal crest of the sphenoid bone to terminate in the deep surface of the temporalis muscle that they innervate.

8. The _____ may begin at the same location as the masseteric nerve and the anterior temporal nerve may be associated at its origin with the buccal nerve.

9. The _____ is an efferent nerve that passes between the sphenoid bone and the superior border of the lateral pterygoid muscle; the nerve then accompanies the masseteric blood vessels through the mandibular notch to innervate the masseter muscle.

10. A small sensory branch from the anterior trunk of the mandibular nerve also goes to the temporomandibular joint; the _____, after a short course the nerve enters the deep surface of the lateral pterygoid muscle between the muscle's two heads of origin and serves as an efferent nerve for that muscle.

masseteric nerve	muscular branches	afferent nerves
buccal nerve	posterior temporal nerve	buccinator muscle
anterior trunk	lateral pterygoid nerve	occlusal plane
deep temporal nerves		

References Chapter 8, Nervous system. In Fehrenbach MJ, Herring SW: *Illustrated anatomy of the head and neck,* ed 6, St. Louis, 2021, Saunders; Chapter 9, Anatomy of local anesthesia. In Fehrenbach MJ, Herring SW: *Illustrated anatomy of the head and neck,* ed 6, St. Louis, 2021, Saunders.

ANSWER KEY 1. anterior trunk, 2. afferent nerves, 3. buccal nerve, 4. buccinator muscle, 5. occlusal plane, 6. muscular branches, 7. deep temporal nerves, 8. posterior temporal nerve, 9. masseteric nerve, 10. lateral pterygoid nerve

FIGURE 8.14 **Mandibular nerve (V$_3$): Anterior trunk (medial view of cut mandible)**

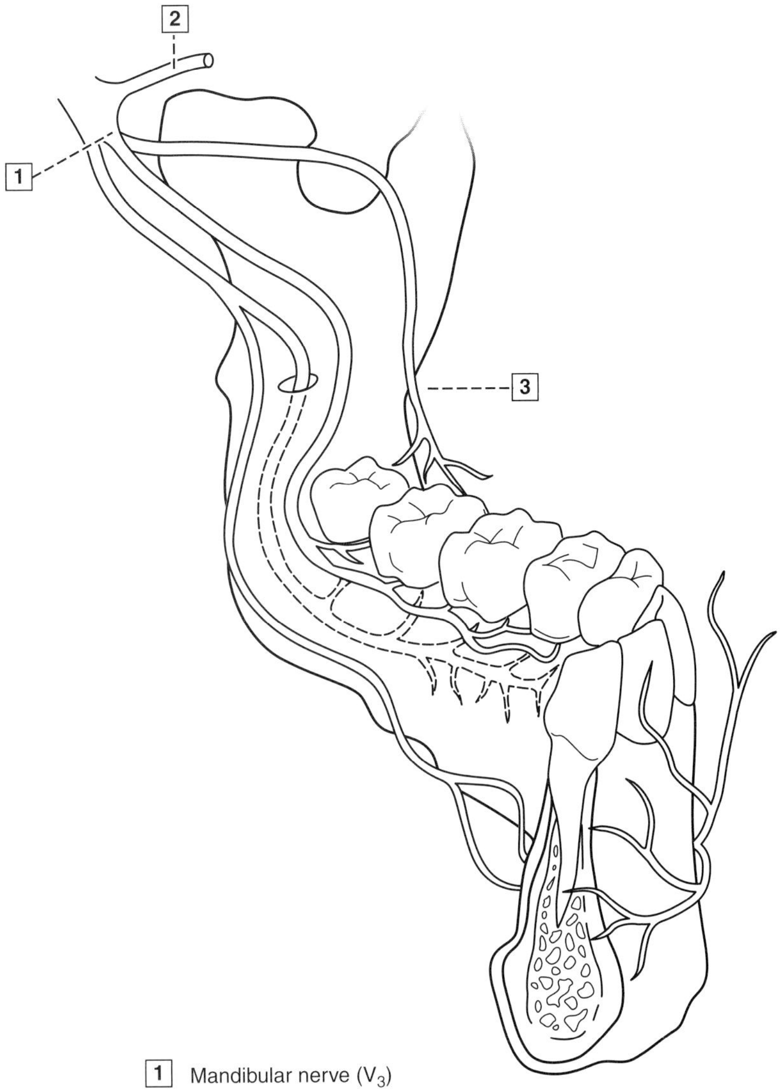

1 Mandibular nerve (V$_3$)

2 Auriculotemporal nerve (cut)

3 Buccal nerve

REVIEW QUESTIONS: Mandibular nerve (V₃): Anterior trunk

Fill in the blanks by choosing the appropriate terms from the list below.

1. The anterior trunk or *anterior division* of the mandibular nerve is formed by the merger of the
_____ and additional muscular nerve branches.

2. The anterior trunk of the mandibular nerve has both afferent nerves and _____.

3. The buccal nerve (or long buccal nerve) serves as a(n) _____ for the skin of the cheek,
buccal mucosa, as well as the associated buccal periodontium and gingiva of the mandibular molars.

4. The buccal nerve is initially located on the surface of the buccinator muscle and then travels posteriorly in
the cheek, deep to the _____.

5. At the level of the occlusal plane of the most distal molar of the mandibular arch, the buccal nerve crosses
anteriorly to the anterior border of the _____ and goes between the two heads of the
lateral pterygoid muscle to join the anterior trunk of V₃, a landmark for the administration of the buccal
nerve block.

6. Several muscle branches are part of the anterior trunk of V₃; they begin off from the
_____ of the trigeminal nerve.

7. The deep temporal nerves, usually two in number with both anterior and posterior nerves, are efferent
nerves that pass between the sphenoid bone and the superior head of the lateral pterygoid muscle and
turn around the infratemporal crest of the sphenoid bone to terminate in the deep surface of the
_____ that they innervate.

8. The posterior temporal nerve may begin at the same location as the masseteric nerve, and the
_____ may be associated at its origin with the buccal nerve.

9. The masseteric nerve is an efferent nerve that passes between the sphenoid bone and the superior border
of the lateral pterygoid muscle; the nerve then accompanies the masseteric blood vessels through the
_____ to innervate the masseter muscle.

10. A small sensory branch from the anterior trunk of the mandibular nerve also goes to the temporomandibular joint; the lateral pterygoid nerve, after a short course, enters the deep surface of the
_____ between the muscle's two heads of origin and serves as an efferent nerve for
that muscle.

motor root	mandibular notch	masseter muscle
buccal nerve	mandibular ramus	anterior temporal nerve
efferent nerves	afferent nerve	lateral pterygoid muscle
temporalis muscle		

References Chapter 8, Nervous system. In Fehrenbach MJ, Herring SW: *Illustrated anatomy of the head and neck,* ed 6,
St. Louis, 2021, Saunders; Chapter 9, Anatomy of local anesthesia. In Fehrenbach MJ, Herring SW: *Illustrated anatomy of the head
and neck,* ed 6, St. Louis, 2021, Saunders.

ANSWER KEY 1. buccal nerve, 2. efferent nerves, 3. afferent nerve, 4. masseter muscle, 5. mandibular ramus, 6. motor root, 7. temporalis muscle, 8. anterior temporal nerve, 9. mandibular notch, 10. lateral pterygoid muscle

FIGURE 8.15   Mandibular nerve (V₃): Posterior trunk (lateral view of cutaway skull)

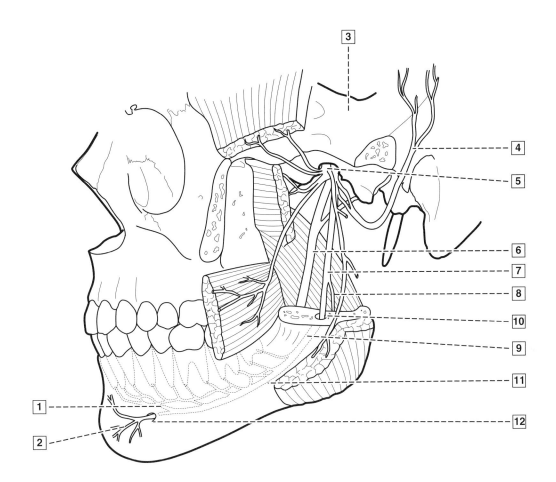

MANDIBULAR NERVE: POSTEROR TRUNK

1	Incisive	5	Mandibular (V₃)
2	Mental	6	Lingual
3	Location of trigeminal ganglion	7	Inferior alveolar
4	Auriculotemporal	8	Mylohyoid
		9	Inferior dental plexus

ASSOCIATED STRUCTURES

10 Mandibular foramen

11 Mandibular canal

12 Mental foramen

Fill in the blanks by choosing the appropriate terms from the list below.

1. The merger of the auriculotemporal, lingual, and inferior alveolar nerves forms the _____ or *posterior division* of the mandibular nerve; the final nerve formed has both afferent nerves and efferent nerves.

2. The _____ travels with the superficial temporal blood vessels and serves as an afferent nerve for the external ear, scalp, and temporomandibular joint; the nerve also carries postganglionic parasympathetic nerve fibers to the parotid salivary gland; the preganglionic parasympathetic fibers begin from the lesser petrosal branch of the glossopharyngeal or ninth cranial nerve, with the postganglionic fibers joining the auriculotemporal nerve only after relaying in the otic ganglion near the foramen ovale.

3. Communication of the auriculotemporal nerve with the _____ near the ear occurs; the auriculotemporal nerve courses deep to the lateral pterygoid muscle and neck of the mandible, splitting to encircle the middle meningeal artery, and finally joins the posterior trunk of V₃, a landmark for the administration of the Gow-Gates mandibular nerve block.

4. The _____ is an afferent nerve formed from the merger of the mental and incisive nerves; after forming, the nerve continues to travel posteriorly through the mandibular canal, along with the inferior alveolar artery and vein, and where the nerve is then joined by dental branches such as the interdental and interradicular branches from the surrounding periodontium to be part of the inferior dental plexus in the mandibular arch.

5. The inferior alveolar nerve exits the mandible through the mandibular foramen after traveling the mandibular canal where it is joined by the nearby _____; the mandibular foramen is an opening of the mandibular canal on the medial surface of the mandibular ramus, approximately two-thirds the distance from the coronoid notch to the posterior border of the mandibular ramus, entirely within the pterygomandibular space, landmarks for the administration of the inferior alveolar nerve block.

6. The _____ is composed of external branches that serve as afferent nerves for the chin, lower lip, and labial mucosa as well as the associated facial periodontium and gingiva of the mandibular anterior teeth and premolars to the midline; the nerve then enters the mental foramen on the lateral surface of the mandible along with the mental blood vessels, usually inferior to the apices of the mandibular premolars; these are landmarks for the administration for both the mental nerve block and the incisive nerve block, the latter which is administered at the same site with deeper anesthesia by using a more local anesthetic agent.

7. The inferior alveolar nerve block, Gow-Gates mandibular nerve block or the Vazirani-Akinosi mandibular nerve block can be used to anesthetize the mental nerve along with other branches of the _____ from other target injection sites; in addition, the incisive nerve can be anesthetized by these three nerve blocks.

8. After entering via the mental foramen and traveling a distance within the mandibular canal, the mental nerve merges with the _____ to form the inferior alveolar nerve within the mandibular canal but before the newly formed nerve exits the canal.

9. The incisive nerve is an afferent nerve composed of dental branches from the mandibular anterior teeth and premolars that originate in the pulp, exit the teeth through the apical foramina, and join with interdental branches from the surrounding periodontium to be part of the _____ in the mandibular arch in the region; the incisive nerve either begins as nerve endings within the mandibular anterior teeth or adjacent bone and soft tissue.

10. The incisive nerve serves as an afferent nerve for the mandibular anterior teeth and premolars and associated facial periodontium and gingiva to the midline; it travels along with the incisive blood vessels within the mandibular incisive canal, which is an anterior continuation of the mandibular canal that runs bilaterally from the mental foramen usually to the region of the ipsilateral lateral incisor teeth, and where the nerve then merges with the mental nerve just posterior to the mental foramen and goes on next to form the inferior alveolar nerve within the _____ before it exits.

inferior alveolar nerve	mandibular canal	inferior dental plexus
posterior trunk	facial nerve	incisive nerve
auriculotemporal nerve	mandibular nerve	mental nerve
mylohyoid nerve		

References Chapter 8, Nervous system. In Fehrenbach MJ, Herring SW: *Illustrated anatomy of the head and neck,* ed 6, St. Louis, 2021, Saunders; Chapter 9, Anatomy of local anesthesia. In Fehrenbach MJ, Herring SW: *Illustrated anatomy of the head and neck,* ed 6, St. Louis, 2021, Saunders.

FIGURE 8.16   Mandibular nerve (V₃): Posterior trunk (medial view of cut mandible)

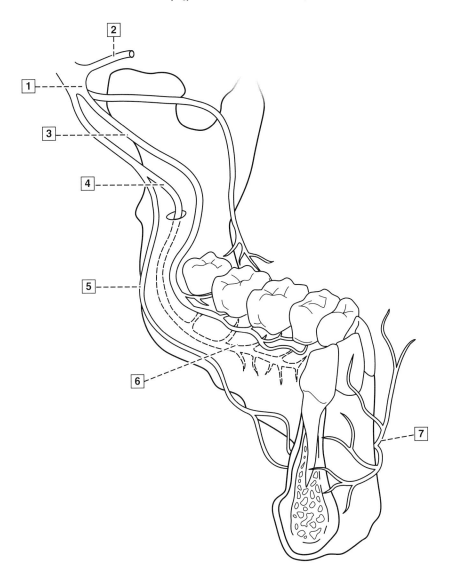

1	Mandibular nerve (V₃)	5	Mylohyoid nerve
2	Auriculotemporal nerve (cut)	6	Inferior dental plexus
3	Lingual nerve	7	Mental nerve
4	Inferior alveolar nerve		

Fill in the blanks by choosing the appropriate terms from the list below.

1. The _____ travels lateral to the medial pterygoid muscle, between the sphenomandibular ligament and mandibular ramus; the nerve is now posterior and slightly lateral to the lingual nerve and then joins the posterior trunk of V_3 as it carries the afferent innervation for the mandibular teeth and associated facial periodontium and gingiva of the mandibular anterior teeth and premolars as well as labial mucosa through its incisive and mental branches to the midline.

2. In some cases, there are two nerves present on the one side, creating _____ inferior alveolar nerves; this situation can occur unilaterally or bilaterally and can be detected on a radiograph by the presence of a double mandibular canal.

3. The _____ is formed from afferent branches from the associated lingual periodontium and gingiva of mandibular teeth and the body of the tongue and then first travels along the lateral surface of the tongue; then the nerve passes posteriorly, passing from the medial to the lateral side of the duct of the submandibular salivary gland by going inferior to the duct where it communicates with the submandibular ganglion located superior to the deep lobe of the gland.

4. The parasympathetic efferent innervation for the sublingual and submandibular salivary glands begins from the _____ (more specifically, a branch of the nerve, the chorda tympani) but both the preganglionic and some of the postganglionic fibers travel along with the lingual nerve.

5. At the base of the tongue, the lingual nerve ascends and runs between the medial pterygoid muscle and the mandible, where it is positioned _____ and slightly medial to the inferior alveolar nerve; thus the lingual nerve is also anesthetized when administering an inferior alveolar nerve block through the diffusion of the local anesthetic agent so that the Gow-Gates or Vazirani-Akinosi mandibular blocks can also be used to anesthetize the lingual nerve.

6. The lingual nerve then continues to travel _____ to join the posterior trunk of V_3; thus the lingual nerve serves as an afferent nerve for general sensation for the body of the tongue, the floor of the mouth, and the associated lingual periodontium and gingiva of the mandibular teeth to the midline.

7. After the inferior alveolar nerve exits the mandibular foramen, a small branch occurs, the _____.

8. The mylohyoid nerve pierces the sphenomandibular ligament and runs inferiorly and anteriorly in the mylohyoid groove and then onto the inferior surface of the _____, which it innervates.

9. The mylohyoid nerve serves as an efferent nerve to the mylohyoid muscle and _____ of the digastric muscle (the posterior belly of the digastric muscle is innervated by a branch from the facial nerve).

10. The mylohyoid nerve may in some cases also serve as an afferent nerve for the _____, which needs to be considered when there is a lack of clinical effectiveness of the inferior alveolar nerve block; the mylohyoid nerve can then be anesthetized by supraperiosteal injection for the tooth on the medial border of the mandible, the Gow-Gates mandibular nerve block or the Vazirani-Akinosi mandibular nerve block.

superiorly	lingual nerve	inferior alveolar nerve
mandibular first molar	bifid	facial nerve
anterior	anterior belly	mylohyoid nerve
mylohyoid muscle		

References Chapter 8, Nervous system. In Fehrenbach MJ, Herring SW: *Illustrated anatomy of the head and neck,* ed 6, St. Louis, 2021, Saunders; Chapter 9, Anatomy of local anesthesia. In Fehrenbach MJ, Herring SW: *Illustrated anatomy of the head and neck,* ed 6, St. Louis, 2021, Saunders.

FIGURE 8.17   Mandibular nerve (V₃): Motor and sensory branches (medial cutaway view of maxilla and mandible)

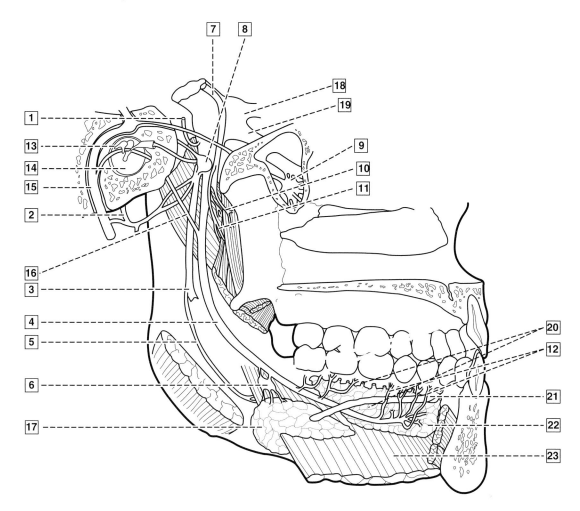

MANDIBULAR NERVE

1 Middle meningeal	7 Motor root of trigeminal nerve (cut)
2 Auriculotemporal	8 Otic ganglion
3 Inferior alveolar	9 Pterygopalatine ganglion
4 Lingual	10 Nerve to tensor veli palatini muscle
5 Mylohyoid	11 Nerve to medial pterygoid muscle
6 Submandibular ganglion	12 Branches to tongue

ASSOCIATED STRUCTURES

13 Ear ossicles	19 Maxillary nerve (V₂)
14 Tympanic membrane	20 Ducts of Rivinus
15 Facial nerve (VII)	21 Submandibular duct
16 Chorda tympani nerve	22 Sublingual salivary gland
17 Submandibular salivary gland	23 Mylohyoid muscle
18 Ophthalmic nerve (V₁)	

REVIEW QUESTIONS: Mandibular nerve (V₃): Motor and sensory branches

Fill in the blanks by choosing the appropriate terms from the list below.

1. The fifth cranial nerve (V) or _____ has both an efferent component for the muscles of mastication, as well as some other cranial muscles, and an afferent component for the teeth, tongue, and oral cavity, as well as most of the skin of the face and head; although the trigeminal nerve has no preganglionic parasympathetic fibers, many postganglionic parasympathetic fibers travel along with its branches.

2. The _____ (V₃) is the largest of the three nerve divisions that form the trigeminal nerve.

3. The mandibular nerve is derived from both the sensory and motor _____ of the cranial nerve; it has both afferent nerves and efferent nerves as well as contains the entire efferent part of the trigeminal nerve.

4. The _____ of the trigeminal nerve accompanies the mandibular nerve of the sensory root and also exits the skull through the foramen ovale of the sphenoid bone.

5. The mandibular nerve has a short main trunk formed by the merger of a smaller anterior and a larger posterior _____.

6. Also from the undivided mandibular nerve is the _____, which is an efferent nerve for the medial pterygoid and tensor tympani muscles as well as a muscle of the middle ear, the tensor veli palatini.

7. The merger of the auriculotemporal, lingual, and inferior alveolar nerves forms the _____ or *posterior division* of the mandibular nerve; the final nerve formed has both afferent nerves and efferent nerves.

8. After the inferior alveolar nerve exits the mandibular foramen, a small branch occurs, the _____.

9. The seventh cranial nerve (VII) or _____ carries both efferent and afferent components; the nerve carries an efferent component for the muscles of the second pharyngeal or branchial arch and for the preganglionic parasympathetic innervation of the lacrimal gland and small nasal and palatal glands (relaying in the pterygopalatine ganglion) as well as the submandibular and sublingual salivary glands (relaying in the submandibular ganglion).

10. The ninth cranial nerve (IX) or _____ carries an efferent component for the pharyngeal muscle, the stylopharyngeus muscle and also provides preganglionic gland parasympathetic innervation for the parotid salivary gland (relaying the otic ganglion); the nerve also carries an afferent component for the oropharynx and for taste and general sensation from the base of the tongue and thus is the afferent limb of the gag reflex.

mandibular nerve	motor root	muscular branches
posterior trunk	facial nerve	trunk
glossopharyngeal nerve	mylohyoid nerve	trigeminal nerve
roots		

Reference Chapter 8, Nervous system. In Fehrenbach MJ, Herring SW: *Illustrated anatomy of the head and neck,* ed 6, St. Louis, 2021, Saunders.

Copyright © 2023 Elsevier Inc. All Rights Reserved.

FIGURE 8.18 Facial (VII) and trigeminal (V) nerves (cutaway medial view of maxilla and mandible)

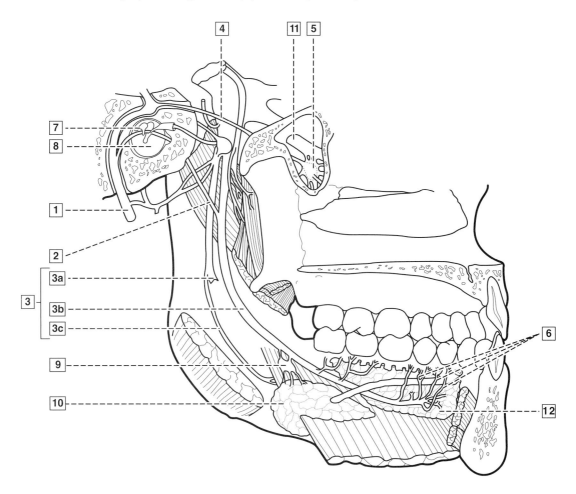

MANDIBULAR NERVE AND FACIAL NERVE

1	**Facial (VII)**	**4**	Greater petrosal
2	Chorda tympani	**5**	Pterygopalatine ganglion
3	**Mandibular nerve (V$_3$)**	**6**	Sensory fibers from tongue
3a	Inferior alveolar		
3b	Lingual		
3c	Mylohyoid		

ASSOCIATED STRUCTURES

7 Ear ossicles

8 Tympanic membrane

9 Submandibular ganglion

10 Submandibular salivary gland

11 Maxillary nerve (V$_2$)

12 Sublingual salivary gland

REVIEW QUESTIONS: Facial (VII) and trigeminal (V) nerves

Fill in the blanks by choosing the appropriate terms from the list below.

1. The seventh cranial nerve (VII) or _____ emerges from the brain and enters the internal acoustic meatus in the petrous part of the temporal bone; within the temporal bone, the nerve gives off a small efferent branch to the muscle in the middle ear (stapedius) and two larger branches, the greater petrosal and chorda tympani nerves, both of which carry parasympathetic fibers.

2. The main trunk of the facial nerve emerges from the skull through the _____ of the temporal bone and gives off two branches, the posterior auricular nerve and a branch to the posterior belly of the digastric and stylohyoid muscles.

3. The facial nerve then passes into the _____ and divides the gland into superficial and deep lobes; the trunk of the facial nerve itself divides into numerous terminal branches to supply the muscles of facial expression but does not innervate the gland itself.

4. The _____ is a branch off the facial nerve before it exits the skull.

5. The greater petrosal nerve carries efferent nerve fibers, which are preganglionic parasympathetic fibers to the _____ in the pterygopalatine fossa.

6. The postganglionic fibers arising in the pterygopalatine ganglion from the greater petrosal nerve then join with branches of the _____ of the trigeminal nerve to be carried to the lacrimal gland (via the zygomatic and lacrimal nerves), nasal cavity, and minor salivary glands of the hard and soft palate; the greater petrosal nerve also carries afferent nerve fibers for a taste sensation in the palate.

7. The _____ is a small branch of the facial nerve that is a parasympathetic efferent nerve for the submandibular and sublingual salivary glands and also serves as an afferent nerve for taste sensation for the anterior two-thirds of the body of the tongue.

8. After branching off the facial nerve within the petrous part of the temporal bone, the chorda tympani nerve crosses the medial surface of the tympanic membrane (eardrum) and then exits the skull by the _____, located immediately posterior to the temporomandibular joint.

9. The chorda tympani nerve then travels with the _____ along the floor of the mouth in the same nerve bundle.

10. In the submandibular triangle, the chorda tympani nerve, appearing as part of the lingual nerve, has communication with the _____ where the parasympathetic fibers synapse; the submandibular ganglion is located superior to the deep lobe of the submandibular salivary gland, for which it supplies parasympathetic efferent innervation and the postganglionic fibers for the sublingual gland rejoin the lingual nerve to reach the gland.

petrotympanic fissure	parotid salivary gland	chorda tympani nerve
lingual nerve	submandibular ganglion	facial nerve
greater petrosal nerve	maxillary nerve	pterygopalatine ganglion
stylomastoid foramen		

Reference Chapter 8, Nervous system. In Fehrenbach MJ, Herring SW: *Illustrated anatomy of the head and neck,* ed 6, St. Louis, 2021, Saunders.

FIGURE 8.19   Facial (VII) nerve (cutaway lateral view with gland sectioned)

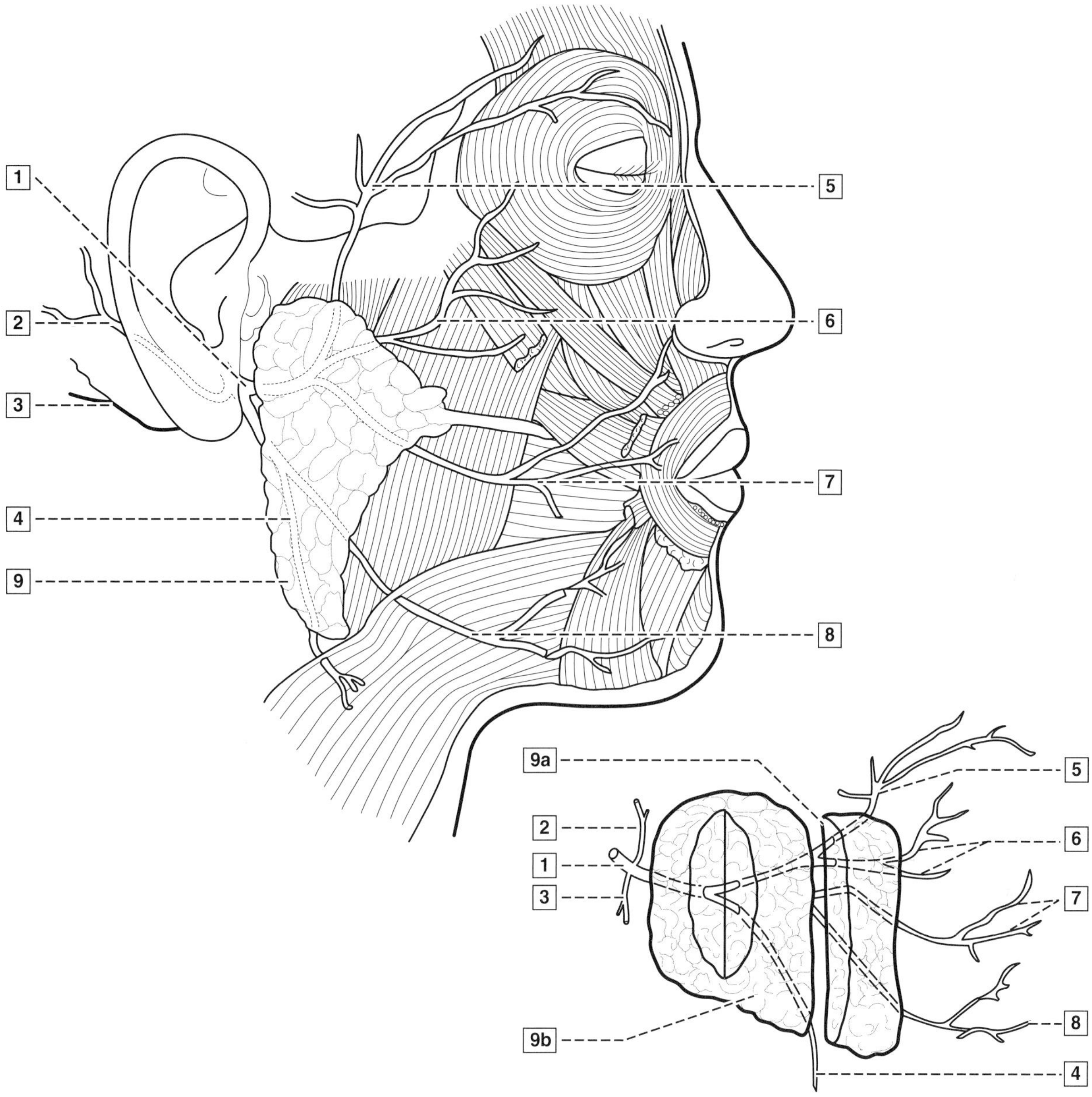

FACIAL NERVE

1 Facial nerve (VII) trunk

2 Posterior auricular

3 Nerve to posterior belly of digastric muscle and to stylohyoid muscle

4 Cervical branch

5 Temporal branches

6 Zygomatic branches

7 Buccal branches

8 Mandibular branch

ASSOCIATED STRUCTURE

9 Parotid salivary gland

9a Deep lobe

9b Superficial lobe

REVIEW QUESTIONS: Facial (VII) nerve

Fill in the blanks by choosing the appropriate terms from the list below.

1. The posterior auricular nerve, stylohyoid nerve, and posterior digastric nerve are branches of the
_____ (VII) after it exits the stylomastoid foramen; all the branches after the nerve exits
from the skull are efferent nerves.

2. The _____ supplies the occipital belly of the epicranial muscle.

3. The _____ supplies the stylohyoid muscle.

4. The _____ supplies the posterior belly of the digastric muscle.

5. Additional efferent nerve branches of the facial nerve originate within the parotid salivary gland and pass to
the _____ that they innervate; these branches to the muscles of facial expression in-
clude the temporal, zygomatic, buccal, (marginal) mandibular, and cervical branches.

6. The _____ supply the muscles anterior to the ear, frontal belly of the epicranial muscle,
superior part of the orbicularis oculi muscle, and corrugator supercilii muscle.

7. The _____ supply the inferior part of the orbicularis oculi muscle and zygomatic major
and minor muscles.

8. The _____ (not to be confused with the sensory [long] buccal nerve from V_3) supply the
muscles of the upper lip and nose and buccinator, risorius, and orbicularis oris muscles; the zygomatic and
buccal branches are usually closely associated, exchanging many fibers.

9. The (marginal) _____ supplies the muscles of the lower lip and mentalis muscle; the
mandibular branch should not be confused with the mandibular nerve or V_3.

10. The _____ runs inferior to the mandible to supply the platysma muscle.

cervical branch	muscles of facial expression	posterior auricular nerve
facial nerve	zygomatic branches	mandibular branch
stylohyoid nerve	temporal branches	posterior digastric nerve
buccal branches		

Reference Chapter 8, Nervous system. In Fehrenbach MJ, Herring SW: *Illustrated anatomy of the head and neck,* ed 6,
St. Louis, 2021, Saunders.

NOTES

FIGURE 8.20 Parotid salivary gland lobes with facial (VII) nerve division (transverse section)

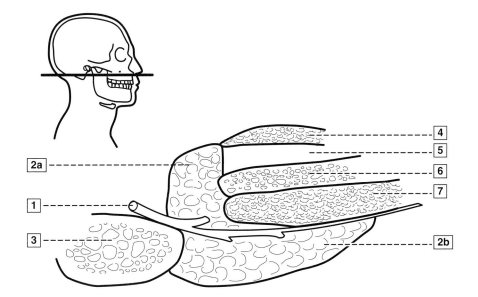

1	Facial nerve (VII) trunk	4	Medial pterygoid muscle
2	Parotid salivary gland	5	Pterygomandibular space
2a	Deep lobe	6	Mandibular ramus
2b	Superficial lobe	7	Masseter muscle
3	Mastoid process		

REVIEW QUESTIONS: Parotid salivary gland lobes with facial (VII) nerve division

Fill in the blanks by choosing the appropriate terms from the list below.

1. The posterior auricular nerve, stylohyoid nerve, and posterior digastric nerve are branches of the facial nerve (VII) after it exits the _____; all the branches after the nerve exits from the skull are efferent nerves.

2. The posterior auricular nerve supplies the occipital belly of the _____.

3. The stylohyoid nerve supplies the _____.

4. The posterior digastric nerve supplies the _____.

5. Additional _____ of the facial nerve originate within the parotid salivary gland and pass to the muscles of facial expression that they innervate; these branches to the muscles of facial expression include the temporal, zygomatic, buccal, (marginal) mandibular, and cervical branches.

6. The temporal branches supply the muscles anterior to the ear, frontal belly of the epicranial muscle, _____ part of the orbicularis oculi muscle, and corrugator supercilii muscle.

7. The zygomatic branches supply the _____ part of the orbicularis oculi muscle and zygomatic major and minor muscles.

8. The buccal branches (not to be confused with the sensory [long] buccal nerve from V₃) supply the muscles of the upper lip and nose and buccinator, risorius, and orbicularis oris muscles; the zygomatic and buccal branches are usually closely associated, exchanging many _____.

9. The (marginal) mandibular branch supplies the muscles of the lower lip and mentalis muscle; the mandibular branch should not be confused with the _____ or V₃.

10. The cervical branch runs inferior to the mandible to supply the _____.

superior	stylohyoid muscle	posterior belly of the digastric muscle
inferior	epicranial muscle	fibers
stylomastoid foramen	mandibular nerve	platysma muscle
efferent nerve branches		

Reference Chapter 8, Nervous system. In Fehrenbach MJ, Herring SW: *Illustrated anatomy of the head and neck,* ed 6, St. Louis, 2021, Saunders.

NOTES

FIGURE 9.1   Upper body lymphatics (frontal view including right and left side indications)

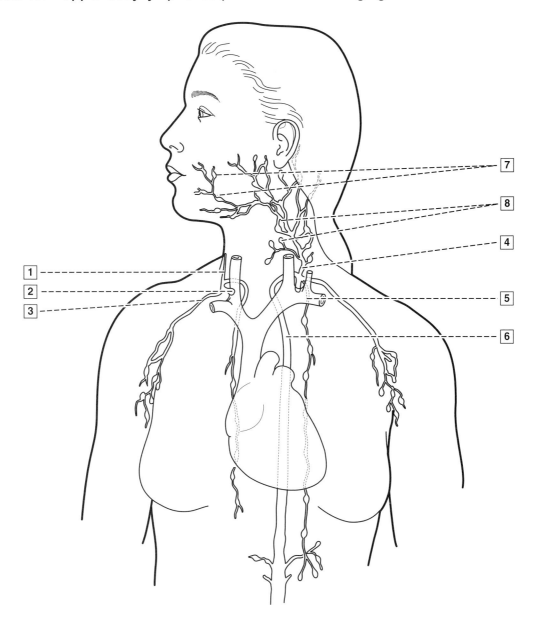

LYMPHATICS

Right side

1	Right jugular trunk
2	Right lymphatic duct
3	Right subclavian trunk

Left side

4	Left jugular trunk
5	Left subclavian trunk
6	Thoracic duct

ASSOCIATED STRUCTURES

| 7 | Facial lymph nodes |
| 8 | Cervical lymph nodes |

REVIEW QUESTIONS: Upper body lymphatics

Fill in the blanks by choosing the appropriate terms from the list below.

1. The _____ of the right side of the head and neck converges by way of the right jugular trunk, joining that of the right arm and thorax (chest) to form the right lymphatic duct.

2. The _____ drains into the venous drainage of the vascular system at the junction of the right subclavian and right internal jugular veins.

3. The lymphatic vessels of the left side of the head and neck converge into the _____, actually a short vessel, and then into the thoracic duct, which joins the venous drainage at the junction of the left subclavian and left internal jugular veins.

4. The lymphatic system from the left arm and thorax also joins the _____, a main duct of the lymphatic system, ascending through the thoracic cavity anterior to the spinal column and discharging the lymph into the blood of the vascular system through the left subclavian vein.

5. The thoracic duct is much larger than the right lymphatic duct because it drains the lymph from the entire _____ of the body for both the right and left sides.

6. Within the tissue located in outer regions of the body, smaller lymphatic vessels containing lymph converge into larger _____.

7. The lymphatic ducts then empty into the venous drainage endpoint of the _____ in the thorax (chest); both lymphatic ducts each have one-way valves at the junction with the venous system and these valves function similarly to other lymphatic valves in the lymphatic vessels by preventing venous blood from flowing into the lymph duct.

8. However, the final drainage endpoint of the lymphatic vessels into the lymphatic ducts depends on which _____ is involved, which mirrors a similar concept in the vascular system.

9. The lymphatic system is part of the _____ that consists of vessels, nodes, ducts, and tonsils.

10. The lymphatic system helps fight _____ such as infection and cancer and also serves other functions in the body.

thoracic duct	lymphatic system	lymphatic ducts	immune system
left jugular trunk	right lymphatic duct	side of the body	disease processes
lower half	vascular system		

References Chapter 10, Lymphatic system. In Fehrenbach MJ, Herring SW: *Illustrated anatomy of the head and neck,* ed 6, St. Louis, 2021, Saunders; Chapter 8, Head and neck. In Drake R, Vogl AW, Mitchell AWM: *Gray's anatomy for students,* ed 4, Philadelphia, 2020, Churchill Livingstone.

ANSWER KEY 1. lymphatic system, 2. right lymphatic duct, 3. left jugular trunk, 4. thoracic duct, 5. lower half, 6. lymphatic ducts, 7. vascular system, 8. side of the body, 9. immune system, 10. disease processes

FIGURE 9.2 Superficial lymph nodes of the head (lateral view)

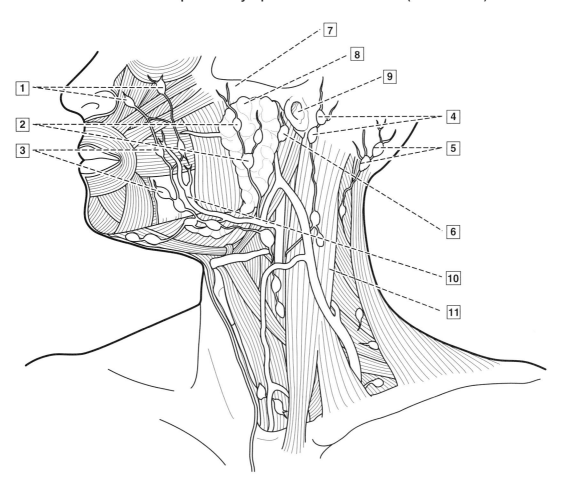

NODES	ASSOCIATED STRUCTURES
1 Facial nodes	**7** Zygomatic arch
2 Superficial parotid nodes	**8** Parotid salivary gland
3 Facial nodes	**9** External acoustic meatus
4 Posterior auricular nodes	**10** Facial vein
5 Occipital nodes	**11** Sternocleidomastoid muscle
6 Anterior auricular node	

REVIEW QUESTIONS: Superficial lymph nodes of the head

Fill in the blanks by choosing the appropriate terms from the list below.

1. The five groups of paired _____ located in the head include the occipital, posterior auricular, anterior auricular, superficial parotid, and facial lymph nodes.

2. The _____ are located on the posterior base of the head in the occipital region and drain this part of the scalp.

3. The _____ (or postauricular) are located posterior to each auricle and the external acoustic meatus, where the sternocleidomastoid muscle inserts on the mastoid process.

4. The _____ (or preauricular) are located immediately anterior to each tragus, and the superficial parotid lymph nodes are located just superficial to each parotid salivary gland.

5. The posterior auricular, anterior auricular, and superficial parotid lymph nodes drain the external ear, lacrimal gland, and adjacent regions of the scalp and face; all of these lymph nodes empty into the _____.

6. The _____ are superficial lymph nodes located along the facial vein with its diagonal course across the side of the face and are usually small and variable in number; these lymph nodes are further categorized into four subgroups, which include the malar, nasolabial, buccal, and mandibular lymph nodes.

7. The lymph nodes in the infraorbital region are the _____ (or infraorbital nodes) and the lymph nodes located along the nasolabial sulcus are the nasolabial lymph nodes.

8. The lymph nodes around the labial commissure and just superficial to the buccinator muscle are the _____.

9. The lymph nodes in the tissue superior to the surface of the mandible and anterior to the masseter muscle are the _____.

10. Each facial lymph node subgroup drains the skin and mucous membranes where the lymph nodes are located; the facial lymph nodes also drain from one to the other superior to inferior and then finally drain together into the deep cervical lymph nodes by way of the _____.

deep cervical lymph nodes	occipital lymph nodes	submandibular lymph nodes
posterior auricular lymph nodes	anterior auricular lymph nodes	buccal lymph nodes
facial lymph nodes	malar lymph nodes	superficial lymph nodes of the head
mandibular lymph nodes		

Reference Chapter 10, Lymphatic system. In Fehrenbach MJ, Herring SW: *Illustrated anatomy of the head and neck,* ed 6, St. Louis, 2021, Saunders.

FIGURE 9.3   Deep lymph nodes of the head (lateral view)

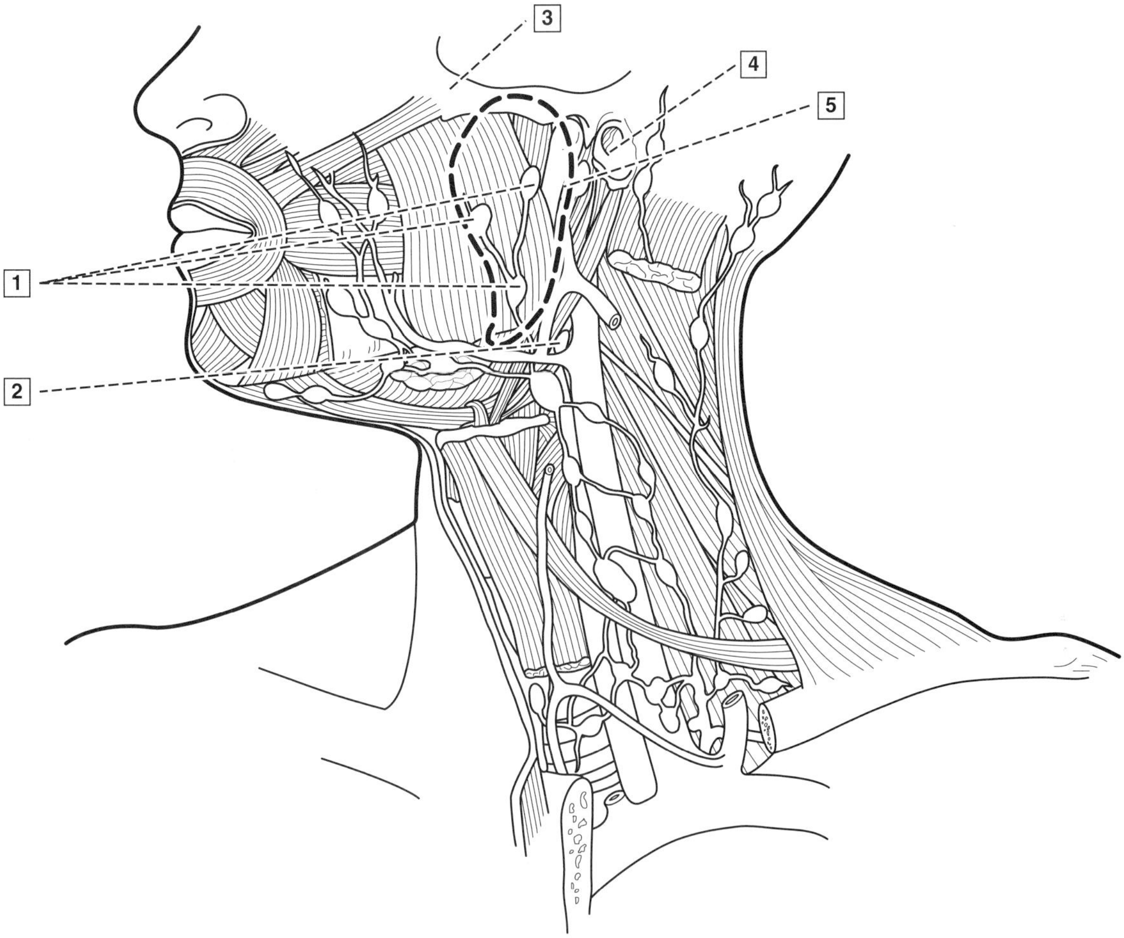

NODES

1 Deep parotid nodes

2 Retropharyngeal node

ASSOCIATED STRUCTURES

3 Zygomatic arch

4 External acoustic meatus

5 Parotid salivary gland location

REVIEW QUESTIONS: Deep lymph nodes of head

Fill in the blanks by choosing the appropriate terms from the list below.

1. The _____ include the paired deep parotid and retropharyngeal lymph nodes.

2. The deep lymph nodes of the head drain into the _____.

3. The _____ are located deep within the parotid salivary gland and drain the middle ear, auditory tube (pharyngotympanic tube), and parotid salivary gland.

4. Located near the deep parotid lymph nodes and at the level of the atlas, the first cervical vertebra, are the _____ of the lymphatic system.

5. The retropharyngeal lymph nodes drain and are _____ to the pharynx, palate, paranasal sinuses, and nasal cavity; they frequently disappear by age 4 to 5.

6. The deep lymph nodes in the head region cannot be palpated during an extraoral examination due to their increased depth in the tissue; however, the deep lymph nodes in the head still communicate with the more _____.

7. The _____ or *retrovisceral space* extends from the base of the skull, where it is posterior to the superior pharyngeal constrictor muscle and inferior to the thorax (chest); the space is divided into two lateral compartments by a fibrous raphe and contains the retropharyngeal lymph nodes in early childhood.

8. The _____ extends to the pterygomandibular raphe, where it is continuous with the infra-temporal and buccal spaces; the space's anterior compartment contains the deep cervical lymph nodes.

9. The deep parotid lymph nodes are within the _____ , which covers the masseter muscle and structures inferior to the zygomatic arch and surrounds the parotid salivary gland.

10. The primary lymph nodes for the scalp are the posterior auricular, anterior auricular, superficial parotid, occipital, and accessory lymph nodes; the _____ for the scalp are the deep cervical and supraclavicular lymph nodes.

retropharyngeal space	deep lymph nodes of the head	superficial regional lymph nodes
retropharyngeal lymph nodes	deep parotid lymph nodes	parapharyngeal space
deep cervical lymph nodes	masseteric-parotid fascia	buccopharyngeal fascia
posterior		

References   Chapter 10, Lymphatic system; Fasciae and spaces. In Fehrenbach MJ, Herring SW: *Illustrated anatomy of the head and neck,* ed 6, St. Louis, 2021, Saunders; Chapter 11, Fasciae and spaces. In Fehrenbach MJ, Herring SW: *Illustrated anatomy of the head and neck,* ed 6, St. Louis, 2021, Saunders.

FIGURE 9.4 Superficial cervical lymph nodes (lateral view)

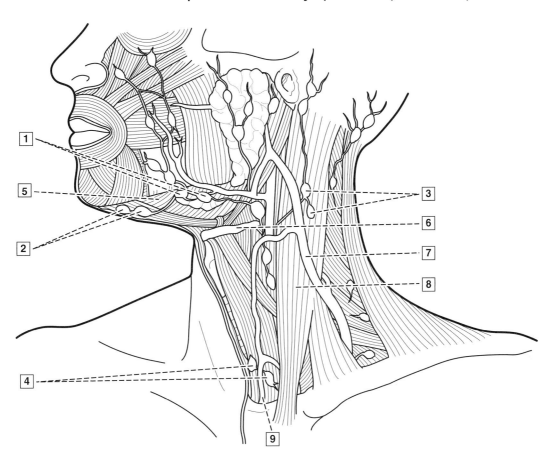

NODES		ASSOCIATED STRUCTURES	
1	Submandibular nodes	5	Mylohyoid muscle
2	Submental nodes	6	Hyoid bone
3	External jugular nodes	7	External jugular vein
4	Anterior jugular nodes	8	Sternocleidomastoid muscle
		9	Anterior jugular vein

REVIEW QUESTIONS: Superficial cervical lymph nodes

Fill in the blanks by choosing the appropriate terms from the list below.

1. The four groups of _____ include the submental, submandibular, external jugular, and anterior jugular lymph nodes.

2. The _____ are located inferior to the chin within the submental fascial space, as well as the submental triangle, which is between the anterior bellies of the digastric muscles; these lymph nodes are near the midline inferior to the mandibular symphysis in the suprahyoid region, and also just superficial to the mylohyoid muscle.

3. The submental lymph nodes bilaterally drain the lower lip, both sides of the chin, the floor of the mouth, the apex of the tongue, and the mandibular incisors and associated periodontium and gingiva; these lymph nodes then empty into the submandibular lymph nodes or directly into the _____.

4. The submandibular lymph nodes are located at the inferior border of the mandibular ramus, just superficial to the _____, and within the submandibular fascial space; the nodes are also posterolateral to the anterior belly of the digastric muscles.

5. The _____ unilaterally drains the cheeks, upper lip, body of the tongue, anterior hard palate, and all teeth with associated periodontium and gingiva, except for the mandibular incisors and maxillary third molars.

6. The submandibular lymph nodes may be _____ for the submental lymph nodes and facial regions.

7. The lymphatic system from both the _____ and submandibular salivary glands drains into the submandibular lymph nodes; these lymph nodes then empty into the deep cervical lymph nodes.

8. The _____ (or superficial cervical nodes) are located on each side of the neck along the external jugular vein, superficial to the sternocleidomastoid muscle.

9. The external jugular lymph nodes may be secondary nodes for the occipital, posterior auricular, anterior auricular, and _____; the external jugular lymph nodes then empty into the deep cervical lymph nodes.

10. The _____ (or anterior cervical nodes) are located on each side of the neck along the length of the anterior jugular vein, anterior to the larynx, trachea, and superficial to the sternocleidomastoid muscle as well as between the superficial layer of deep cervical fascia and the infrahyoid muscles; these lymph nodes drain the infrahyoid region of the neck and then empty into the deep cervical lymph nodes.

anterior jugular lymph nodes	submandibular lymph nodes	submental lymph nodes
deep cervical lymph nodes	superficial cervical lymph nodes	sublingual salivary gland
submandibular salivary gland	secondary nodes	superficial parotid lymph nodes
external jugular lymph nodes		

Reference Chapter 10, Lymphatic system. In Fehrenbach MJ, Herring SW: *Illustrated anatomy of the head and neck,* ed 6, St. Louis, 2021, Saunders.

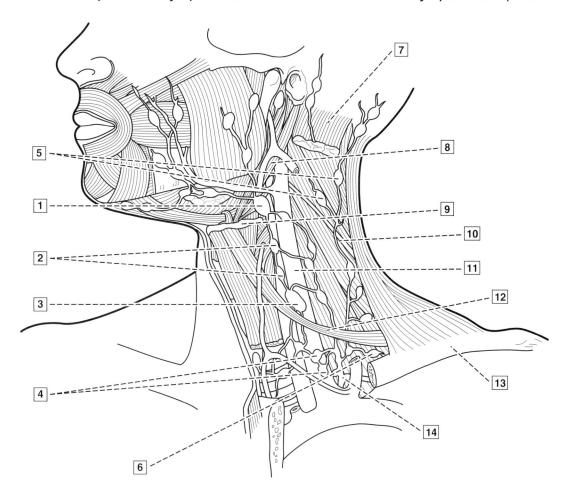

FIGURE 9.5 Deep cervical lymph nodes and associated cervical lymph nodes (lateral view)

NODES

1 Jugulodigastric node
2 Superior deep cervical nodes
3 Jugulo-omohyoid node
4 Inferior deep cervical nodes
5 Accessory nodes
6 Supraclavicular node

ASSOCIATED STRUCTURES

7 Sternocleidomastoid muscle (cut)
8 Digastric muscle
9 Hyoid bone
10 Accessory nerve
11 Internal jugular vein
12 Omohyoid muscle
13 Clavicle (cut)
14 Thoracic duct

Fill in the blanks by choosing the appropriate terms from the list below.

1. The _____ are located along the length of the internal jugular vein on each side of the neck, deep to the sternocleidomastoid muscle; these lymph nodes extend from the base of the skull to the root of the neck, adjacent to the pharynx, esophagus, and trachea and can be divided into two groups, the superior and inferior deep cervical lymph nodes, based on the vertical anatomic position of the lymph nodes to the point where omohyoid muscle crosses the internal jugular vein.

2. The _____ are located deep underneath the sternocleidomastoid muscle, superior relative to the point where the omohyoid muscle crosses the internal jugular vein; these lymph nodes are primary nodes for draining the posterior nasal cavity, posterior hard palate, soft palate, base of the tongue, maxillary third molars with associated periodontium and gingiva, temporomandibular joint, esophagus, trachea, and thyroid gland.

3. The superior deep cervical lymph nodes may be _____ for all other lymph nodes of the head and neck, except inferior deep cervical lymph nodes; the superior deep cervical nodes empty into the inferior deep cervical lymph nodes or directly into the jugular trunk.

4. A possibly prominent and palpable lymph node of the superior deep cervical lymph nodes, the _____ or *tonsillar node* is located inferior to the posterior belly of the digastric muscle and posterior to the angle of the mandible; the lymph node drains the palatine tonsils.

5. The _____ are a continuation of the superior deep cervical group; these lymph nodes are also located deep to the sternocleidomastoid muscle, but inferior relative to the point where the omohyoid muscle crosses the internal jugular vein, extending into the supraclavicular fossa, superior to each clavicle.

6. The inferior deep cervical lymph nodes are _____ that drain the posterior part of the scalp and neck, the superficial pectoral region, and a part of the arm.

7. A possibly prominent and palpable lymph node of the inferior deep cervical nodes, the _____, is located at the angle created by the actual crossing of the omohyoid muscle and internal jugular vein; this lymph node drains the tongue and submental region as well as associated structures and regions.

8. The inferior deep cervical lymph nodes may be secondary nodes for the superficial lymph nodes of the head and superior deep cervical lymph nodes; their efferent vessels form the _____, which is one of the tributaries of the right lymphatic duct on the right side and the thoracic duct on the left, allowing communication with the axillary lymph nodes that drain the breast region.

9. The _____ are located along the eleventh cranial nerve or accessory nerve in the most inferior part of the neck; these lymph nodes drain the scalp and neck regions and then drain into the supraclavicular lymph nodes.

10. The _____ are located superiorly along the clavicle close to where the sternum joins it and drain the lateral cervical triangles in the most inferior part of the neck; these lymph nodes may empty into one of the jugular trunks or directly into the right lymphatic duct or thoracic duct and are located in the final endpoint of lymphatic drainage from the entire body.

jugular trunk	deep cervical lymph nodes	superior deep cervical lymph nodes
primary nodes	supraclavicular lymph nodes	jugulodigastric lymph node
inferior deep cervical lymph nodes	jugulo-omohyoid lymph node	accessory lymph nodes
secondary nodes		

References Chapter 10, Lymphatic system. In Fehrenbach MJ, Herring SW: *Illustrated anatomy of the head and neck,* ed 6, St. Louis, 2021, Saunders; Chapter 11, Head and neck structures. In Fehrenbach MJ, Popowics T: *Illustrated dental embryology, histology, and anatomy,* ed 5, St. Louis, 2020, Saunders.

FIGURE 9.6 **Tonsils (sagittal section)**

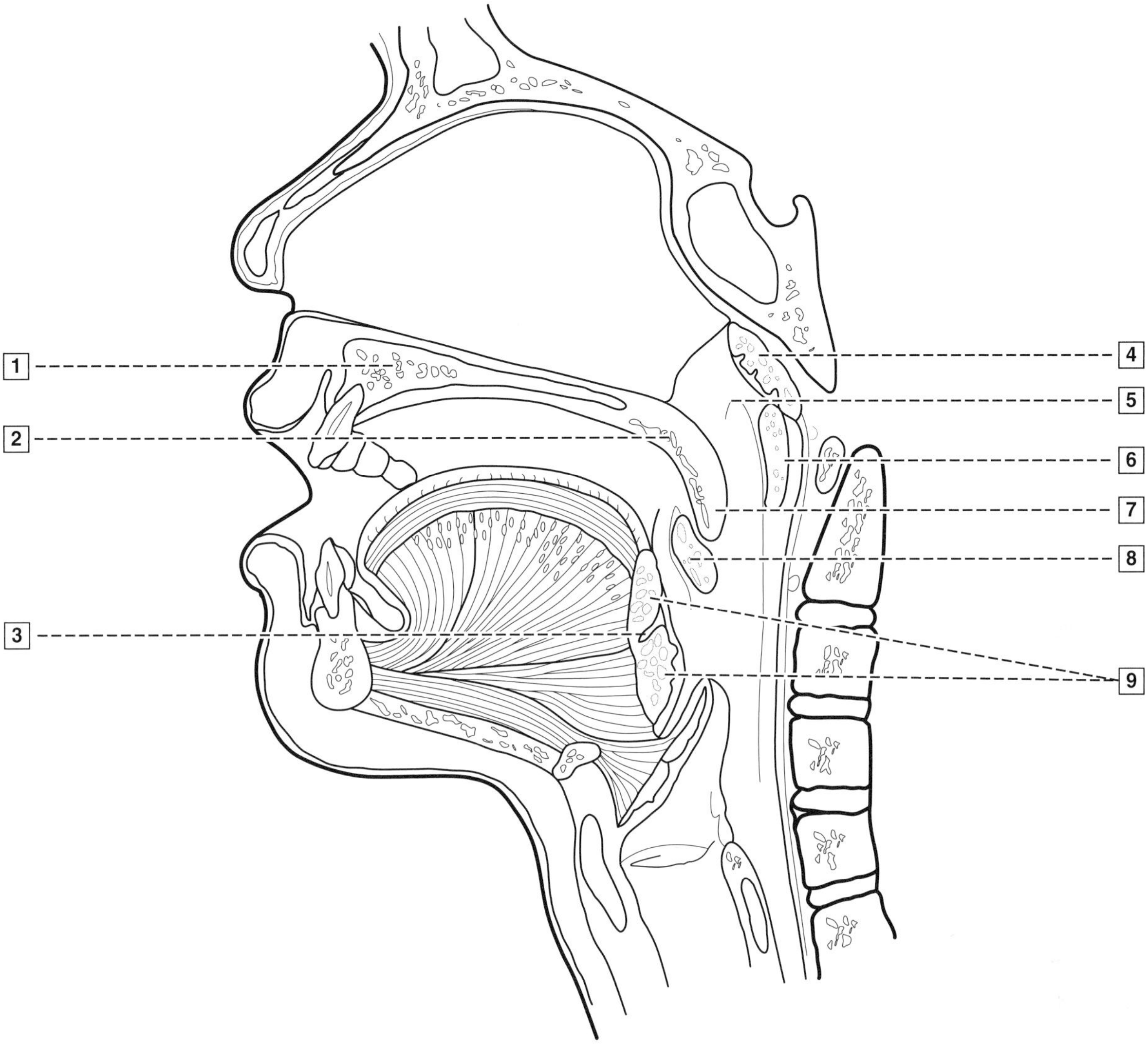

1	Hard palate	6	Tubal tonsil
2	Soft palate	7	Uvula
3	Foramen cecum	8	Palatine tonsil
4	Pharyngeal tonsil	9	Lingual tonsil
5	Opening of auditory tube		

REVIEW QUESTIONS: Tonsils

Fill in the blanks by choosing the appropriate terms from the list below.

1. The _____ are lymphoid tissue that drain as a group into the superior deep cervical lymph nodes, particularly affecting the jugulodigastric lymph node, which is considered the tonsillar node.

2. The _____, what patients call their "tonsils," are two rounded masses of variable size located in the oral cavity between the anterior and posterior faucial pillars on each side of the fauces and within the tonsillar fossa.

3. The _____ is an indistinct layer of lymphoid nodules located intraorally on the dorsal surface of the base of the tongue, posterior to the circumvallate lingual papillae; its lymphoid tissue consists of many lymphatic nodules, usually each with a germinal center and only one associated tonsillar crypt.

4. The _____ or *adenoids* location is on the midline of superior and posterior walls or roof of the nasopharynx behind the uvula, which forms an incomplete ring of lymphoid tissue along with the other tonsils, the Waldeyer ring.

5. The _____ is also located in the lateral wall of the nasopharynx, posterior to the openings of the auditory tube (pharyngotympanic tube).

6. The two vertical folds of the faucial pillars are formed by muscles of the soft palate with the palatine tonsils located between the anterior and posterior faucial pillars on each side of the fauces; the _____ forms the anterior faucial pillar while the palatopharyngeus muscle forms the posterior faucial pillar.

7. The major blood supply to the palatine tonsil is from the tonsillar branch of the _____, which penetrates the superior constrictor muscle.

8. Because sensory innervation of the oropharynx is by the _____, this nerve carries sensory innervation from the palatine tonsil.

9. The mucosa covering the pharyngeal surface of the tongue is irregular in contour because of the many small nodules of _____ in the submucosa, which collectively make up the lingual tonsil.

10. A network of veins is associated with the palatine tonsil, which drains into the _____ or directly into the facial vein.

tubal tonsil	lingual tonsil	facial artery	glossopharyngeal nerve
tonsils	pharyngeal tonsil	pharyngeal plexus of veins	lymphoid tissue
palatine tonsils	palatoglossus muscle		

References   Chapter 10, Lymphatic system. In Fehrenbach MJ, Herring SW: *Illustrated anatomy of the head and neck,* ed 6, St. Louis, 2021, Saunders; Chapter 11, Head and neck structures. In Fehrenbach MJ, Popowics T: *Illustrated dental embryology, histology, and anatomy,* ed 5, St. Louis, 2020, Saunders; Chapter 8, Head and neck. In Drake R, Vogl AW, Mitchell AWM: *Gray's anatomy for students,* ed 4, Philadelphia, 2020, Churchill Livingstone.

ANSWER KEY 1. tonsils, 2. palatine tonsils, 3. lingual tonsil, 4. pharyngeal tonsil, 5. tubal tonsil, 6. palatoglossus muscle, 7. facial artery, 8. glossopharyngeal nerve, 9. lymphoid tissue, 10. pharyngeal plexus of veins

FIGURE 9.7   Palatine tonsil (microanatomic view)

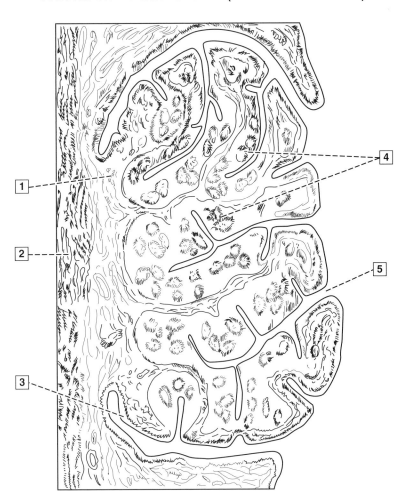

1 Connective tissue
   (lamina propria)

2 Skeletal muscle

3 Stratified squamous
   epithelium (oral epithelium)

4 Lymphatic nodules
   with germinal centers

5 Tonsillar crypt

REVIEW QUESTIONS: Palatine tonsil

Fill in the blanks by choosing the appropriate terms from the list below.

1. Intraoral tonsillar tissue, such as the palatine tonsils, consists of nonencapsulated masses of _____ located in the lamina propria of the oral mucosa.

2. The _____ are two rounded masses of lymphoid tissue of variable size located between the anterior faucial pillar and posterior faucial pillar, with each mass containing fused-together lymphatic nodules that generally have germinal centers.

3. The intraoral tonsillar tissue, such as the palatine tonsils, is covered by stratified squamous epithelium that is continuous with the surrounding oral mucosa; like lymph nodes, the tonsils contain _____, the white blood cells that remove toxic products and then move to the epithelial surface as they mature.

4. Each palatine tonsil also has 10 to 20 epithelial invaginations, or grooves, which penetrate deeply into the tonsil to form _____; these contain shed epithelial cells, mature lymphocytes, and oral bacteria.

5. Unlike lymph nodes, _____ such as the palatine tonsils is not located along lymphatic vessels but is situated near airway and food passages to protect the body against disease processes from the related toxic.

6. The lingual tonsil is an indistinct layer of diffuse lymphoid tissue located on the base of the _____ of the tongue, posterior to the circumvallate lingual papillae.

7. The lymphoid tissue of the lingual tonsil consists of many lymphatic nodules, usually each with a(n) _____ and only one associated tonsillar crypt.

8. During prenatal development, the _____ are also largely obliterated by the development of the palatine tonsil; however, a part persists as the tonsillar fossa between the tonsillar pillars.

9. The tonsils have on their cellular surface specialized antigen-capture cells, the M cells, that allow for the uptake of antigens produced by the pathogens; these M cells then alert the underlying B cells and T cells to produce a(n) _____.

10. The B cells are activated and proliferate in the germinal centers in the tonsil, where B memory cells are created to _____ since they are associated with IgA.

lymphocytes	immune response	secretory antibody
tonsillar crypts	lymphoid tissue	germinal center
intraoral tonsillar tissue	palatine tonsils	second pharyngeal pouches
	dorsal surface	

References Chapter 11, Head and neck structures. In Fehrenbach MJ, Popowics T: *Illustrated dental embryology, histology, and anatomy,* ed 5, St. Louis, 2020, Saunders; Chapter 2, Embryology of the head, face, and oral cavity. In Nanci A: *Ten Cate's Oral Histology,* ed 9, St. Louis, 2018, Mosby.

ANSWER KEY 1. lymphoid tissue, 2. palatine tonsils, 3. lymphocytes, 4. tonsillar crypts, 5. intraoral tonsillar tissue, 6. dorsal surface, 7. germinal center, 8. second pharyngeal pouches, 9. immune response, 10. secretory antibody

FIGURE 10.1   Fasciae: Face (coronal section of head)

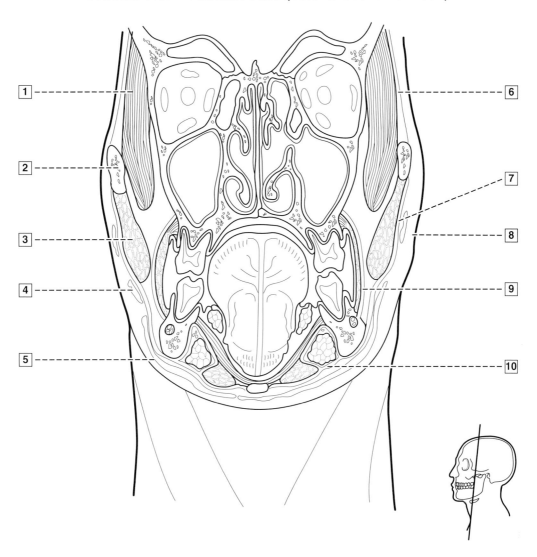

1	Temporalis muscle	6	Temporal fascia
2	Zygomatic bone	7	Masseteric-parotid fascia
3	Masseter muscle	8	Superficial fascia
4	Risorius muscle	9	Buccopharyngeal part of visceral fascia
5	Platysma muscle	10	Investing fascia

REVIEW QUESTIONS: Fasciae: Face

Fill in the blanks by choosing the appropriate terms from the list below.

1. The _____ consists of layer upon layer of fibrous connective tissue.

2. The fascia lies just deep to and connected to the _____ that surrounds the much deeper muscles, bones, vessels, nerves, organs, and other structures; the fasciae of the head and neck and other areas of the body can be divided into either the superficial fasciae or the deep fasciae.

3. Potential spaces are created between the layers of fascia of the body because of the sheetlike nature of fasciae; these potential spaces are termed _____ or *fascial planes*.

4. Layers of superficial fascia are found just deep to and attached to the skin in most cases, the layers of superficial fascia separate skin from deeper structures, allowing the skin to _____ independently of these deeper structures.

5. The layers of superficial fascia vary in thickness in different parts of the body and are composed of fat tissue as well as irregularly arranged _____.

6. The blood vessels and _____ of the skin also travel in the superficial fascia.

7. In contrast to superficial fascia, the layers of _____ cover the deeper structures of the body including the head and neck such as the bones, muscles, nerves, and vessels.

8. The layers of deep fascia consist of a dense and inelastic fibrous tissue forming _____ around the deeper structures of the body.

9. The layers of superficial fasciae of the body do not usually enclose _____, except for the superficial fasciae of the face and neck.

10. The superficial fascia of the face encloses most of the _____, a group of striated muscles innervated by the seventh cranial or facial nerve that among other things control facial expression.

deep fascia	sheaths	muscles of facial expression
nerves	fascial spaces	move
fascia	muscles	connective tissue
skin		

Reference Chapter 11, Fasciae and spaces. In Fehrenbach MJ, Herring SW: *Illustrated anatomy of the head and neck*, ed 6, St. Louis, 2021, Saunders.

NOTES

FIGURE 10.2   Fasciae: Face, jaws, and cervical (transverse sections of oral cavity and neck)

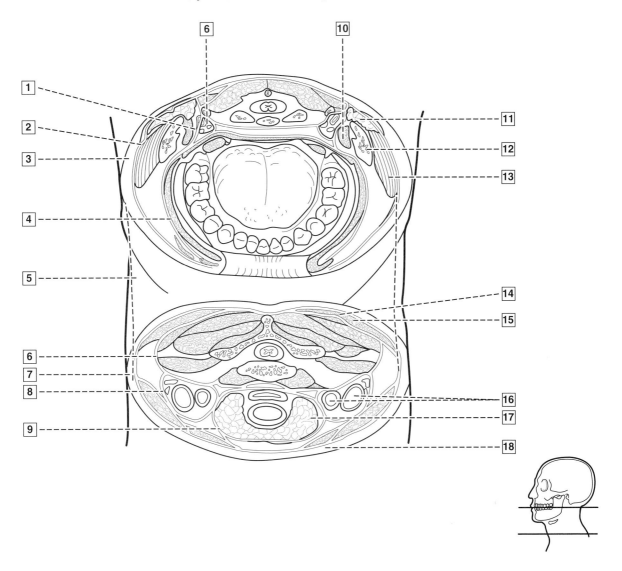

1	Pterygoid fascia	**7**	Investing fascia	**13**	Masseter muscle
2	Masseteric-parotid fascia	**8**	Carotid sheath	**14**	Trapezius muscle
3	Superficial fascia	**9**	Visceral fascia	**15**	Vertebral muscle
4	Buccopharyngeal visceral fascia	**10**	Medial pterygoid muscle	**16**	Internal carotid artery and internal jugular vein
5	Continuous layer	**11**	Parotid salivary gland	**17**	Thyroid gland
6	Vertebral fascia	**12**	Mandible	**18**	Platysma muscle

REVIEW QUESTIONS: Fasciae: Face, jaws, and cervical

Fill in the blanks by choosing the appropriate terms from the list below.

1. The _____ of the neck contains the platysma muscle, which covers most of the anterior cervical triangle as well as parts of the anterior and external jugular veins.

2. The layers of _____ associated with the face and jaws are divided into the temporal, the masseteric-parotid, and the pterygoid fasciae, which are continuous with each other.

3. The _____ of the deep fasciae of the face and jaws covers the temporalis muscle and structures superior to the zygomatic arch.

4. The _____ of the deep fasciae of the face and jaws covers the masseter muscle and structures inferior to the zygomatic arch and surrounds the parotid salivary gland.

5. The _____ of the deep fasciae of the face and jaws is located on the medial surface of the medial pterygoid muscle.

6. The layers of _____ include the investing fascia, the carotid sheath, the visceral fascia, the buccopharyngeal fascia, and the vertebral fascia.

7. The layers of the various regions of deep cervical fascia are _____ with each other.

8. The investing fascia or *superficial layer of the deep cervical fascia* is the most _____ layer of deep cervical fascia.

9. The investing fascia of deep cervical fascia surrounds the _____, continuing onto the masseteric-parotid fascia.

10. The _____ of deep cervical fascia splits around two salivary glands (submandibular and parotid) and two superficial cervical muscles (sternocleidomastoid and trapezius), enclosing them completely; the branching laminae from this fascia provide the deep fasciae that surround the infrahyoid muscles, running from the hyoid bone inferiorly to the sternum.

neck	temporal fascia	superficial cervical fascia
investing fascia	continuous	deep fasciae
masseteric-parotid fascia	pterygoid fascia	deep cervical fasciae
external		

Reference Chapter 11, Fasciae and spaces. In Fehrenbach MJ, Herring SW: *Illustrated anatomy of the head and neck*, ed 6, St. Louis, 2021, Saunders.

NOTES

FIGURE 10.3   **Fasciae: Deep cervical (midsagittal section of head and neck)**

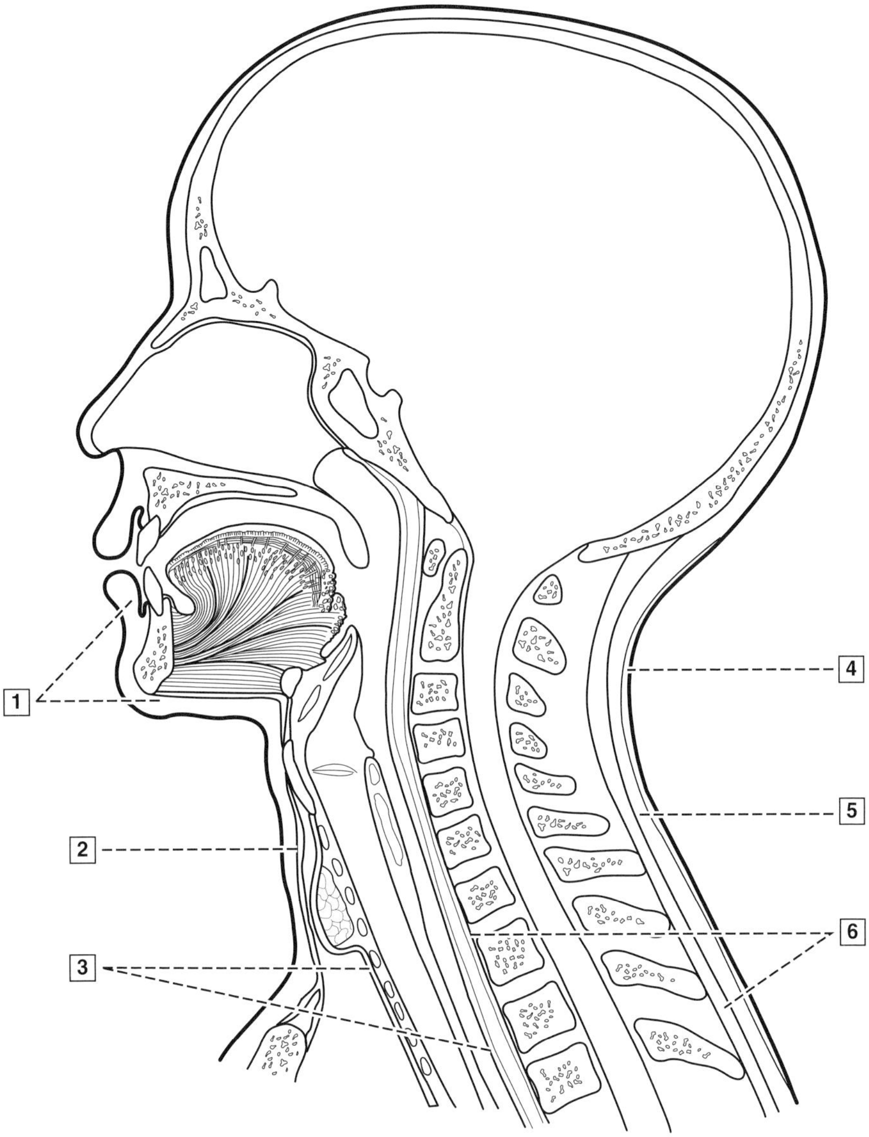

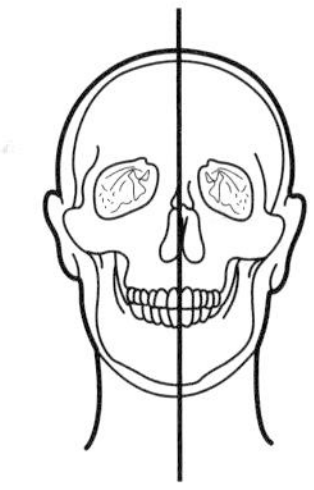

1 Superficial fascia
(contains muscles of facial expression)

2 Investing fascia

3 Visceral fascia

4 Superficial fascia

5 Investing fascia

6 Vertebral fascia

REVIEW QUESTIONS: Fasciae: Deep cervical

Fill in the blanks by choosing the appropriate terms from the list below.

1. The layers of _____ include the investing fascia, the carotid sheath, the visceral fascia, the buccopharyngeal fascia, and the vertebral fascia.

2. The investing fascia or *superficial layer of the deep cervical fascia* is the most external layer of deep cervical fascia, surrounding the neck, and continuing onto the _____.

3. The _____ also splits around two salivary glands (submandibular and parotid) and two superficial cervical muscles (sternocleidomastoid and trapezius), enclosing them completely; branching laminae from this fascia also provide the deep fasciae that surround the infrahyoid muscles, running from the hyoid bone inferiorly to the sternum.

4. The _____ is a bilateral tube of deep cervical fascia deep to the investing fascia and sternocleidomastoid muscle; it runs inferiorly along each side of the neck from the base of the skull to the thorax (chest) and borders the vascular compartments of the neck.

5. The carotid sheath contains the _____, the common carotid artery, and the internal jugular vein, as well as the tenth cranial or vagus nerve; all of these contents travel between the braincase and the thorax (chest) within the sheath.

6. Deep and parallel to the carotid sheath is the _____ or *pretracheal fascia*, which is a single midline tube of deep cervical fascia running inferiorly along the neck and covering the floor of the anterior cervical triangle.

7. The visceral fascia of the deep cervical fascia contains the _____, esophagus, and thyroid gland; the visceral fascia also borders the visceral compartment of the neck.

8. Nearer to the skull, the layer of visceral fascia located posterior and lateral to the pharynx is the _____.

9. The buccopharyngeal fascia of the visceral fascia encloses the entire superior part of the alimentary canal and is continuous with the fascia covering the buccinator muscle at a location where that muscle and the superior pharyngeal constrictor muscle come together at the _____, which is present in the oral cavity as the pterygomandibular fold.

10. The deepest layer of the deep cervical fascia, the _____ or *prevertebral fascia*, covers the spinal cord, cervical vertebrae, and associated vertebral muscles; the fascia borders the vertebral compartment of the neck.

carotid sheath	vertebral fascia	pterygomandibular raphe
internal carotid artery	buccopharyngeal fascia	masseteric-parotid fascia
deep cervical fasciae	visceral fascia	investing fascia
trachea		

Reference Chapter 11, Fasciae and spaces. In Fehrenbach MJ, Herring SW: *Illustrated anatomy of the head and neck*, ed 6, St. Louis, 2021, Saunders.

FIGURE 10.4   Fasciae: Deep cervical (transverse section of neck)

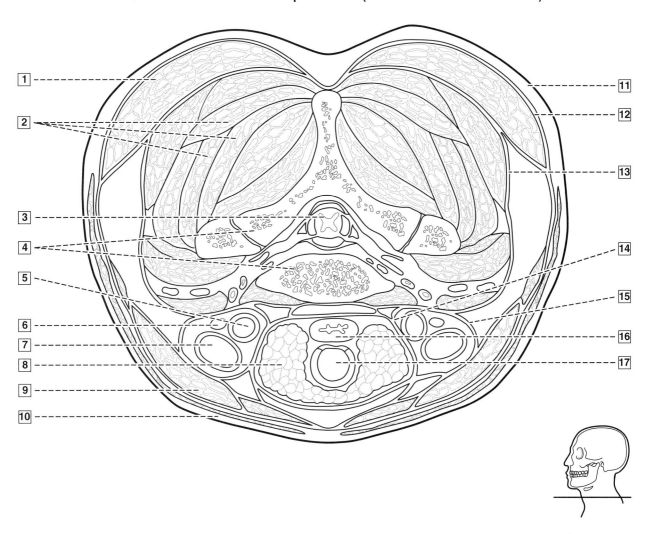

1	Trapezius muscle	7	Internal jugular vein	13	Vertebral fascia
2	Vertebral muscles	8	Thyroid gland	14	Visceral fascia
3	Spinal cord	9	Sternocleidomastoid muscle	15	Carotid sheath
4	Cervical vertebra	10	Platysma muscle	16	Esophagus
5	Common carotid artery	11	Superficial fascia	17	Trachea
6	Vagus nerve	12	Investing fascia		

REVIEW QUESTIONS: Fasciae: Deep cervical

Fill in the blanks by choosing the appropriate terms from the list below.

1. The carotid sheath is a bilateral tube of deep cervical fascia deep to the investing fascia and _____, a major superficial cervical muscle; this sheath runs inferiorly along each side of the neck from the base of the skull to the thorax (chest) and borders the vascular compartments of the neck.

2. The carotid sheath contains the internal carotid artery, the common carotid artery, and the _____, as well as the tenth cranial nerve or vagus nerve; all of these structures travel between the braincase and the thorax (chest) within the sheath.

3. Deep and parallel to the carotid sheath is the _____ or *pretracheal fascia*, which is a single midline tube of deep cervical fascia running inferiorly along the neck and covering the floor of the anterior cervical triangle that contains the trachea, esophagus, and thyroid gland.

4. Nearer to the skull, the layer of visceral fascia located posterior and lateral to the pharynx is the _____; this deep cervical fascia encloses the entire superior part of the alimentary canal and is continuous with the fascia covering the buccinator muscle, a location where that muscle and the superior pharyngeal constrictor muscle come together at the pterygomandibular raphe, which is present in the oral cavity as the pterygomandibular fold.

5. The pterygomandibular raphe or fold is a(n) _____ for the administration of the inferior alveolar nerve block.

6. The deepest layer of the deep cervical fascia, the _____ or *prevertebral fascia*, covers the spinal cord, cervical vertebrae, and associated vertebral muscles; the fascia borders the vertebral compartment of the neck.

7. The two carotid sheaths border each two bilateral _____ of the neck (or lateral compartments) that are located lateral and posterior to the pharynx.

8. The visceral fascia borders the single _____ of the neck (or anterior compartment).

9. The vertebral fascia borders the single _____ of the neck (or posterior compartment).

10. Some anatomists distinguish a separate layer of the vertebral fascia called the _____, which runs from the base of the skull to connect with the visceral fascia inferiorly in the neck.

vertebral compartment	vertebral fascia	visceral compartment
sternocleidomastoid muscle	buccopharyngeal fascia	landmark
internal jugular vein	vascular compartments	alar fascia
visceral fascia		

Reference Chapter 11, Fasciae and spaces. In Fehrenbach MJ, Herring SW: *Illustrated anatomy of the head and neck*, ed 6, St. Louis, 2021, Saunders.

FIGURE 10.5   Spaces: Face, jaws, and vestibular (coronal section of head and neck)

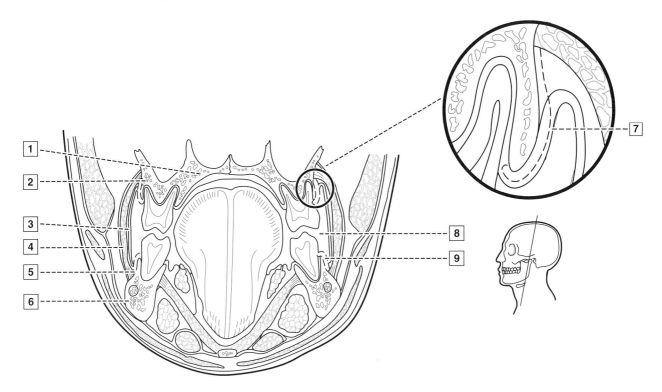

1	Palatine process of maxilla	**6**	Body of mandible
2	Alveolar process of maxilla	**7**	Vestibular space of maxilla
3	Oral mucosa	**8**	Vestibule of mouth
4	Buccinator muscle	**9**	Vestibular space of mandible
5	Alveolar process of mandible		

REVIEW QUESTIONS: Spaces: Face, jaws, and vestibular

Fill in the blanks by choosing the appropriate terms from the list below.

1. Potential spaces are created between the layers of fascia of the body because of the sheetlike nature of fasciae and are termed _____ or *fascial planes*.

2. Unlike the neck, the spaces of the face and jaws are often defined by the arrangement of _____ forming borders, in addition to the surrounding fasciae; thus, many of the major spaces located in the head are not strictly considered fascial spaces.

3. The spaces of the face and jaws can communicate with each other directly and with the _____.

4. The major spaces of the _____ include the vestibular space of the maxilla, vestibular space of the mandible, canine space, parotid space, buccal space, masticator space, space of the body of the mandible, submental space, submandibular space, and sublingual space.

5. The space of the upper jaw, the _____, is located medial to the buccinator muscle and inferior to the attachment of this muscle along the alveolar process of the maxilla.

6. The vestibular space of the maxilla lateral wall is the _____.

7. The vestibular space of the maxilla communicates with the _____ and associated periodontium and gingiva.

8. The space of the lower jaw, the _____, is located between the buccinator muscle and overlying oral mucosa.

9. The vestibular space of the mandible is bordered by the attachment of the buccinator muscle onto the _____.

10. The vestibular space of the mandible communicates with the _____ and associated periodontium and gingiva, as well as the space of the body of the mandible.

oral mucosa	vestibular space of the mandible	face and jaws
muscles and bones	alveolar process of the mandible	cervical fascial spaces
vestibular space of the maxilla	fascial spaces	mandibular posterior teeth
maxillary molars		

Reference Chapter 11, Fasciae and spaces. In Fehrenbach MJ, Herring SW: *Illustrated anatomy of the head and neck*, ed 6, St. Louis, 2021, Saunders.

NOTES

FIGURE 10.6 Spaces: Canine and buccal (frontal and cutaway views of head)

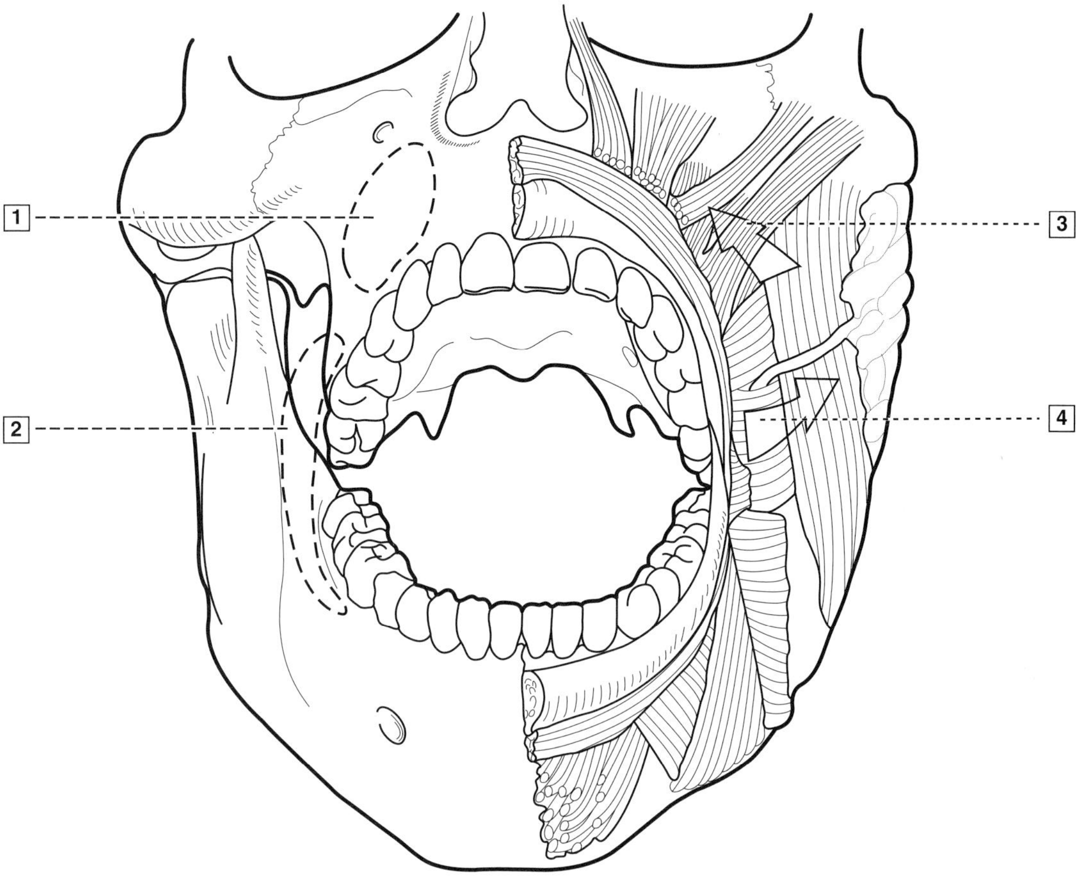

1 Canine space

2 Buccal space

3 Arrow entering canine space (deep to muscles that elevate lip)

4 Arrow entering buccal space (deep to masseter muscle)

REVIEW QUESTIONS: Spaces: Canine and buccal

Fill in the blanks by choosing the appropriate terms from the list below.

1. The _____ as a space of the face and jaws is located superior to the upper lip and lateral to the apex of the maxillary canine, deep to the overlying skin and muscles of facial expression that elevate the upper lip, levator labii superioris, and zygomaticus minor muscles.

2. The floor of the canine space is the depression of the _____ on the maxilla, which is covered by the periosteum and is bordered anteriorly by the orbicularis oris muscle and posteriorly by the levator anguli oris muscle.

3. The canine space contains the angular artery and vein as well as the _____ nerve and vessels.

4. The _____ as a fascial space of the face and jaws is formed between the buccinator muscle (actually the buccopharyngeal fascia) and masseter muscle; therefore, it is inferior to the zygomatic arch, superior to the mandible, lateral to the buccinator muscle, and medial and anterior to the masseter muscle.

5. The bilateral buccal space is partially covered by the platysma muscle, as well as by an extension of fascia from the parotid salivary gland capsule; the space contains the _____, parotid duct, and facial artery.

6. The canine space and buccal space communicate with each other, and the buccal space also communicates with the _____ and the space of the body of the mandible.

7. The buccal space contains the buccal fat pad, parotid duct, and _____.

8. Inferior to the infraorbital foramen is an elongated depression, the canine fossa, which is just posterosuperior to each of the roots of the _____.

9. The _____ covers a dense pad of inner tissue, the buccal fat pad.

10. The duct associated with the parotid salivary gland is the _____ (or Stenson); this long duct emerges from the anterior border of the gland, superficial to the masseter muscle, which then pierces the buccinator muscle, and then opens up into the oral cavity on the inner surface of the buccal mucosa of the cheek, usually opposite the maxillary second molar.

canine space	buccal fat pad	maxillary canines
canine fossa	facial artery	buccal mucosa
pterygomandibular space	infraorbital	parotid duct
buccal space		

Reference Chapter 11, Fasciae and spaces. In Fehrenbach MJ, Herring SW: *Illustrated anatomy of the head and neck*, ed 6, St. Louis, 2021, Saunders.

FIGURE 10.7   Spaces: Parotid (transverse section of head and neck)

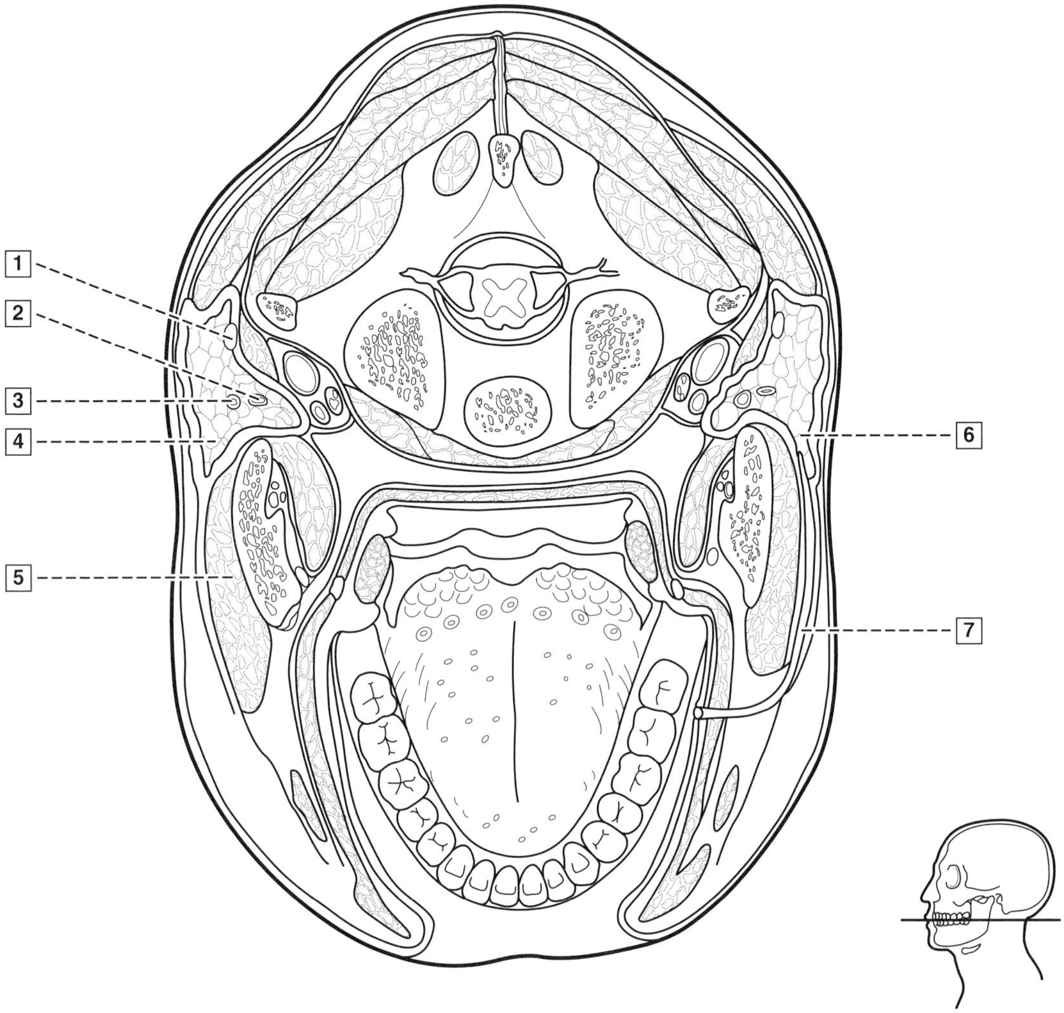

1	Facial nerve
2	Retromandibular vein
3	External carotid artery
4	Parotid salivary gland
5	Masseter muscle
6	Parotid space
7	Parotid duct

REVIEW QUESTIONS: Spaces: Parotid

Fill in the blanks by choosing the appropriate terms from the list below.

1. The parotid salivary gland extends irregularly from the _____ to the angle of the mandible.

2. The parotid space is created inside the investing fascial layer of the _____ as it envelops the entire parotid salivary gland.

3. The parotid space contains the entire _____, the largest of the major salivary glands.

4. The parotid space contains part of the seventh cranial nerve or _____, external carotid artery, and retromandibular vein.

5. The fascial _____ of the parotid space help to keep pathology associated with the parotid salivary gland (such as cancer) from spreading to other sites.

6. Communication by the parotid space occurs with _____, which is a bilateral fascial space lateral to the pharynx and medial to the medial pterygoid muscle, parallel to the carotid sheath, with connections to the retropharyngeal space.

7. The parotid salivary gland occupies the parotid space, an area posterior to the _____, anterior and inferior to the ear.

8. The parotid salivary gland is the largest encapsulated _____ salivary gland but does not contribute the most to the total salivary volume.

9. The seventh cranial nerve or facial nerve (VII) then passes into the parotid salivary gland and divides the gland into larger superficial and smaller deep lobes; the trunk of the facial nerve itself divides into numerous branches to supply the _____, but does not innervate the parotid salivary gland itself.

10. The seventh cranial nerve or facial nerve (VII) within the parotid salivary gland can also become _____ by both an incorrectly administered inferior alveolar or Vazirani-Akinosi mandibular nerve blocks with an overreaching needle that does not contact the medial surface of the mandibular ramus.

major	deep cervical fascia	mandibular ramus
facial nerve	parotid salivary gland	muscles of facial expression
zygomatic arch	parapharyngeal space	anesthetized
borders		

References Chapter 7, Glandular tissue. In Fehrenbach MJ, Herring SW: *Illustrated anatomy of the head and neck*, ed 6, St. Louis, 2021, Saunders; Chapter 11, Fasciae and spaces. In Fehrenbach MJ, Herring SW: *Illustrated anatomy of the head and neck*, ed 6, St. Louis, 2021, Saunders.

ANSWER KEY 1. zygomatic arch, 2. deep cervical fascia, 3. parotid salivary gland, 4. facial nerve, 5. borders, 6. parapharyngeal space, 7. mandibular ramus, 8. major, 9. muscles of facial expression, 10. anesthetized

FIGURE 10.8   Spaces: Temporal and infratemporal (coronal section of head)

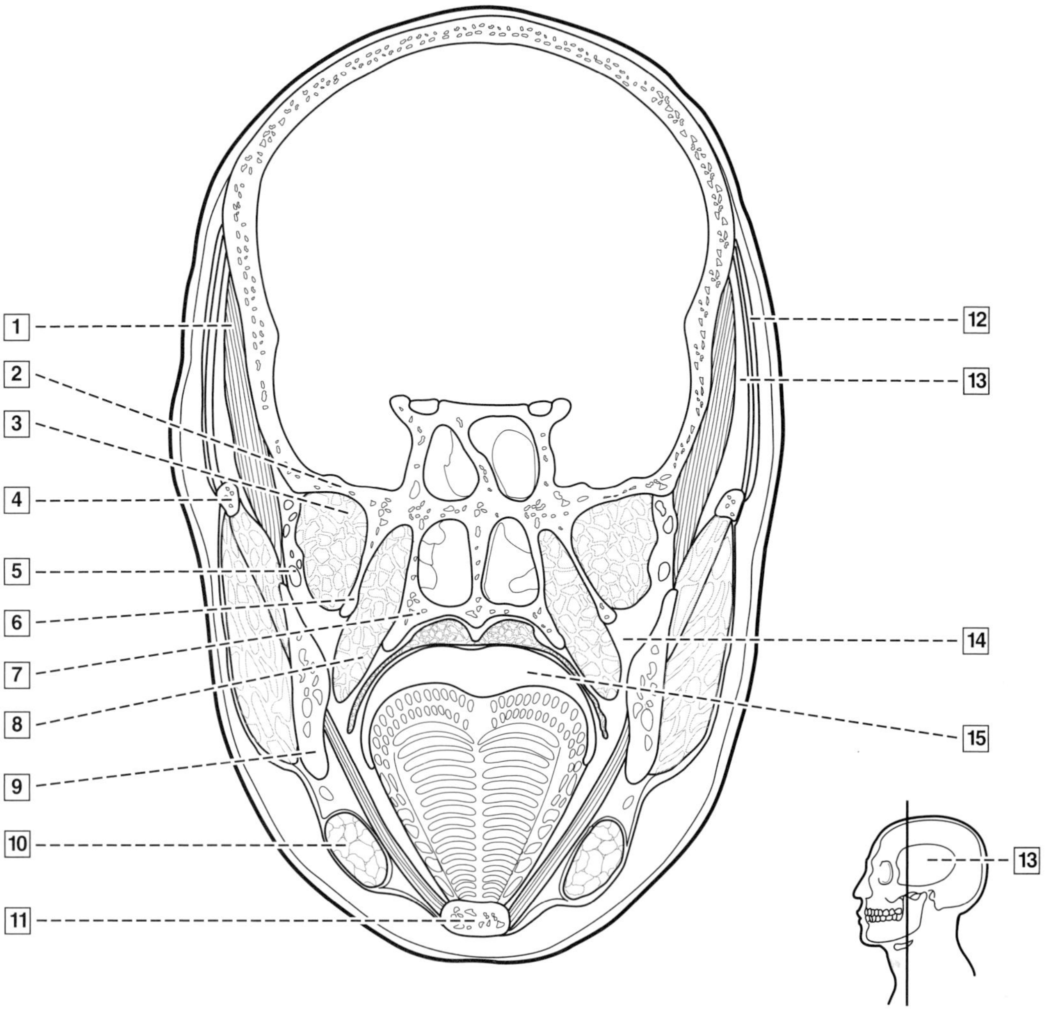

1	Temporalis muscle	**9**	Mandible
2	Infratemporal crest	**10**	Submandibular salivary gland
3	Lateral pterygoid muscle	**11**	Hyoid bone
4	Zygomatic bone	**12**	Temporal fascia
5	Maxillary artery	**13**	Temporal space
6	Lateral pterygoid plate	**14**	Infratemporal space
7	Medial pterygoid plate	**15**	Oral cavity
8	Medial pterygoid muscle		

REVIEW QUESTIONS: Spaces: Temporal and infratemporal

Fill in the blanks by choosing the appropriate terms from the list below.

1. The _____ is a general designation used to include the entire area of the mandible and associated muscles of mastication.

2. The masticator space includes the temporal, infratemporal, and submasseteric spaces, as well as one of the muscles of mastication, the _____ and both the mandibular ramus and the body of the mandible.

3. A part of the masticator space is the _____, which is formed by the temporal fascia anterior to the temporalis muscle; it can be divided into either superficial or deep temporal spaces.

4. The temporal space is between the temporal fascia and temporalis muscle and therefore extends from the _____ inferiorly to the zygomatic arch and infratemporal crest.

5. The temporal space contains fat tissue and communicates with the infratemporal space and the _____.

6. The infratemporal space is a part of the masticator space and occupies the _____, an area adjacent to the lateral pterygoid plate of the sphenoid bone and maxillary tuberosity of the maxilla.

7. The infratemporal space is bordered laterally by the medial surface of the _____ and the temporalis muscle, with its roof formed by the infratemporal surface of the greater wing of the sphenoid bone; medially, the space is bordered anteriorly by the lateral pterygoid plate and posteriorly by the pharynx with its visceral layer of deep fascia.

8. There is no border inferiorly and posteriorly for the infratemporal space, where the space is continuous with a more inferior and deep cervical fascial space, the _____.

9. The infratemporal space contains a part of the _____ as it branches (such as the inferior alveolar artery), the mandibular nerve and its branches, and the pterygoid plexus of veins; it also contains the medial and lateral pterygoid muscles.

10. The infratemporal space communicates with the temporal space and submasseteric space, as well as with the _____ and parapharyngeal space of the neck.

submandibular space	maxillary artery	mandible
parapharyngeal space	masseter muscle	submasseteric space
superior temporal line	masticator space	infratemporal fossa
temporal space		

Reference Chapter 11, Fasciae and spaces. In Fehrenbach MJ, Herring SW: *Illustrated anatomy of the head and neck*, ed 6, St. Louis, 2021, Saunders.

FIGURE 10.9 Spaces: Infratemporal and pterygomandibular (midsagittal section of head)

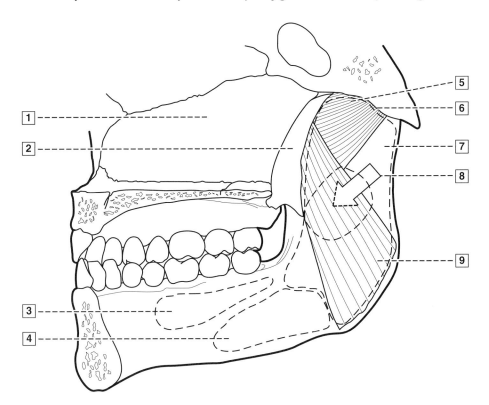

1 Vomer		**6** Infratemporal crest	
2 Medial pterygoid plate		**7** Infratemporal space	
3 Area of sublingual space		**8** Arrow entering pterygomandibular space (outlined)	
4 Area of submandibular space		**9** Medial pterygoid muscle	
5 Lateral pterygoid muscle			

REVIEW QUESTIONS: Spaces: Infratemporal and pterygomandibular

Fill in the blanks by choosing the appropriate terms from the list below.

1. The _____ is a space that is part of the masticator space and occupies the infratemporal fossa, an area adjacent to the lateral pterygoid plate of the sphenoid bone and maxillary tuberosity of the maxilla, bordered laterally by the medial surface of the mandible and the temporalis muscle, with its roof formed by the infratemporal surface of the greater wing of the sphenoid bone; medially, the space is bordered anteriorly by the lateral pterygoid plate and posteriorly by the pharynx with its visceral layer of deep fascia.

2. There is no border inferiorly and posteriorly for the infratemporal space, where the space is continuous with a more inferior and deep cervical fascial space, the _____.

3. The _____ is a space that is part of the infratemporal space and is bordered by the medial pterygoid muscle medially and the medial surface of the mandibular ramus laterally; posteriorly, the parotid salivary gland curves medially around the posterior border of the mandibular ramus, while anteriorly the buccinator and superior constrictor muscles come together to form a tendinous band, the medially located pterygomandibular raphe or pterygomandibular fold intraorally.

4. The pterygomandibular space contains the _____ and blood vessels as well as the lingual nerve and is the target area for the inferior alveolar nerve block as well as the Vazirani-Akinosi mandibular nerve block.

5. The pterygomandibular space communicates with both the _____ and the parapharyngeal space of the neck.

6. The infratemporal space contains a part of the _____ as its branches, the mandibular nerve and its branches, and the pterygoid plexus of veins; it also contains the medial and lateral pterygoid muscles.

7. The infratemporal space communicates with the _____ and submasseteric space, as well as with the submandibular space and parapharyngeal space.

8. The infratemporal fossa is a paired depression that is inferior to the anterior part of the _____.

9. The infratemporal crest on the greater wing of the _____ contributes to both the adjoining temporal fossa and infratemporal fossa.

10. The infratemporal fossa also contains a part of the _____ (or third division) of the fifth cranial or trigeminal nerve (V) including the inferior alveolar and lingual nerves; the mandibular nerve enters by way of the foramen ovale, passing between the cranial cavity and oral cavity.

sphenoid bone	maxillary artery	temporal space
inferior alveolar nerve	parapharyngeal space	temporal fossa
infratemporal space	pterygomandibular space	
submandibular space	mandibular nerve	

Reference   Chapter 11, Fasciae and spaces. In Fehrenbach MJ, Herring SW: *Illustrated anatomy of the head and neck*, ed 6, St. Louis, 2021, Saunders.

FIGURE 10.10   Spaces: Pterygomandibular (transverse section of head and neck)

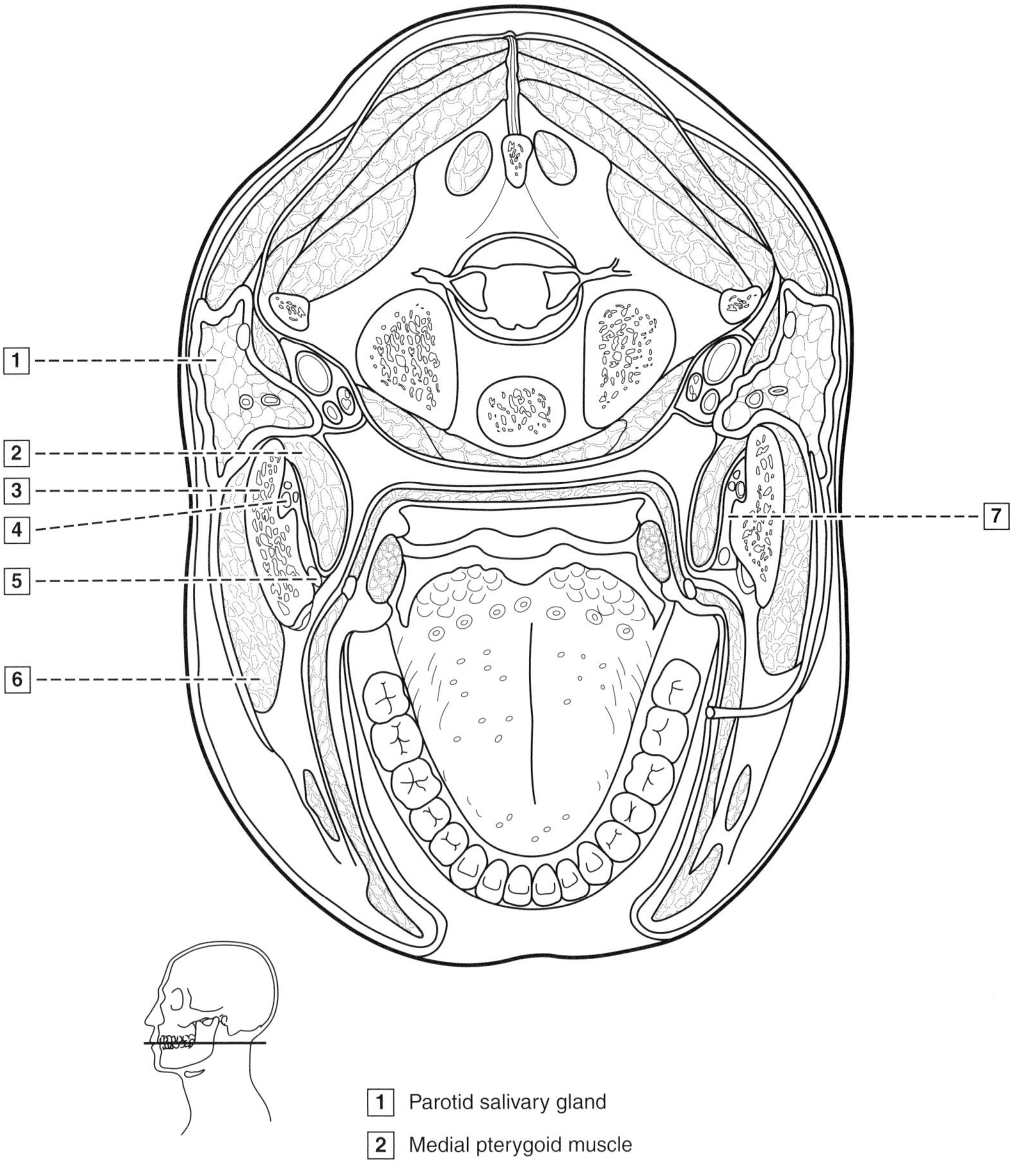

1 Parotid salivary gland

2 Medial pterygoid muscle

3 Mandible

4 Inferior alveolar nerve

5 Lingual nerve

6 Masseter muscle

7 Pterygomandibular space

REVIEW QUESTIONS: Spaces: Pterygomandibular

Fill in the blanks by choosing the appropriate terms from the list below.

1. The _____ is a space that is a part of the infratemporal space, which is a masticator space.

2. The pterygomandibular space is bordered by the _____ medially and the medial surface of the mandibular ramus laterally.

3. The pterygomandibular space is a small fascial-lined cleft containing mostly _____.

4. The pterygomandibular space contains the inferior alveolar nerve and _____ as well as the lingual nerve; it serves as the target area for the inferior alveolar nerve block as well as the Vazirani-Akinosi mandibular nerve block.

5. The pterygomandibular space communicates with both the submandibular space and the _____ of the neck.

6. The _____ is anesthetized when administering an inferior alveolar nerve block through diffusion of the local anesthetic agent.

7. The position of the _____ is approximately two-thirds the distance from the coronoid notch to the posterior border of the mandibular ramus, entirely within the pterygomandibular space.

8. The _____ is anesthetized by the inferior alveolar nerve block within the pterygomandibular space.

9. The injection site of the inferior alveolar nerve block is within the depth of the pterygomandibular space, lateral to both the _____ and the sphenomandibular ligament.

10. For the inferior alveolar nerve block, the needle is inserted into the soft tissue and advanced within the depth of the pterygomandibular space until gentle contact with the bony medial surface of the _____, and then the injection is administered.

blood vessels	parapharyngeal space	mandibular foramen
mandibular ramus	pterygomandibular space	inferior alveolar nerve
medial pterygoid muscle	pterygomandibular fold	loose connective tissue
lingual nerve		

References   Chapter 9, Anatomy of local anesthesia. In Fehrenbach MJ, Herring SW: *Illustrated anatomy of the head and neck*, ed 6, St. Louis, 2021, Saunders; Chapter 11, Fasciae and spaces. In Fehrenbach MJ, Herring SW: *Illustrated anatomy of the head and neck*, ed 6, St. Louis, 2021, Saunders.

NOTES

FIGURE 10.11 Spaces: Submasseteric (lateral views of head and mandible)

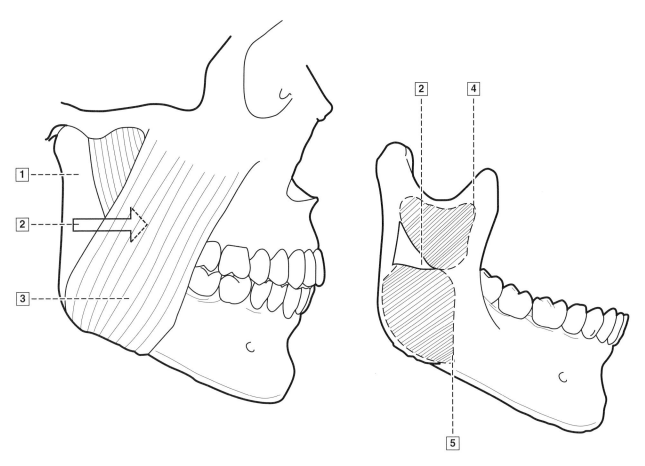

1 Mandibular ramus

2 Arrow entering (or where it entered) submasseteric space

3 Masseter muscle

4 Insertion of deep head of masseter muscle

5 Insertion of superficial head of masseter muscle

REVIEW QUESTIONS: Spaces: Submasseteric

Fill in the blanks by choosing the appropriate terms from the list below.

1. The general designation of _____ is used to describe a space that includes the entire area of the mandible and associated muscles of mastication, which includes the masseter and temporalis muscles, as well as the medial and lateral pterygoids.

2. The masticator space includes the temporal space, infratemporal space, and _____.

3. The masticator space also includes the masseter muscle and both the mandibular ramus and body of the _____.

4. The submasseteric space is located between the _____ and the external surface of the vertical mandibular ramus.

5. The submasseteric space communicates with both the _____ and the infratemporal space.

6. The submasseteric space contains the masseteric artery and _____.

7. The _____ supplies the masseter muscle.

8. All parts of the masticator space communicate with each other, as well as with the _____ and a nearby cervical fascial space, the parapharyngeal space.

9. The spaces of the head and neck communicate with each other directly, as well as through the associated _____ and lymph vessels contained within the space.

10. The communication between spaces may allow the spread of _____ (or odontogenic) from an initial superficial area in the face and jaws to more vital deeper structures in the neck or even travel to the brain.

blood vessels	masseteric artery	submandibular space
submasseteric space	masseter muscle	dental infection
mandible	masticator space	
temporal space	masseteric vein	

Reference Chapter 11, Fasciae and spaces. In Fehrenbach MJ, Herring SW: *Illustrated anatomy of the head and neck*, ed 6, St. Louis, 2021, Saunders.

NOTES

FIGURE 10.12 Spaces: Body of the mandible (coronal section of head and neck)

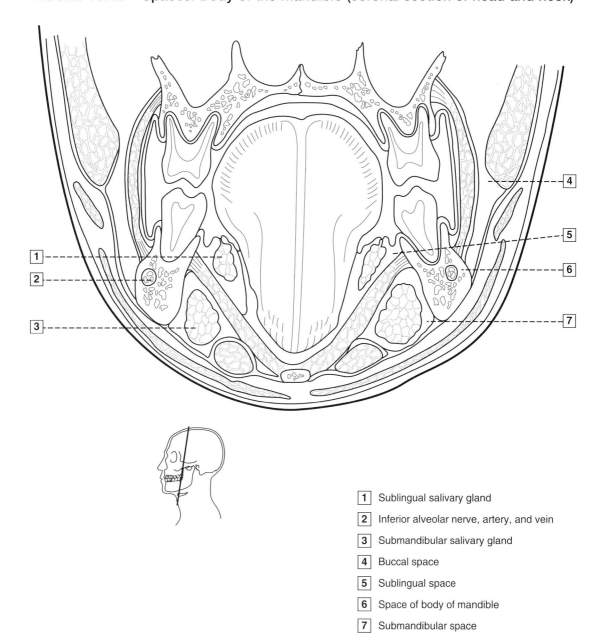

1 Sublingual salivary gland

2 Inferior alveolar nerve, artery, and vein

3 Submandibular salivary gland

4 Buccal space

5 Sublingual space

6 Space of body of mandible

7 Submandibular space

REVIEW QUESTIONS: Spaces: Body of the mandible

Fill in the blanks by choosing the appropriate terms from the list below.

1. The _____ is formed by the periosteum covering part of the bony surface of the mandible, which is a specialized connective tissue membrane that lines the outer surface of all bones.

2. The space of the body of the mandible is anterior to the body of the _____, from its symphysis to the anterior borders of both the masseter and medial pterygoid muscles.

3. The space of the body of the mandible contains the mandible and a part of the _____, a branch of the mandibular nerve.

4. The space of the body of the mandible also contains the _____, and the dental and alveolar branches of these blood vessels, as well as the mental and incisive branches.

5. The space of the body of the mandible communicates with the _____ of the mandible.

6. The space of the body of the mandible also communicates with the _____, submental space, submandibular space, and sublingual space.

7. In the midline on the anterior surface of the mandible is a faint ridge, an indication of the _____, demonstrating the fusion of right and left mandibular processes during the embryologic development of the mandible.

8. The mandible is a single facial bone that forms the lower jaw and is the only freely movable bone of the skull; the mandible has its movable articulation with the _____ at each temporomandibular joint.

9. The _____ is a broad and thick flat rectangular muscle (almost quadrilateral) of mastication on each side of the face that is anterior to the parotid salivary gland.

10. Deeper, yet similar in its rectangular form to the more superficial masseter muscle, is another muscle of mastication, the _____.

temporal bone	masseter muscle	medial pterygoid muscle
vestibular space	inferior alveolar artery and vein	buccal space
inferior alveolar nerve	space of the body of the mandible	mandibular symphysis
mandible		

References Chapter 4, Muscular system. In Fehrenbach MJ, Herring SW: *Illustrated anatomy of the head and neck*, ed 6, St. Louis, 2021, Saunders; Chapter 11, Fasciae and spaces. In Fehrenbach MJ, Herring SW: *Illustrated anatomy of the head and neck*, ed 6, St. Louis, 2021, Saunders.

NOTES

FIGURE 10.13 Spaces: Submental and submandibular (anterolateral view with skin and platysma muscle removed, leaving superficial cervical fasciae)

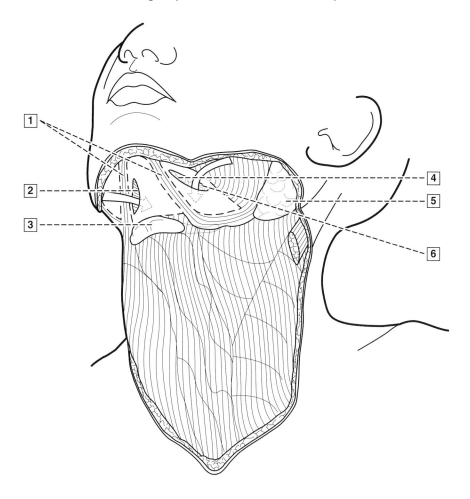

1	Anterior bellies of digastric muscle
2	Superficial cervical fascia (cut to demonstrate entrance) with arrow entering submental space
3	Hyoid bone
4	Submandibular salivary gland
5	Parotid salivary gland
6	Superficial cervical fascia (cut to demonstrate entrance) with arrow entering submandibular space

REVIEW QUESTIONS: Spaces: Submental and submandibular

Fill in the blanks by choosing the appropriate terms from the list below.

1. The _____ is located in the midline between the mandibular symphysis and the hyoid bone; the space coincides with the anatomic region of the submental triangle, which is part of the anterior cervical triangle.

2. The floor of the submental space is the _____ covering the suprahyoid muscles, with the mylohyoid muscle as its roof covered by the investing fascia.

3. Forming the lateral borders of the submental space are the diverging anterior bellies of the _____.

4. The submental space contains the _____ and the origin of the anterior jugular vein.

5. The submental space communicates with the _____, submandibular space, and sublingual space.

6. The _____ is a space located lateral and posterior to the submental space on each side of the jaws; the space coincides with the anatomic region of the submandibular triangle, part of the anterior cervical triangle.

7. The cross-sectional shape of the bilateral submandibular space is triangular, with the _____ of the mandible being its superior border, which is the origin of the mylohyoid muscle.

8. The _____ forms the medial borders of the submandibular space and the hyoid bone creates its medial apex.

9. The submandibular space contains the _____, most of the submandibular salivary gland, and parts of the facial artery, which is a branch of the external carotid artery that supplies structures of the superficial face.

10. The submandibular space communicates with the infratemporal space, submental space, and _____, as well as the parapharyngeal space of the neck.

submental lymph nodes	mylohyoid muscle	digastric muscles
superficial cervical fascia	submandibular lymph nodes	space of the body of the mandible
mylohyoid line	sublingual space	submandibular space
submental space		

Reference   Chapter 11, Fasciae and spaces. In Fehrenbach MJ, Herring SW: *Illustrated anatomy of the head and neck*, ed 6, St. Louis, 2021, Saunders.

FIGURE 10.14   Spaces: Submandibular and sublingual (coronal section of head and neck)

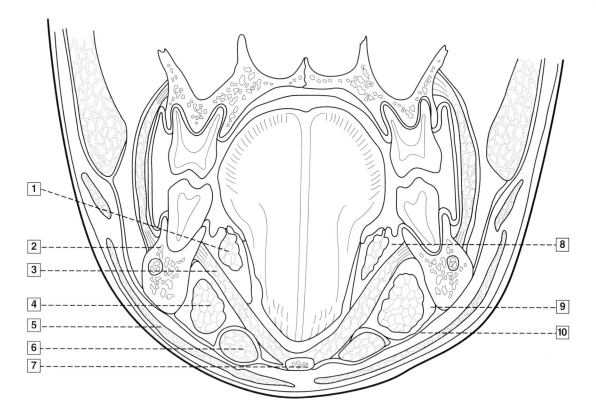

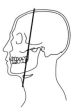

1 Sublingual salivary gland
2 Mandible
3 Mylohyoid muscle
4 Submandibular salivary gland
5 Platysma muscle
6 Digastric muscle
7 Hyoid bone
8 Sublingual space
9 Submandibular space
10 Investing fascia

REVIEW QUESTIONS: Spaces: Submandibular and sublingual

Fill in the blanks by choosing the appropriate terms from the list below.

1. The _____ is located lateral and posterior to the submental space on each side of the jaws; the space coincides with the anatomic region termed the submandibular triangle, part of the anterior cervical triangle.

2. The cross-sectional shape of the bilateral submandibular space is triangular, with the mylohyoid line on the medial surface of the _____ being its superior border, which is the origin of the mylohyoid muscle.

3. The mylohyoid muscle forms the medial border of the submandibular space, and the _____ creates its medial apex.

4. The submandibular space contains the submandibular lymph nodes, most of the _____, and parts of the facial artery, which is a branch of the external carotid artery that supplies structures of the superficial face.

5. The submandibular space communicates with the infratemporal space, submental space, and sublingual space, as well as the _____ of the neck.

6. The sublingual space is located deep to the _____, with the oral mucosa its roof.

7. The floor of the sublingual space is the _____; thus, this muscle creates the division between the submandibular and sublingual spaces with the sublingual space superior to the more inferior submandibular space.

8. The _____ and its intrinsic muscles form the medial border of the sublingual space, and the mandible forms its lateral wall.

9. The sublingual space contains the _____ and ducts, the duct of the deep lobe of the submandibular salivary gland, a part of the lingual nerve and artery, and the twelfth cranial nerve or hypoglossal nerve.

10. The sublingual space communicates with the _____ and submandibular space, as well as with the space of the body of the mandible.

submental space	tongue	sublingual salivary gland
mylohyoid muscle	oral mucosa	parapharyngeal space
submandibular salivary gland	submandibular space	mandible
hyoid bone		

Reference   Chapter 11, Fasciae and spaces. In Fehrenbach MJ, Herring SW: *Illustrated anatomy of the head and neck*, ed 6, St. Louis, 2021, Saunders.

FIGURE 10.15 Spaces: Previseral and retropharyngeal (midsagittal section of head and neck)

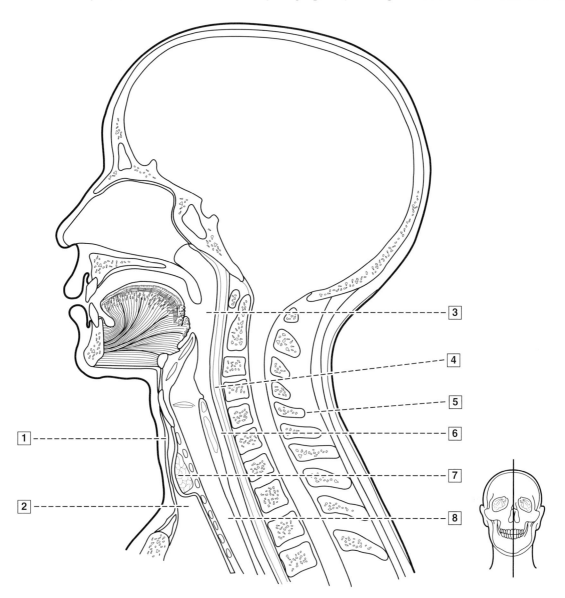

1 Investing fascia
2 Previsceral space
3 Pharynx
4 Retropharyngeal space
5 Cervical vertebrae with prevertebral space
6 Esophagus
7 Thyroid gland
8 Trachea

REVIEW QUESTIONS: Spaces: Previseral and retropharyngeal

Fill in the blanks by choosing the appropriate terms from the list below.

1. The _____ include the previsceral space, parapharyngeal space, retropharyngeal space, and perivertebral space.

2. The _____ or *visceral space* is located between the visceral and investing fasciae.

3. The previsceral space is anterior to the _____.

4. The previsceral space encases the _____ of the neck.

5. The visceral compartment of the neck, which is encased by the previsceral space, contains the _____, larynx, trachea, and esophagus.

6. The previsceral space _____ with the parapharyngeal spaces.

7. The _____ or *retrovisceral space* is a fascial space located immediately posterior to the pharynx, between the vertebral and visceral fasciae.

8. The retropharyngeal space extends from the base of the _____, where it is posterior to the superior pharyngeal constrictor muscle and inferior to the thorax (chest).

9. The retropharyngeal space is divided into two lateral compartments by a fibrous raphe and contains the _____ in early childhood.

10. The retropharyngeal space communicates with the _____ since it is continuous with them.

communicates	skull	trachea
retropharyngeal lymph nodes	retropharyngeal space	visceral compartment
parapharyngeal spaces	previsceral space	pharynx
cervical spaces		

Reference   Chapter 11, Fasciae and spaces. In Fehrenbach MJ, Herring SW: *Illustrated anatomy of the head and neck*, ed 6, St. Louis, 2021, Saunders.

NOTES

FIGURE 10.16 Spaces: Previseral and retropharyngeal (transverse section of neck)

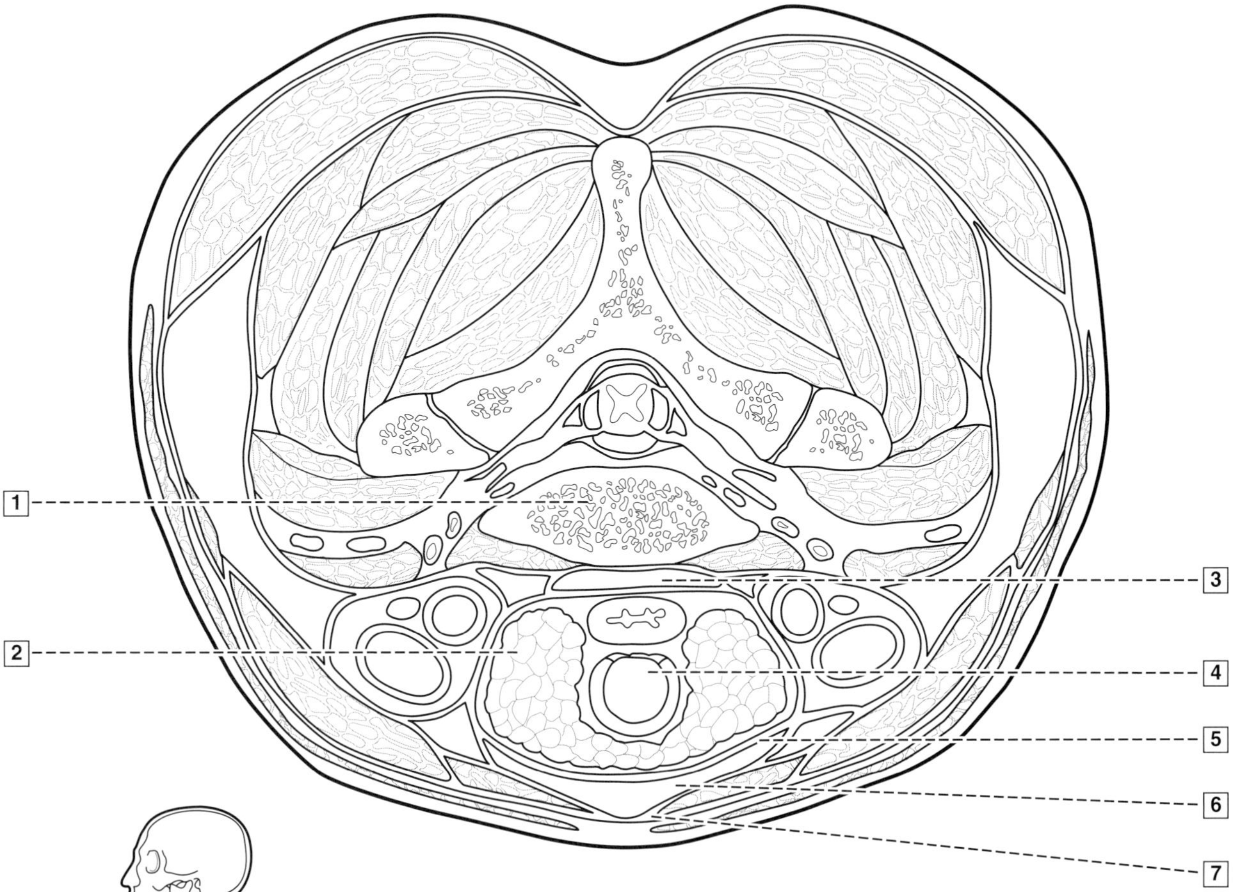

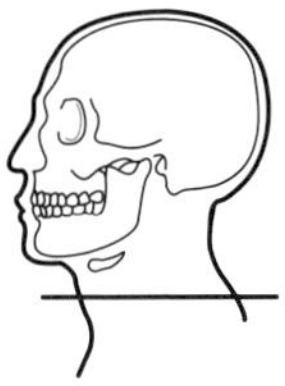

1 Cervical vertebra with perivertebral space

2 Thyroid gland

3 Retropharyngeal space

4 Trachea

5 Visceral fascia

6 Previsceral space

7 Investing fascia

REVIEW QUESTIONS: Spaces: Previseral and retropharyngeal

Fill in the blanks by choosing the appropriate terms from the list below.

1. The _____ within the neck connect the spaces of the face and jaws with those of the thorax (chest).

2. The retropharyngeal space or *retrovisceral space* is a fascial space located immediately posterior to the _____, between the vertebral and visceral fasciae.

3. The retropharyngeal space extends from the base of the skull, where it is posterior to the _____, inferior to the thorax (chest).

4. The _____ is located between the visceral and investing fasciae, anterior to the trachea.

5. Both the retropharyngeal space and previsceral space communicate with the _____.

6. Posterior to the retropharyngeal space is the _____ that contains the cervical vertebrae and associated structures.

7. The perivertebral space is a cylinder-shaped space surrounded by the _____ and extends from the skull base to the lower spine.

8. The perivertebral space can be divided into the _____ anteriorly and the paravertebral space posteriorly.

9. The cervical spaces within the neck can communicate with the _____, as well as with each other.

10. Most importantly, the cervical spaces connect the spaces of the face and jaws with those of the _____.

spaces of the face and jaws	cervical spaces	deep cervical fasciae
previsceral space	superior pharyngeal muscle	prevertebral space
parapharyngeal spaces	perivertebral space	thorax
pharynx		

Reference   Chapter 11, Fasciae and spaces. In Fehrenbach MJ, Herring SW: *Illustrated anatomy of the head and neck*, ed 6, St. Louis, 2021, Saunders.

NOTES

FIGURE 10.17 Spaces: Parapharyngeal and retropharyngeal (transverse section of oral cavity and neck)

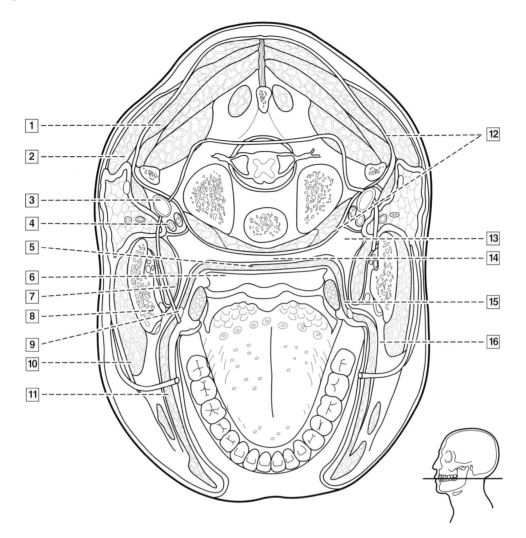

1	Vertebral muscles	**9**	Pterygomandibular raphe
2	Sternocleidomastoid muscle	**10**	Masseter muscle
3	Internal jugular vein	**11**	Buccinator muscle
4	Internal carotid artery	**12**	Vertebral fascia
5	Superior pharyngeal constrictor muscle	**13**	Parapharyngeal space
6	Pharynx	**14**	Retropharyngeal space
7	Medial pterygoid muscle	**15**	Buccopharyngeal fascia
8	Mandible	**16**	Buccal space

REVIEW QUESTIONS: Spaces: Parapharyngeal and retropharyngeal

Fill in the blanks by choosing the appropriate terms from the list below.

1. The _____ are spaces located within the neck that can communicate with the spaces of the face and jaws, as well as with each other.

2. The cervical spaces connect the _____ of the head with those of the thorax (chest).

3. The cervical spaces include the previsceral space, parapharyngeal space, retropharyngeal space, and _____.

4. The _____ or *visceral space* is located between the visceral and investing fasciae, anterior to the trachea; this space encases the visceral compartment of the neck, which contains the pharynx, larynx, trachea, and esophagus, and communicates with the parapharyngeal spaces.

5. The _____ or *lateral pharyngeal space*, is a bilateral fascial space lateral to the pharynx with its superior pharyngeal constrictor muscle and medial to the medial pterygoid muscle as well as parallel to the carotid sheath.

6. The bilateral parapharyngeal space in its posterior compartment is adjacent to the _____, which contains the internal and common carotid arteries and the internal jugular vein, as well as the tenth cranial nerve or vagus nerve.

7. The parapharyngeal space also adjacent to the _____, which are the ninth, eleventh, and twelfth as they exit the cranial cavity.

8. Anteriorly, the parapharyngeal space extends to the _____, where it is continuous with the infratemporal and buccal spaces; the space is shaped like an inverted pyramid, with the skull base superiorly and inferiorly to the greater cornu of the hyoid bone at its apex.

9. The anterior compartment of the parapharyngeal space contains the _____.

10. Posteriorly, the posterior compartment of the parapharyngeal space extends around the _____, where it is continuous with another cervical fascial space, the retropharyngeal space; the parapharyngeal space communicates only with the retropharyngeal space.

pharynx	previsceral space	pterygomandibular raphe
spaces of the face and jaws	carotid sheath	deep cervical lymph nodes
posterior cranial nerves	parapharyngeal space	perivertebral space
cervical spaces		

Reference Chapter 11, Fasciae and spaces. In Fehrenbach MJ, Herring SW: *Illustrated anatomy of the head and neck*, ed 6, St. Louis, 2021, Saunders.

FIGURE 10.18   Cervical compartments with contents and borders (transverse section of neck)

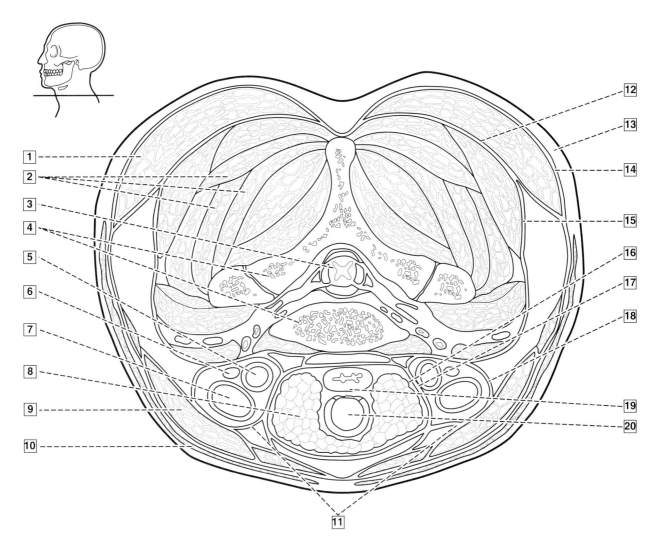

1	Trapezius muscle	**8**	Thyroid gland	**15**	Vertebral fascia
2	Vertebral muscles	**9**	Sternocleidomastoid muscle	**16**	Visceral fascia
3	Spinal cord	**10**	Platysma muscle	**17**	VISCERAL COMPARTMENT
4	Cervical vertebra	**11**	VASCULAR COMPARTMENTS	**18**	Carotid sheath
5	Common carotid artery	**12**	VERTEBRAL COMPARTMENT	**19**	Esophagus
6	Vagus nerve	**13**	Superficial fascia	**20**	Trachea
7	Internal jugular vein	**14**	Investing fascia		

REVIEW QUESTIONS: Cervical compartments with contents and borders

Fill in the blanks by choosing the appropriate terms from the list below.

1. The single _____ (or posterior compartment) contains the spinal cord, cervical vertebrae, and associated vertebral muscles that support and move the head and neck.

2. The vertebral compartment is bordered by the _____ in the neck.

3. The single _____ (or anterior compartment) contains the thyroid, thymus, and parathyroid glands as well as the hyoid bone, larynx, trachea, esophagus, and pharynx.

4. The visceral compartment is a continuation of the _____ and respiratory systems.

5. The visceral compartment is more _____ in comparison to the other compartments since it changes its overall shape during swallowing or speech.

6. The visceral compartment is bordered by the _____ in the neck.

7. The two bilateral _____ (or lateral compartments) are located lateral and posterior to the pharynx.

8. The vascular compartments consist of two _____ bordered by each vascular compartment in the neck.

9. Each vascular compartment contains major _____.

10. The major blood vessels within the vascular compartments include the internal carotid and common carotid arteries as well as the _____.

gastrointestinal	internal jugular veins
visceral compartment	movable
vertebral compartment	vascular compartments
vertebral fascia	blood vessels
carotid sheaths	visceral fascia

Reference   Chapter 11, Fascia and spaces. In Fehrenbach MJ, Herring SW: *Illustrated anatomy of the head and neck*, ed 6, St. Louis, 2021, Saunders.

NOTES

1. How many erupted primary teeth does a 4-year-old child have?
   A. 10
   B. 12
   C. 16
   D. 18
   E. 20

2. Which of the following are considered functions of the incisors?
   A. Biting and tearing
   B. Grinding and cutting
   C. Biting and cutting
   D. Tearing and grinding

3. Which of the following structures or features are found in numbers of four in the oral cavity but ONLY during the permanent dentition period?
   A. Molars
   B. Dental arches
   C. Canine cusp slopes
   D. Maxillary premolars
   E. Quadrants

4. When viewed from the proximal, the crown of the permanent mandibular first molar is inclined
   A. buccally.
   B. lingually.
   C. mesially.
   D. distally.

5. Which of the following BEST describes the groove pattern on the occlusal table of the permanent mandibular second molar?
   A. Linear
   B. Snake eyes
   C. Crescent
   D. Cross-shaped

6. Which tooth is considered succedaneous?
   A. #13 (#25)
   B. #14 (#26)
   C. #18 (#37)
   D. #19 (#36)

7. Which of the following features is located on the lateral surface of the mandible?
   A. Lingula
   B. Submandibular fossa
   C. Genial tubercles
   D. Sublingual fossa
   E. Mental foramen

8. Which of the following bones of the skull is paired?
   A. Sphenoid
   B. Ethmoid
   C. Occipital
   D. Vomer
   E. Parietal

9. Which of the following bones of the skull is considered a facial bone?
   A. Occipital
   B. Parietal
   C. Sphenoid
   D. Zygomatic
   E. Frontal

10. Which of the following landmarks of the temporomandibular joint is located on the mandible?
    A. Articular eminence
    B. Coronoid process
    C. Articular fossa
    D. Postglenoid process

11. Which of the following lymph nodes are FIRST affected in a patient who develops an infection in the lower lip after trauma from an accident?
    A. Submandibular
    B. Deep cervical
    C. Submental
    D. Buccal
    E. Malar

12. Which of the following nerves that serve the parotid salivary gland can also be affected by medication and thus be involved in xerostomia?
    A. Facial
    B. Trigeminal
    C. Glossopharyngeal
    D. Chorda tympani

13. Which of the following arteries of the head and neck provides the MOST reliable arterial pulse of the body?
    A. Internal carotid
    B. Common carotid
    C. Lingual
    D. Facial
    E. Superior thyroid

14. Which muscle can become enlarged in the presence of the parafunctional habit of bruxism?
- **A.** Mentalis
- **B.** Masseter
- **C.** Orbicularis oris
- **D.** Risorius
- **E.** Epicranial

15. Which of the following muscles is palpated during an extraoral examination of the posterior cervical triangle?
- **A.** Suprahyoid
- **B.** Infrahyoid
- **C.** Sternocleidomastoid
- **D.** Temporalis

16. Which permanent teeth may cause sensations that suggest a carious or endodontic situation when ONLY a sinus infection is diagnosed?
- **A.** Maxillary anterior teeth
- **B.** Maxillary posterior teeth
- **C.** Mandibular anterior teeth
- **D.** Mandibular posterior teeth

17. Which of the following salivary glands is MOST commonly involved in stone formation?
- **A.** Parotid
- **B.** Submandibular
- **C.** Sublingual
- **D.** Submandibular and sublingual

18. Which of the following structures divides the tongue into its body and the base?
- **A.** Circumvallate lingual papilla
- **B.** Sulcus terminalis
- **C.** Foramen cecum
- **D.** Median lingual sulcus
- **E.** Lingual tonsil

19. Which of the following teeth are contained within the secondary palate?
- **A.** Maxillary central and lateral incisors
- **B.** Maxillary canines and posterior teeth
- **C.** Mandibular central and lateral incisors
- **D.** Mandibular canines and posterior teeth

20. Which is the MOST common type of epithelium found in the oral cavity?
- **A.** Stratified squamous
- **B.** Cuboidal
- **C.** Transitional
- **D.** Simple squamous

21. Which of the following nerves or branches of the nerve causes discomfort during infection of the external ear noted upon extraoral examination?
- **A.** Lingual
- **B.** Auriculotemporal
- **C.** Inferior alveolar
- **D.** Buccal

22. Which pair of bones form the floor of the nasal cavity?
- **A.** Frontal and ethmoid
- **B.** Ethmoid and lacrimal
- **C.** Lacrimal and maxillary
- **D.** Maxillary and palatine
- **E.** Zygomatic and palatine

23. Which of the following methods is MOST commonly used in the United States for the designation of teeth?
- **A.** Universal Numbering System
- **B.** Palmer Notation Method
- **C.** International Numbering System
- **D.** World Health Organization System

24. Which of the following statements is CORRECT concerning the pterygoid plexus of veins?
- **A.** Surrounds the infrahyoid muscles
- **B.** Protects the superficial temporal artery
- **C.** Drains only the superficial parts of the face
- **D.** Injury can lead to hematoma

25. Which of the following permanent teeth has an oblique ridge?
- **A.** Mandibular second molar
- **B.** Maxillary first molar
- **C.** Mandibular third molar
- **D.** Maxillary third molar

26. Which permanent tooth has a buccal pit that is susceptible to caries?
- **A.** Mandibular first molar
- **B.** Maxillary first molar
- **C.** Mandibular second molar
- **D.** Maxillary second molar

27. Which of the following structures is located just posterior to the MOST distal molar of the permanent mandibular dentition?
   A. Maxillary tuberosity
   B. Median palatine suture
   C. Incisive foramen
   D. Greater palatine foramen
   E. Retromolar triangle

28. The permanent mandibular third molar, compared with the mandibular second molar, is
   A. larger in the crown.
   B. more "wrinkled" on the occlusal surface.
   C. less variable overall in form.
   D. longer in the roots.

29. Which of the following nerves supplies the muscles of mastication?
   A. Hypoglossal
   B. Vagus
   C. Facial
   D. Chorda tympani
   E. Trigeminal

30. The submandibular duct opens into the oral cavity
   A. opposite the permanent maxillary second molar.
   B. onto the sublingual caruncle.
   C. onto the buccal mucosa.
   D. at the base of the mandibular labial frenum.

31. Which of the following permanent teeth has two roots?
   A. Maxillary first molar
   B. Maxillary second premolar
   C. Maxillary first premolar
   D. Maxillary third molar

32. Which of the following permanent teeth has two pulp canals?
   A. Maxillary first premolar
   B. Mandibular first premolar
   C. Maxillary first molar
   D. Mandibular first molar

33. Which of the following muscles, when fully contracted, helps close the jaws?
   A. Lateral pterygoid
   B. Platysma
   C. Mentalis
   D. Buccinator
   E. Temporalis

34. Accumulation of food in the left mandibular vestibule might suggest malfunction of which of the following muscles?
   A. Buccinator
   B. Risorius
   C. Orbicularis oris
   D. Medial pterygoid
   E. Levator anguli oris

35. Rank the following tooth tissue from MOST to LEAST resistant to abrasion.
   A. Dentin, enamel, cementum
   B. Enamel, cementum, dentin
   C. Enamel, dentin, cementum
   D. Cementum, enamel, dentin

36. Which of the following structures are NOT found within the pterygomandibular space?
   A. Inferior alveolar nerve
   B. Hypoglossal nerve
   C. Inferior alveolar artery
   D. Sphenomandibular ligament

37. Which of the following are contained within the sheath of the lingual nerve as it passes medial to the mandible and anterior to the mandibular foramen?
   A. Sensory fibers to the lip
   B. Motor fibers to the masseter muscle
   C. Parasympathetic motor secretory fibers to the submandibular salivary gland
   D. Special sense fibers to the anterior two-thirds of the tongue
   E. Somatic sensory fibers to the posterior one-third of the tongue

38. The floor of the mouth and the tongue BOTH receive their blood supply by way of which of the following arteries?
   A. Facial
   B. Lingual
   C. Mylohyoid
   D. Maxillary

39. Which of the following nerves exits the cranium through the foramen ovale?
   A. Facial
   B. Maxillary

C. Ophthalmic

D. Mandibular

E. Glossopharyngeal

40. Which of the following arteries is a branch off the maxillary artery?

 A. Facial

 B. Lingual

 C. Superior thyroid

 D. Inferior alveolar

 E. Ascending pharyngeal

41. Which of the following lymph nodes receives lymphatic drainage from maxillary teeth?

 A. Buccal

 B. Submental

 C. Infraorbital

 D. Submandibular

42. Which of the following nerves innervates the pulp of the permanent mandibular posterior teeth?

 A. Mental

 B. Buccal

 C. Incisive

 D. Inferior alveolar

43. Which nerve listed is affected if a patient complains of being unable to experience touch, pain, hot, cold, or pressure on the anterior two-thirds of the tongue?

 A. Vagus

 B. Lingual

 C. Hypoglossal

 D. Chorda tympani

 E. Glossopharyngeal

44. The nasopalatine nerve enters the oral cavity by way of which of the following foramen (foramina)?

 A. Mental

 B. Incisive

 C. Pterygopalatine

 D. Lesser palatine

 E. Greater palatine

45. Which of the following structures is supplied by the hypoglossal nerve?

 A. Sublingual salivary gland

 B. Muscles of the tongue

C. Mucous membrane of the floor of the oral cavity

D. Muscles of facial expression

46. The supporting alveolar bone is made of

 A. compact and cancellous bone.

 B. cortical and spongy bone.

 C. cancellous and spongy bone.

 D. cortical, cancellous, and spongy bone.

47. Which of the following nerves or branches of a nerve contains pain fibers affected by disturbances of the temporomandibular joint?

 A. Chorda tympani

 B. Auriculotemporal

 C. Zygomaticotemporal

 D. Temporal branch of the facial nerve

48. The parotid duct pierces which of the following muscles before entry into the oral cavity?

 A. Masseter

 B. Mylohyoid

 C. Buccinator

 D. Medial pterygoid

49. The lateral pterygoid muscle inserts into the

 A. coronoid process.

 B. articular eminence.

 C. mandibular condyle.

 D. angle of the mandible.

 E. internal oblique line.

50. The pain impulses from the periodontal ligament are carried by which of the following cranial nerves?

 A. I

 B. II

 C. V

 D. VII

 E. IX

51. The permanent mandibular teeth are vascularized by branches of which of the following arteries?

 A. Facial

 B. Labial

 C. Lingual

 D. Maxillary

52. During the exploration of the root, longitudinal developmental grooves would probably be noted on which of the following root surfaces of a permanent maxillary first premolar?
    A. Lingual
    B. Mesial
    C. Facial
    D. Palatal

53. The roots of which of the following permanent premolars present the GREATEST difficulty during endodontic therapy?
    A. Maxillary first
    B. Maxillary second
    C. Mandibular first
    D. Mandibular second

54. Which structure becomes the dentinoenamel junction of the fully formed tooth?
    A. Outer enamel epithelium
    B. Stellate reticulum
    C. Basement membrane
    D. Dental papilla

55. Which of the following descriptors does NOT pertain to the alveolar mucosa?
    A. Nonkeratinized
    B. Found beyond the mucogingival junction
    C. Flexible tissue
    D. Component of gingivae

56. Which of the following permanent premolars often has three cusps?
    A. Maxillary first
    B. Maxillary second
    C. Mandibular first
    D. Mandibular second

57. The permanent tooth that has the longest crown is the
    A. maxillary lateral incisor.
    B. maxillary central incisor.
    C. mandibular canine.
    D. maxillary first molar.

58. Which of the following statement is CORRECT when considering the vessels in the head and neck?
    A. Blood vessels are MORE numerous than lymphatic vessels in the head and neck.
    B. Venous vessels are NOT parallel to the lymphatic vessels in location.
    C. Blood vessels are LESS numerous than lymphatic vessels in the head and neck.
    D. Blood vessels are NOT involved in the spreading of cancer to distant sites.

59. Which of the following permanent premolars frequently lacks a transverse ridge?
    A. Maxillary first
    B. Maxillary second
    C. Mandibular first
    D. Mandibular second

60. How does the permanent mandibular second premolar differ in related structural numbers from the permanent mandibular first molar?
    A. Cusps
    B. Roots
    C. Lingual grooves
    D. Marginal ridges

61. Which of the following is CORRECT concerning where is the cingulum usually located on the teeth indicated?
    A. Incisal third of the lingual surface of anterior teeth
    B. Middle third of the lingual surface of posterior teeth
    C. Cervical third of the lingual surface of anterior teeth
    D. Occlusal third of the lingual surface of posterior teeth

62. Which of the following determines the shape of the tooth's root(s)?
    A. Rests of Malassez
    B. Stellate reticulum
    C. Hertwig epithelial root sheath
    D. Dental lamina

63. Where is the mesial and distal contact of the permanent mandibular first molar located?
    A. Junction of the occlusal and middle thirds
    B. Center of tooth surface
    C. Junction of the cervical and middle thirds
    D. Lingual of tooth surface

64. An extrinsic tongue muscle that retracts the tongue is the
    A. palatoglossus muscle.
    B. inferior longitudinal muscle.
    C. styloglossus muscle.
    D. genioglossus muscle.

65. The circulating white blood cells which are the FEWEST in number are the
    A. monocytes.
    B. neutrophils.
    C. basophils.
    D. lymphocytes.

66. Where is the soft palate located?
    A. Dorsal aspect of the oral cavity
    B. Just posterior to the hard palate
    C. Center of the hard palate
    D. Between the faucial pillars

67. Which of the following develops into the posterior one-third of the tongue?
    A. Meckel cartilage
    B. Copula
    C. Tuberculum impar
    D. Lingual swellings

68. Where is the lingual tonsil located?
    A. Posterior to the circumvallate lingual papillae
    B. Posterolateral border of the tongue
    C. Along the sulcus terminalis on the tongue
    D. Dorsal surface tongue but not near the sulcus terminalis

69. Colloid is a substance associated with which of the following glands?
    A. Sublingual
    B. Thyroid
    C. Thymus
    D. Parotid

70. Which of the following glands is unencapsulated?
    A. Submandibular
    B. Thyroid
    C. Parotid
    D. Sublingual

71. All of the following structures may be found in oral mucosa EXCEPT
    A. lamina propria.
    B. basal lamina.
    C. keratohyaline granules.
    D. myofibers.

72. Which one of the following is NOT ectodermal in origin?
    A. Reduced enamel epithelium
    B. Dentin
    C. Hertwig epithelial root sheath
    D. Enamel

73. Which is the CORRECT series that lists the parts of the mature tooth in the order of increasing inorganic content?
    A. Enamel, dentin, cementum, pulp
    B. Cementum, dentin, enamel, pulp
    C. Cementum, pulp, dentin, enamel
    D. Pulp, cementum, dentin, enamel

74. The formation of bone in the absence of a preexisting cartilage framework considered
    A. lamellar.
    B. nonlamellar.
    C. intramembranous.
    D. endochondral.

75. Which of the following is NOT part of the reduced enamel epithelium?
    A. Outer enamel epithelium
    B. Stratum intermedium
    C. Ameloblasts
    D. Epithelial diaphragm

COMPREHENSIVE TEST ANSWER KEY AND RATIONALES

1. (E) All of 4-year-old child's primary teeth would have erupted into the oral cavity because the average age for primary (or deciduous) dentition completion is approximately age 3. There are 20 teeth within the primary dentition.

2. (C) Incisors function as instruments for biting and cutting food during mastication because of the incisal ridge, triangular proximal form, and arch position. There are eight incisors, two of each type, the central and lateral.

3. (D) Only during the permanent dentition period are four maxillary premolars (or bicuspids) present, two of each type, the first and

second. The two types of molars, the first and second molars, are only found during the primary dentition period. The three types of molars are found during the permanent dentition period. Only two arches are found in both the primary and permanent dentition periods. Only two canine cusp slopes per tooth are found during both periods. There are four quadrants, which are present during both primary and permanent dentition periods.

4. (B) All permanent mandibular molars, including the first molar, show strong lingual inclination when viewed proximally. This inclines the crown lingually on the root base, bringing the cusps into proper occlusion with the maxillary antagonists and the distributing forces along the long axis.

5. (D) A cross-shaped groove pattern is formed on the occlusal table of the permanent mandibular second molar when the well-defined central groove is crossed by the buccal groove and lingual groove, dividing the occlusal table into four parts that are nearly equal.

6. (A) Tooth #13 (or #25), the permanent second premolar, is succedaneous for the primary second molar. All others noted are permanent molars, and all molars are nonsuccedaneous because they do not have any primary predecessors and thus erupt distally to the primary second molar.

7. (E) The mental foramen is located on the lateral (or outer) surface of the mandible. All other structures are located on the medial (or inner) surface of the mandible.

8. (E) The parietal bone is the only paired bone of the skull. Other bones listed are single bones of the skull.

9. (D) The zygomatic bone is considered a facial bone because it helps create facial features and serves as a base for the dentition of the skull. Vomer, lacrimal bones, maxillae, and mandible as well as the zygomatic bones, nasal bones, and inferior nasal conchae are also facial bones of the skull. The palatine bones are not strictly considered facial bones.

All others are listed as cranial bones because they form the cranium of the skull. Cranial bones include the occipital bone, frontal bone, parietal bones, temporal bones, sphenoid bone, and ethmoid bone.

10. (B) The coronoid process is located on the mandible and is part of the temporomandibular joint. All others listed are part of the joint but are located on the temporal bone. The coronoid process is a thin triangular eminence, flattened from side to side.

11. (C) The lower lip drains directly into the submental lymph nodes, which serve as the primary lymph nodes during an infection, which would mean that they were first affected by an infection. The submandibular and deep cervical lymph nodes would serve as the secondary nodes if the infection progressed since the submental lymph nodes drain into the submandibular lymph nodes or directly into the deep cervical lymph nodes. The buccal and malar lymph nodes drain the upper and middle cheek, respectively.

12. (C) The parotid salivary gland is supplied by the ninth cranial nerve (or glossopharyngeal [IX], with preganglionic parasympathetic innervation). Even though the seventh cranial nerve (or facial [VII]) travels through the parotid salivary gland, it does not supply it. The chorda tympani a branch of the facial seventh cranial nerve supplies both the submandibular and sublingual salivary glands but not the parotid salivary gland, which may also be affected by drugs to produce xerostomia (dry mouth). The trigeminal (or fifth cranial nerve [V]) serves many other oral cavity structures but not the parotid salivary gland.

13. (B) The common carotid artery provides the most reliable carotid pulse from the carotid sinus, the swelling of the common carotid before it bifurcates into the internal and external carotid arteries. Other branches listed are from the internal carotid artery after bifurcation. The carotid pulse should be used only by trained emergency personnel; however, the radial pulse can be used when taking the vital sign of a baseline pulse.

14. (B) The masseter muscle can become enlarged or hypertrophied in a patient who habitually has bruxism or grinds and/or clenches the teeth. The action of the masseter muscle during bilateral contraction of the entire muscle is to raise or elevate the mandible, thus raising the lower jaw. Elevation of the mandible occurs during the closing of the jaws or grinding of the teeth. All others listed are muscles of facial expression and not muscles of mastication.

15. (C) The sternocleidomastoid muscle divides each side or lateral surface of the neck into the anterior and posterior cervical triangles. The posterior cervical triangle is located on the side or lateral surface of the neck and the anterior cervical triangle corresponds to the anterior region or front of the neck that contains both the suprahyoid and infrahyoid muscles. The temporalis muscle is located in the temporal region on the lateral surface (or side) of the skull.

16. (B) Discomfort from maxillary sinusitis can be confused with tooth-related discomfort from the maxillary posterior teeth because the roots of the maxillary posterior teeth are in close proximity to the maxillary sinus. Others listed are not near the maxillary sinus, which is the sinus most commonly involved in sinus infections.

17. (B) The duct for the submandibular salivary gland is the submandibular duct (or Wharton duct); the long duct travels along the anterior floor of the mouth. The tortuous upward travel of the submandibular salivary gland for a considerable distance during its course may be the reason that the gland is most commonly involved in salivary stone formation.

18. (B) Sulcus terminalis divides the tongue into its posterior base and anterior body. The dorsum (top) surface is convex and marked by the sulcus terminalis; this sulcus ends posteriorly, about 2.5 cm from the root of the tongue, in a pit-like depression, the foramen cecum, from which a shallow groove, the sulcus terminalis, runs lateralward and forward on either side to the margin of the tongue. Others listed are also on the dorsal surface of the tongue.

19. (B) The secondary palate will form the posterior two-thirds of the hard palate and contains the maxillary canines and posterior teeth, such as the premolars and molars, and not central and lateral incisors, which are anterior teeth and would be then contained instead within the primary palate, which makes up the anterior one-third of the hard palate. No mandibular teeth are contained within the secondary palate.

20. (A) Stratified squamous epithelium is the most common type of soft tissue found in the oral cavity. Cuboidal, simple squamous, and transitional epithelia are not found in the oral cavity.

21. (B) The auriculotemporal nerve serves as an afferent nerve for the external ear and scalp near the temporomandibular joint. The auriculotemporal nerve is a branch of the mandibular nerve that runs with the superficial temporal artery and vein and provides sensory innervation to various regions on the side of the head. All others listed are afferent for oral structures but not for that area of the head.

22. (D) The horizontal plates of the palatine bones and the palatine process of the maxilla together form the floor of the nasal cavity. These two sets of bones also form the anterior part of the hard palate (roof) of the oral cavity. All others form the orbital walls.

23. (A) The Universal Numbering System is the most used system in the United States for the designation of both dentitions because it is adaptable to electronic data transfer. The Palmer Notation Method is used during orthodontic therapy. The International Numbering System is mainly used internationally.

24. (D) The pterygoid plexus of veins is surrounded by the lateral pterygoid muscle and also surrounds the maxillary artery on each side of the face within infratemporal fossa. These veins protect the maxillary artery from being compressed during mastication. When the pterygoid plexus of veins is pierced, a small amount of blood escapes and enters the tissue, causing a hematoma. The pterygoid plexus of veins can be pierced when the posterior superior alveolar nerve block is incorrectly administered with the needle being overinserted. The pterygoid plexus of veins drains the veins from the deep parts of the face and then drains into the maxillary vein.

25. (B) The permanent maxillary first molar has an oblique ridge that is formed by the union of the triangular ridge of the distolingual cusp and the distal cusp ridge of the mesiolingual cusp, crossing the occlusal table obliquely. All other teeth do not have oblique ridges.

26. (A) The permanent mandibular first molar's mesiobuccal groove almost always ends in a buccal pit, which is susceptible to caries because of increased dental biofilm retention and because of the thin enamel that forms the walls of the pit. Enamel sealants or other restorative materials can be placed in the buccal pit to protect the tooth from caries. All other teeth do not have buccal pits.

27. (E) The retromolar triangle is located just posterior to the most distal molar of the permanent mandibular dentition. All other structures are found on the maxilla and are associated with the maxillary dentition. The retromolar pad is the clinical manifestation of the retromolar triangle.

28. (B) Generally, the more posterior the tooth, the more supplemental grooves are present, causing the occlusal table to appear more "wrinkled." Thus the permanent mandibular third molar has a more "wrinkled" occlusal surface than that of the second molar of the same arch, the mandibular arch. The other descriptors listed refer to the permanent mandibular second molar and not the permanent mandibular third molar.

29. (E) The muscles of mastication are four paired muscles attached to the mandible; they include the masseter, temporalis, medial pterygoid, and lateral pterygoid muscles. The mandibular division of the fifth (V) cranial nerve, trigeminal, innervates all muscles of mastication. The seventh (VII) cranial nerve is the facial nerve. The tenth (X) cranial nerve is the vagus

nerve. The twelfth (XII) cranial nerve is the hypoglossal nerve. The chorda tympani is a branch of the facial nerve (seventh [VII] cranial nerve). However, the other nerves innervate important structures of the oral cavity.

30. (C) The submandibular duct opens up into the oral cavity from the sublingual caruncle on the floor of the mouth. The parotid duct opens opposite the maxillary second molar onto the buccal mucosa. The mandibular labial frenum has only minor salivary gland ducts nearby within the labial mucosa.

31. (C) The permanent maxillary first premolar has two roots. All maxillary molars have three roots (or trifurcated); however, sometimes the roots of the third molar are so close together that they are fused roots, either partially or fully, giving the appearance of one root. The permanent maxillary second premolar has one root and only occasionally has two roots (or bifurcated).

32. (A) The pulp cavity for permanent maxillary first premolar has two pulp canals (or root canals), even if there is only one undivided root. The permanent mandibular first premolar has one pulp canal. Both maxillary and mandibular first molars mostly have three pulp canals.

33. (E) Both the lateral pterygoid and temporalis muscles are muscles of mastication that affect the movement of the jaws. If the entire temporalis muscle has a bilateral contraction, its action is to elevate the mandible, thus raising the lower jaw. Elevation of the mandible occurs during the closing of the jaws. The main action with bilateral contraction of the lateral pterygoid muscles is to bring the lower jaw forward, thus causing mainly protrusion of the mandible, with a slight depression of the mandible during the opening of the jaws. If only unilateral contraction of the lateral pterygoid muscle occurs, the lower jaw shifts to the contralateral side, causing a lateral deviation of the mandible. All other muscles listed are considered the muscles of facial expression.

34. (A) The buccinator muscle is the muscle of the cheek and aids in the clearing of food from the oral cavity's vestibules; the muscle also helps retain food in the mouth during mastication. Because the buccinator muscle is innervated by the buccal branch of the facial nerve (or seventh cranial nerve [VII]), any injury to the nerve will affect the action of the muscle (e.g., Bell palsy).

35. (C) Enamel is the hardest at 96% mineralized and therefore most abrasion-resistant tissue, followed by dentin at 70% mineralization and cementum at 65% mineralization. The strength of enamel as the covering of the tooth is important in the longevity of tooth structure.

36. (B) The following structures are found within the pterygomandibular space, which is part of the infratemporal space between the medial pterygoid muscle and the mandibular ramus: the inferior alveolar nerve, inferior alveolar artery (as well as the vein), and sphenomandibular ligament. This space is an important landmark for the injection site for the administration of the inferior alveolar nerve block. The lingual nerve is also included within this space but the lingual artery will be superficial to this site. The hypoglossal nerve, which is the twelfth (XIII) cranial nerve, exits the skull through the hypoglossal canal within the occipital bone and is not found within the pterygomandibular space.

37. (D) Special sense fibers to the anterior two-thirds of the tongue are contained within the sheath of the lingual nerve as it passes medial to the mandible (as well as the inferior alveolar nerve), anterior to the mandibular foramen. The part of the tongue thus becomes anesthetized as the local anesthetic agent diffuses to the lingual nerve initially during the administration of the inferior nerve block. Lingual nerve shock can also occur when the needle contacts the lingual nerve during this injection.

38. (B) Both the floor of the mouth and the tongue receive blood supply by way of the lingual artery. The facial artery with its major branches supplies the face in the oral, buccal, zygomatic, nasal, infraorbital, and orbital regions. The mylohyoid artery supplies the floor of the mouth and the mylohyoid muscle. The maxillary artery has branches near the muscles supplied.

39. (D) The mandibular nerve is the third of the three divisions of the fifth cranial nerve (or trigeminal). The first division (or ophthalmic) exits through the superior orbital fissure, the second division (or maxillary) through the foramen rotundum (meaning round-shaped), and the third (or mandibular) through the foramen ovale (meaning oval-shaped). The fissure and foramina are all located within the sphenoid bone. This fissure also carries the third, fourth, and sixth cranial nerves and the ophthalmic vein.

40. (D) The maxillary artery is one of the two terminal branches of the external carotid artery. Branches of the maxillary artery supply the teeth and supporting structures of both arches of the dentition. Blood supply to the mandibular teeth and the supporting structures is mainly from the inferior alveolar branch of the maxillary artery.

41. (D) The submandibular lymph nodes receive lymphatic drainage from the maxillary teeth. The facial lymph nodes are positioned along the length of the facial vein to drain the area and include both the buccal and infraorbital lymph nodes. However, these two node groups drain into each other and then into the submandibular lymph nodes. The submental lymph nodes drain both sides of the chin, lower lip, floor of the mouth, apex of the tongue, and the mandibular incisors and then empty into the submandibular lymph nodes or directly into the deep cervical lymph nodes.

42. (D) The inferior alveolar nerve innervates the pulp of the permanent mandibular posteriors. The buccal (or long buccal) nerve is afferent to the skin of the cheek, area of the buccal oral mucosa, and associated buccal periodontium and gingiva of the permanent mandibular posterior teeth. The mental nerve is composed of external branches that are afferent to the chin, lower lip, and labial mucosa near the permanent mandibular anterior teeth.

43. (B) The lingual nerve is affected if a patient complains of being unable to experience touch, pain, heat, cold, or pressure on the anterior two-thirds of the tongue; the lingual nerve is a branch of the mandibular nerve from the fifth (V) cranial nerve (or trigeminal). The ninth (IX) cranial nerve (or glossopharyngeal nerve) covers the general sensation from the base of the tongue to the posterior one-third of the tongue. The tenth (X) cranial nerve (or vagus nerve) is efferent for muscles of the soft palate, pharynx, and larynx. The chorda tympani is a branch of the facial nerve (or seventh cranial nerve [VII]) and afferent for taste sensation for the body of the tongue.

44. (B) The nasopalatine nerve enters the oral cavity by way of the incisive foramen on the midline of the anterior of the hard palate formed from the maxillae. The lesser palatine nerve enters the lesser palatine foramen in each of the palatine bones. The mental nerve enters the mental foramen on each lateral side of the mandible. The greater palatine nerve enters the greater palatine foramen in each of the palatine bones.

45. (B) Muscles of the tongue are supplied by the hypoglossal nerve (or twelfth cranial nerve [XII]), which is efferent for the intrinsic and extrinsic muscles of the tongue and exits the skull through the hypoglossal canal. The facial (seventh cranial nerve [VII]) serves the muscles of facial expression. The lingual nerve serves the floor of the mouth, as well as the submandibular salivary gland (by way of parasympathetic efferent innervation), which is a branch of the mandibular nerve.

46. (A) Supporting alveolar bone is made up of both compact and cancellous bone. Both the facial and lingual cortical plates are made up of compact bone; the spongy bone between these plates is cancellous bone.

47. (B) The auriculotemporal nerve contains pain fibers affected by disturbances of the temporomandibular joint, such as those occurring with temporomandibular disorders (TMDs). This nerve also serves as an afferent nerve for the external ear and scalp near the temporomandibular joint. The chorda tympani is a branch of the facial nerve (or seventh cranial nerve [VII]) and afferent for taste sensation for the body of the tongue. The zygomatic nerve is composed of the union of zygomaticofacial and zygomaticotemporal in the orbit and is afferent; it conveys the postganglionic parasympathetic fibers to the lacrimal gland.

48. (C) The buccinator muscle is pierced by the parotid duct before entry into the oral cavity and after it emerges from the anterior border of the parotid salivary gland. The parotid duct (or Stensen) serves the parotid salivary gland; the duct opens up into the oral cavity at the parotid papilla on the buccal mucosa, opposite the permanent maxillary first molar.

49. (C) The lateral pterygoid muscle inserts into the mandibular condyle; this includes both heads. The superior head inserts on the anterior surface of the neck of the mandibular condyle at pterygoid fovea of the mandible as well as the temporomandibular joint disc and capsule, while the inferior head inserts on the anterior surface of the neck of the mandibular condyle at pterygoid fovea of the mandible. The superior head of the lateral pterygoid muscle originates from the infratemporal surface and infratemporal crest of the greater wing of the sphenoid bone, while the inferior head of the muscle originates from the lateral pterygoid plate of the sphenoid bone. Temporalis muscle inserts on the coronoid process of the mandibular ramus. The masseter muscle's superficial head inserts on the angle of the mandible and the deep head on the mandibular ramus. The medial pterygoid muscle has both its deep and superficial heads inserted on the medial surface of the mandibular ramus and the angle of the mandible. All are muscles of mastication.

50. (C) The fifth (V) cranial nerve (or trigeminal) carries pain impulses from the periodontal ligament of all the teeth to the brain by its two major nerve branches, the maxillary and mandibular nerves, which serve the maxillary and mandibular teeth, respectively.

51. (D) The mandibular teeth are vascularized by branches of the maxillary arteries, by way of the inferior alveolar artery, as well as the maxillary teeth. The inferior alveolar artery arises from the maxillary artery within the infratemporal fossa, turns inferiorly to enter the mandibular foramen, and then enters the mandibular canal with the inferior alveolar nerve; it then branches into the mylohyoid artery before this main artery enters the mandibular canal. In the mandibular canal, the inferior alveolar artery branches into the mandibular posterior and alveolar (or dental) branches to supply the associated periodontium and gingiva of these teeth as well as the pulp of these teeth by way of their apical foramina.

52. (B) Longitudinal developmental grooves or root concavity would probably be noted on mesial root surfaces of permanent maxillary first premolar (#5/#12 or #14/#24). Because of its depth, there may be increased tooth deposits in this area that may require instrumentation or an increased risk of root caries if exposed by way of gingival recession or periodontal disease with pathologic pocket formation.

53. (A) The roots of the permanent maxillary first premolar (#5/#12 or #14/#24) present the greatest difficulty during endodontic therapy compared with all the other premolars, whether first or second or even mandibular, because of its two roots; has one buccal and one lingual (palatal) root so it is bifurcated. The tooth may also be fused or laminated. In addition, its crown is the widest mesiodistally of all premolars.

54. (C) The basement membrane marks the junction where dentin and enamel will meet. The outer enamel epithelium and stellate reticulum are cell layers of the enamel organ. The dental papilla forms the pulp.

55. (D) The alveolar mucosa is a nonkeratinized flexible (mobile) tissue of the oral cavity and is located beyond the mucogingival junction. However, the alveolar mucosa is a separate part of the oral mucosa and is not classified as a component of the gingivae.

56. (D) The permanent mandibular second premolar (#20/#29 or #35/#45) has three cusps for one of its two types. Its tricuspidate form has one large buccal cusp and two smaller lingual cusps; its grooves form a distinctive Y-shaped pattern on the occlusal table so it resembles a small molar. The other premolars have two cusps.

57. (C) The permanent mandibular canine (#22/#27 or #33/#43) has the longest crown in the permanent dentition; the crown of the mandibular canine can be as long as or even longer than the maxillary canine.

58. (C) The blood vessels in the head and neck are less numerous than the lymphatic vessels. Venous vessels are parallel to the lymphatic vessels in location. Blood vessels are also involved in the spread of cancer to distant sites, which is considered metastasis.

59. (B) The permanent mandibular second premolar (#20/#29 or #35/#45) has either two or three cusps (or tricuspidate form). The two-cusp type has a transverse ridge, while the more common three-cusp type does not. The bicuspidate form (or two cusp form) is similar to that of the mandibular first premolars; it has one larger buccal cusp and one smaller lingual cusp; the central groove is crescent or U-shaped; it also appears rounded from the occlusal.

60. (A) Mandibular second premolar (#20/#29 or #35/#45) differs in structural numbers from the mandibular first molar (#19/#30 or #36/#46) by the number of cusps; has either two (or bicuspidate form) or three cusps (or tricuspidate form). The mandibular first molar has five cusps. Both teeth have two roots and two marginal ridges, and both have a lingual groove that cuts the occlusal outline on the lingual surface, if the premolar has the bicuspidate form (or two cusps).

61. (C) The cingulum is usually located in the cervical third of the lingual surface of the anterior teeth. This structure is noted on incisors and canines for both maxillary and mandibular teeth. Thus the cingulum is a raised rounded

area, with varying degrees of development depending on the tooth type.

62. (C) The shape of the developing root is determined by the Hertwig epithelial root sheath, which forms when the outer and inner epithelial tissue join together. The rests of Malassez are the epithelial remnants of the Hertwig epithelial root sheath and become trapped in the periodontal ligament. The dental lamina and stellate reticulum are structures associated with the developing tooth and are not responsible for the shape of the root.

63. (A) The mesial and distal contact of the permanent mandibular first molar (#19/#30 or #36/#46) is located at the junction of the occlusal and middle thirds of the tooth.

64. (C) The styloglossus muscle moves the tongue both superiorly and posteriorly, thus retracting the tongue. The palatoglossus muscle elevates the tongue against the soft palate during swallowing. The inferior longitudinal muscles are intrinsic tongue muscles and the genioglossus muscle acts to protrude the tongue.

65. (C) The circulating white blood cells that are fewest in number are the basophils (less than 1%) but within the blood the monocytes (2%–10%), neutrophils (54%–62%), lymphocytes (25%–33%) are all more common. Basophils are involved in the hypersensitivity response by releasing bioactive products.

66. (B) The soft palate is just posterior to the hard palate. The location of the hard palate is on the dorsal surface of the oral cavity. The median palatal raphe is in the center or midline of the hard palate. The palatine tonsils, which are lymphoid tissue, lie between the anterior and posterior faucial pillars. The soft palate is the soft tissue forming the back of the roof of the mouth; the soft palate is distinguished from the hard palate at the front of the mouth in that it does not contain bone beneath the oral mucosa.

67. (B) The copula is posterior swelling that forms the base of the tongue, its posterior one-third. The lingual swellings and tuberculum impar form the anterior two-thirds of the tongue or body of the tongue. The first branchial arch (or mandibular arch) is responsible for the formation of the maxilla, mandible, and middle part of the face. Meckel cartilage is important in the formation of the alveolar process of the mandible.

68. (A) The lingual tonsil is located on the dorsal surface of the tongue, posterior to the circumvallate lingual papillae. The lingual tonsil is an irregular mass of tonsillar tissue. The location of the foliate lingual papillae is on the posterolateral border of the tongue. The location of circumvallate lingual papillae is along the sulcus terminalis on the tongue. The fungiform lingual papillae are mostly located on the dorsal surface of the tongue but not near the sulcus terminalis.

69. (B) Colloid is a substance associated with the thyroid gland. Saliva production is associated with both the sublingual and parotid salivary glands. The thymus gland is associated with the production of T-cell lymphocytes for the immune system. Each follicle of the thyroid gland consists of a layer of simple cuboidal epithelium enclosing a cavity that is usually filled with colloid, a stiff material reserved for the future production of thyroxine.

70. (D) The sublingual salivary gland is not capsulated; the other glands, such as the submandibular, thyroid, and parotid glands, are encapsulated. The sublingual salivary gland is located in the sublingual fossa in the sublingual space at the floor of the mouth. The sublingual salivary gland is superior to the mylohyoid muscle, medial to the body of the mandible, and anterior to the submandibular salivary gland.

71. (D) Certain structures may be found in oral mucosa such as lamina propria, basal lamina, and keratohyaline granules but not myofibers; myofibers are found associated with skeletal muscle, which is not found in the oral mucosa. Each muscle is composed of numerous muscle bundles or fascicles, such as bundles of fibers that go together to create a rope, which are then composed of numerous muscle cells or myofibers.

72. (B) The dentin of the tooth is not ectodermal in origin but mesenchymal. Most mesenchyme derives from the middle embryological germ layer, the mesoderm. The reduced enamel epithelium, Hertwig epithelial root sheath, and enamel are instead ectodermal in origin. The ectoderm is the outermost of the three primary germ layers of an embryo, from which the epidermis, nervous tissue, and sense organs develop as well as tooth parts.

73. (D) The correct series that lists the parts of the mature tooth in the order of increasing inorganic content is pulp, cementum, dentin, and enamel. One of the ways to classify compounds is by identifying them as either organic or inorganic. In general, an organic compound is a type of compound that contains a carbon atom or is sometimes viewed as a living matter. Conversely, an inorganic compound would be one that does not contain carbon or is not a living matter.

74. (C) The formation of bone in the absence of a preexisting cartilage framework is considered intramembranous. Intramembranous ossification is the formation of osteoid between two dense connective tissue sheets, which then eventually replaces the outer connective tissue. Intramembranous ossification uses a method of appositional growth similar to that of cartilage with layers of osteoid being produced. The osteoid later becomes mineralized to form bone.

75. (D) Included in the reduced enamel epithelium is the outer enamel epithelium, stratum intermedium, and ameloblasts but not the epithelial diaphragm. After enamel appositional growth ceases in the crown of each primary or permanent tooth, the ameloblasts place an acellular dental cuticle on the newly formed outer enamel surface. In addition, the layers of the enamel organ become compressed, forming the reduced enamel epithelium (REE).